DEPRESSION PREVENTION

THE SERIES IN CLINICAL AND COMMUNITY PSYCHOLOGY

CONSULTING EDITORS

Charles D. Spielberger and Irwin G. Sarason

Auerbach and Stolberg Crisis Intervention with Children and Families
Burchfield Stress: Psychological and Physiological Interactions
Cohen and Ross Handbook of Clinical Psychobiology and Pathology, volume 1
Cohen and Ross Handbook of Clinical Psychobiology and Pathology, volume 2
Diamant Male and Female Homosexuality: Psychological Approaches
Froehlich, Smith, Draguns, and Hentschel Psychological Processes in Cognition and Personality
Hobfoll Stress, Social Support, and Women
Janisse Pupillometry: The Psychology of the Pupillary Response
Krohne and Laux Achievement, Stress, and Anxiety
London Personality: A New Look at Metatheories
London The Modes and Morals of Psychotherapy, Second Edition
Manschreck and Kleinman Renewal in Psychiatry: A Critical Rational Perspective
Morris Extraversion and Introversion: An Interactional Perspective
Muñoz Depression Prevention: Research Directions
Olweus Aggression in the Schools: Bullies and Whipping Boys
Reitan and Davison Clinical Neuropsychology: Current Status and Applications
Rickel, Gerrard, and Iscoe Social and Psychological Problems of Women: Prevention and Crisis Intervention
Smoll and Smith Psychological Perspectives in Youth Sports
Spielberger and Diaz-Guerrero Cross-Cultural Anxiety, volume 1
Spielberger and Diaz-Guerrero Cross-Cultural Anxiety, volume 2
Spielberger and Diaz-Guerrero Cross-Cultural Anxiety, volume 3
Spielberger and Sarason Stress and Anxiety, volume 1
Sarason and Spielberger Stress and Anxiety, volume 2
Sarason and Spielberger Stress and Anxiety, volume 3
Spielberger and Sarason Stress and Anxiety, volume 4
Spielberger and Sarason Stress and Anxiety, volume 5
Sarason and Spielberger Stress and Anxiety, volume 6
Sarason and Spielberger Stress and Anxiety, volume 7
Spielberger, Sarason, and Milgram Stress and Anxiety, volume 8
Spielberger, Sarason, and Defares Stress and Anxiety, volume 9
Spielberger and Sarason Stress and Anxiety, volume 10: A Sourcebook of Theory and Research
Spielberger, Sarason, and Defares Stress and Anxiety, volume 11
Strelau, Farley, and Gale The Biological Bases of Personality and Behavior, volume 1: Theories, Measurement Techniques, and Development
Strelau, Farley, and Gale The Biological Bases of Personality and Behavior, volume 2: Psychophysiology, Performance, and Applications
Ulmer On the Development of a Token Economy Mental Hospital Treatment Program
Williams and Westermeyer Refugee Mental Health in Resettlement Countries

IN PREPARATION

Burstein and Loucks A Comprehensive Scoring Manual for Rorschach's Test
Spielberger and Hackfort Anxiety in Sports: An International Perspective
Spielberger and Vagg The Assessment and Treatment of Test Anxiety

DEPRESSION PREVENTION
Research Directions

Edited by
Ricardo F. Muñoz
University of California, San Francisco

⬤ HEMISPHERE PUBLISHING CORPORATION
A member of the Taylor & Francis Group

New York   Washington   Philadelphia   London

DEPRESSION PREVENTION: Research Directions

2 3 4 5 6 7 8 9 0   B R B R   8 9 8

This book was set in Times Roman by Hemisphere Publishing Corporation. The editors were Christine Flint Lowry and Eleana Cornejo-de-Villanueva; the production supervisor was Peggy M. Rote; and the typesetter was Anahid Alvandian.
Braun-Brumfield, Inc. was printer and binder.

Library of Congress Cataloging-in-Publication Data

Depression prevention.

    (The series in Clinical and Community psychology)
    Bibliography: p.
    Includes index.
    1. Depression, Mental—Prevention. I. Muñoz,
Ricardo F. II. Series.
RC537.D445   1987   616.85'2705   86-14874
ISBN 0-89116-452-9
ISSN 0146-0846

To
Rodrigo Alberto
and
Aubrey Elizabeth Luz

Contents

IV
FUTURE DIRECTIONS FOR DEPRESSION
PREVENTION RESEARCH

Contributors

HAGOP S. AKISKAL, University of Tennessee College of Medicine, Memphis, Tennessee

REGINA ARMAS, University of California, San Francisco, California

SANDRA M. BASS, University of Wisconsin Medical School, Madison, Wisconsin

JAMES N. BRECKENRIDGE, Veterans Administration Medical Center, Palo Alto, California

JULIA STEINMETZ BRECKENRIDGE, Veterans Administration Medical Center, Palo Alto, California

FLORENTIUS CHAN, University of California, San Francisco. Presently at the Long Beach Asian Pacific Mental Health Program, Long Beach, California

PAULA J. CLAYTON, University of Minnesota, Minneapolis, Minnesota

SHEILA D. GINSBURG, University of Rochester, Rochester, New York

JOHN H. GREIST, University of Wisconsin Medical School, Madison, Wisconsin

ROBERTO GURZA, University of California, San Francisco, California. Presently at the University of California, Berkeley, California

RICHARD HOUGH, San Diego State University, San Diego, California

MARJORIE H. KLEIN, University of Wisconsin Medical School, Madison, Wisconsin

BOHDAN KOLODY, San Diego State University, San Diego, California

PETER M. LEWINSOHN, University of Oregon, Eugene, Oregon

MARY JANE LOHR, University of Wisconsin, Madison, Wisconsin

RICARDO F. MUÑOZ, University of California, San Francisco, California

LYNN P. REHM, University of Houston, Houston, Texas

ROBERT E. ROBERTS, The University of Texas Health Science Center, Houston, Texas

MARK SANSTEAD, University of Nebraska, Lincoln, Nebraska

WESLEY E. SIME, University of Nebraska, Lincoln, Nebraska

BETTY TABLEMAN, Michigan Department of Mental Health, Lansing, Michigan

CYNTHIA TELLES, University of California, Los Angeles, California
LARRY W. THOMPSON, Veterans Administration Medical Center, Palo Alto, California
CRAIG T. TWENTYMAN, University of Hawaii, Honolulu, Hawaii
RAMON VALLE, San Diego State University, San Diego, California
WILLIAM A. VEGA, San Diego State University, San Diego, California
YU WEN YING, University of California, San Francisco. Presently at the University of California, Berkeley, California
ANTONETTE M. ZEISS, Veterans Administration Medical Center, Palo Alto, California

Preface

Depression is one of the most prevalent psychiatric disorders. Our purpose here is to consider the proposition that clinical depression *can* be prevented. The book contains contributions from researchers, as well as research-oriented theorists and practitioners, who are actively engaged in studying depression prevention.

Scientific knowledge about depression is growing at a tremendous rate; however, prevention intervention research is still in its infancy. I believe that a concerted effort should be made to rigorously study ways to prevent this common human affliction. I hope that the ideas and the research findings provided here will aid the development of the depression prevention research field.

My interest in the prevention of depression has been influenced by many mentors, colleagues, and friends. Richard C. Ingraham introduced me to the concept of primary prevention in mental health; Albert Bandura to social learning theory (which I find readily applicable to preventive interventions); and Ed Lichtenstein to community psychology, the area of psychology that has been the most supportive of prevention efforts. James G. Kelly generously nurtured my early interests in prevention and actively brought me into the community psychology field by inviting me to collaborate with him on a number of publications. Peter M. Lewinsohn taught me to understand and treat depression and to carry out clinical research. My current work in depression prevention, including this book, combines aspects of all these concepts and methods.

Lonnie Snowden, Rhona Weinstein, Phil and Carolyn Cowan, and the other members of the Community Psychology Interest Group, which meets at the University of California, Berkeley, have been a source of moral support for many years. The members of the University of California, San Francisco, Depression Seminar, and the core group that created the Depression Clinic at San Francisco General Hospital (Jackie Persons, Chuck Garrigues, Jeannie Miranda, and Sergio Aguilar-Gaxiola), have also helped shape my ideas about the nature of depression.

The leadership of the University of California, San Francisco, Department of Psychiatry at the San Francisco General Hospital campus, namely John Hopkin, Frank Johnson, and Mike Rossi, have consistently given substantive support to prevention research and prevention activities, especially those directed at low-income and minority populations. In addition, colleagues such as Guillermo Bernal, Bill Hargreaves, Eliseo Perez-Stable, Mark Perl, Jim Sorensen, and Yu Wen Ying have collaborated and consulted with me on implementing depression prevention research. Laurel Koepernik has provided unfailing administrative support to make the research possible.

The present book owes its existence to a suggestion by Steve Goldston, former Director of the Office of Prevention at the National Institute of Mental Health, to hold a state-of-the-art conference on depression prevention. He was able to arrange funding from NIMH to implement the conference at San Francisco General Hospital. All the conference participants agreed to submit chapters to create this book, and additional research projects, not in existence at the time of the conference, were also added. I am happy to acknowledge the major role that Steve Goldston played in setting in motion the process that brought this book to fruition. It is one of the many contributions he has made to the field of prevention.

A number of people helped make the conference a reality. I want to especially thank Roberto Gurza and Guillermo Bernal. Flo Hurley, Suzanne Thompson, Paul Deloria, Alicia Carranza, Nickie Dunne, Winnie Ho, Hilde Innis, and Wendy King were also very helpful in making it a success.

My wife, Pat, and my parents, Clara and Alberto, have helped in many practical ways to make it possible to spend the time necessary to put this book together. Their loving support has been immeasurable.

Ricardo F. Muñoz

I

A CONTEXT FOR DEPRESSION PREVENTION RESEARCH

The goal of prevention intervention research is to develop methods which will reduce the incidence of depression, that is, the development of new cases of depression. As we begin to consider this objective, it is important to specify its scope, and to bring to bear to this new research effort knowledge from related areas such as epidemiology, clinical research, pharmacological approaches, genetics, personality, and so on.

In the first chapter, I underline the urgency behind efforts to prevent depression. I also discuss the terms to be used throughout the book, such as depression, prevention, and prevention intervention research, the state of the science regarding depression, the feasibility of beginning a concerted preventive effort at this time, the elements of a prevention intervention research project, and high-risk factors in depression.

Paula Clayton devotes the second chapter to clarifying the many types of "depression" that have been studied. She uses data from her own research program on bereavement to illustrate the prevalence of depressive symptoms in individuals who have been exposed to traumatic life events. The implications of her remarks are important in terms of specifying the target of prevention programs, identifying high risk populations, and choosing reasonable criteria for success of a prevention intervention.

One of the important pieces of information needed to decide where to focus prevention efforts is the distribution of depression in the population. Robert E. Roberts presents a review of the epidemiological knowledge presently available. He focuses primarily on the prevalence of depressive symptomatology, and discusses the high risk factors that have been identified in this very active field of investigation. His chapter raises interesting questions regarding whether clinical depression alone is a logical target for prevention, or whether subclinical manifestations of this phenomenon are also reasonable targets for intervention. If depressive symptoms become a target for prevention, he points out that we must seriously consider the implications of the consistent relationship that is found between socioeconomic status and high scores on depression scales.

Depression prevention research must build upon the knowledge that other areas of depression research have developed. The first three chapters address aspects of this knowledge that are important to keep in mind in order not to reinvent the wheel and to effectively pursue promising leads. Prevention research must be an integral part of the research enterprise focused on depression. I fully expect that, in a few years, it will begin to influence older areas of research in important ways. To best prepare for this role, it must embed itself into the fabric of ongoing research efforts, and contribute to the continuing progress of the combined depression field.

1

Depression Prevention Research: Conceptual and Practical Considerations

Ricardo F. Muñoz
University of California, San Francisco

INTRODUCTION

One of the most exciting and largely unmet challenges in the mental health arena is the prevention of psychological problems and mental disorders (Albee & Joffe, 1977; Caplan, 1964; Klein & Goldston, 1977; Muñoz & Kelly, 1975; Muñoz, 1976).

As we near the end of the twentieth century, we find that the mental health field has successfully demonstrated that a number of human maladies can be usefully construed as psychological or psychiatric disorders. The centuries-long struggle to classify these disorders in ways that reflect some type of orderly process, or that, at least, are therapeutically useful, has been advanced greatly in the last two decades. This has occurred both in terms of describing psychological symptoms carefully, and setting up more reliable methods to cluster the symptoms into syndromes. In addition, the classification of psychological disorders has become a collaborative endeavor across the planet, thus beginning to decrease the insularity of former diagnostic systems.

Treatment methods have also progressed in terms of their documented effectiveness. Standards for evaluating the efficacy of psychological and somatic interventions now exist, and there is a growing consensus about the types of treatments that are appropriate for specific symptoms and disorders (Williams & Spitzer, 1984). Though there is clearly much more progress to be made in both identification and treatment of psychological problems, measurable advances have been made.

The prevention of psychological problems, however, is an area of endeavor which is still in its infancy. A few pioneering practitioners are attempting preventive interventions, and an even smaller number of researchers are studying preventive interventions experimentally. Yet, the very question of whether prevention is feasible at this time is a most controversial one. If those who are charting the possibilities of prevention in the mental health area are able to develop the resources to continue their work, the twenty-first century will see advances in prevention as great as those we are seeing now in the area of diagnosis and treatment.

This chapter will provide an analysis of the prospects for the prevention of

The writing of this chapter was supported in part by National Institute of Mental Health Grant MH37992 and a Biomedical Research Support Grant from Langley Porter Institute. I also wish to thank A. Michael Rossi, Jacqueline Persons, Jeanne Miranda, Sergio Aguilar-Gaxiola, and Yu Wen Ying for their editorial suggestions.

depression, one of the most prevalent psychological disorders. I will address the significance of the problem, consider the advisability of engaging in depression prevention activities in the late 1980's, define key terms, describe the practical considerations involved in doing depression prevention research, and discuss high risk factors for depression and their implications for prevention. It is my hope that this chapter will contribute to the building of a solid conceptual base for the field of prevention intervention research and practice.

THE COST OF DEPRESSION AND THE NEED FOR PREVENTION

Depression costs the United States an estimated $16.5 billion per year. Of this amount, approximately $3 billion are treatment costs, and the rest indirect costs, such as lost productivity (Frank, Kamlet, & Stoudemire, 1985).

The cost in terms of human suffering is reflected in the high prevalence rates for depressive disorders: the NIMH Epidemiological Catchment Area Project found lifetime prevalence rates ranging from 6% to 10% across its three first sites (between 2% and 4% for dysthymia, and between 4% and 7% for major depressive episode) (Robins et al., 1984). Other epidemiological studies have shown even higher rates. For example, Weissman and Myers (1978) reported a combined lifetime rate of 26.7% for major and minor depression.

The number of persons suffering from depressive disorders at any one point in time is also very large. Six month prevalence rates reported by the Epidemiological Catchment Area Project range from 4.6% to 6.5% for affective disorders (Myers et al., 1984). Weissman and Myers (1978) reported point prevalence rates of 6.8% for major and minor depression combined.

These figures indicate that between one tenth and one fourth of the adult population of the United States suffers from depression at least once during their lifetime. At any one point in time, somewhere between one out of fifteen and one out of twenty adults is depressed enough to meet diagnostic criteria. Moreover, it has been suggested that the rates of depression may be actually increasing (Gershon, 1985; Klerman et al., 1985).

Yet, only between 16.3% and 19.2% of those who meet diagnostic criteria for affective disorders go to a mental health specialist for treatment (Shapiro et al., 1984). Over 75% do use some kind of health care provider, which suggests that most depressed persons consult with non-psychiatric physicians. However, these physicians generally do not recognize depression. For example, primary care internists in one study recognized only 37% of clinically depressed patients as having a depressive disorder (Perez-Stable, Muñoz, Chan, & Ying, 1985).

The total impact of depression on our communities is hard to measure. There are no accurate estimates of the effects of depression on general productivity, absenteeism, marital harmony, parental care of children, or the effects of prolonged depression on physical health. Clinical speculation attributes some undetermined portion of high-risk behaviors (such as reckless driving, violent crimes, substance abuse, as well as explicitly self-destructive acts) to depression-engendered desperation. The long-term risk of suicide in affective disorders is between 10 and 15 percent (Teuting, Koslow, & Hirschfeld, 1981); and more people die by suicide than by murder (U.S. Bureau of the Census, 1984).

Depression is a costly disorder in terms of individual human suffering and aggregate social cost. It is a disorder that often goes untreated perhaps because it is not recognized as such either by the persons afflicted or by their primary care providers, or because mental health treatment is considered too stigmatizing.

The magnitude of the problem demands that some action be taken. Increases in treatment resources alone are unlikely to be the answer: the number of new clinicians required would be staggering, and most of those afflicted may still choose to go without treatment. An alternative is to establish a concerted program to develop effective depression prevention interventions. The next section addresses the question of whether now is the right time to begin such a concerted effort.

DO WE KNOW ENOUGH TO BEGIN DEPRESSION PREVENTION RESEARCH

From a certain point of view, we have already begun to engage in depression prevention research. After all, any information gathered about depression has the potential to be helpful in the prevention of the disorder. Thus, one could conceive of epidemiological studies, treatment outcome studies, as well as correlational studies investigating factors which are related to depression as being of potential use to the depression prevention enterprise.

The purpose of this chapter, however, is to encourage the implementation of studies which are expressly designed to produce prevention effects. From this standpoint, the most desirable type of study would be a randomized, controlled prevention intervention study in which a specific method to reduce the incidence of depressive symptoms or depressive episodes is evaluated.

Critics of the area of prevention believe that we must wait until we know what causes depression before we can put forward interventions that will have a reasonable chance to prevent it. The standard objection to prevention intervention work is that we do not know enough yet.

How Much Do We Need to Know?

Bloom (1965) has made the argument that, throughout history, a number of successful public health campaigns have been conducted without the correct understanding of the etiological mechanisms which controlled the targeted problem. For example, miasma theory held that infectious diseases were caused by the noxious, odoriferous substances stemming from soil polluted with waste products. Malaria (which means "bad air") was successfully reduced in many communities by cleaning nearby swamps which gave off marsh gases. Now we know that this method was successful because it eliminated breeding grounds for the mosquito which carries the disease. Had the early public health activists waited for this knowledge before acting, many more people would have fallen victim to the disease.

The key element here was noticing a relationship between the prevalence of a health problem and surrounding conditions. Then a hypothesis was made which led to specific action. Finally, the results of the action were observed to determine whether the action produced the desired result, namely, reduction of the target problem. It must be noted that, although such a reduction can support the working hypothesis, it does not in itself prove that the hypothesis is correct.

A similar process was followed by John Snow (MacMahon & Pugh, 1970) in 19th-century London in trying to reduce the number of new cases of cholera. He was able to show that cases of cholera were related to the use of specific water pumps. By limiting access to the water from these pumps, he was able to effect a measurable drop in new cases. This intervention did not involve knowledge of the specific etiologic agents of cholera.

Although these examples are intriguing, we must also recognize that many such hypotheses which led to action probably produced no major preventive effect, and thus were not saved for posterity. This implies that it would be wise to consider the evidence very carefully before interventions are carried out. The more expensive or risky the intervention, of course, the more evidence should be required before it is implemented.

The lack of etiological knowledge regarding depression has not been an obstacle to progress in the treatment of depression. Both psychological and pharmacological approaches have been successful (Steinbrueck, Maxwell, & Howard, 1983). Although there are many theories about how these approaches produce their beneficial effects, there is no conclusive evidence to support them. For example, Baldessarini (1983) points out that: "The short answer to the difficult question of how antidepressants work is that no one knows" (p. 90). He goes on to say that "there is, as yet no compelling general theory of the mechanism of antidepressant action, in part due to the lack of a compelling neurobiological or metabolic theory of depression itself" (p. 131).

Cognitive behavioral therapies, which have been repeatedly shown to be effective in the treatment of depression, are based on rich and varied theoretical frameworks. Patterns of thinking and behavior are hypothesized to influence depressional level. Interventions designed to change them do reduce depression. But other interventions, such as pharmacotherapy, also produce these changes (Simons, Garfield, & Murphy, 1984). Critics of the cognitive behavioral theories rightly point out that the thoughts and behavioral patterns may be part of the syndrome of depression, much like sleeplessness and fatigue, and these patterns go away automatically once the disorder remits (Silverman, Silverman, & Eardley, 1984).

We know that pharmacotherapy and cognitive behavioral therapies are effective treatments for depression. The fact that cognitive behavioral therapies are effective raises the question of whether the biological abnormalities are at the heart of the disorder, or whether they are the byproducts of psychological and environmental factors. The fact that pharmacotherapeutic approaches are effective demonstrates that psychological interventions designed to change specific cognitions or behaviors are not necessary to ameliorate depression.

The knowledge that both psychological and pharmacological treatments work well gives us important information regarding the nature of depression. Future understanding of this disorder will probably not fit neatly into theories biased toward either a primarily biological or psychological explanation. But both of these approaches will have contributed much to our progress. Analogously, efforts to study the prevention of depression will provide a competing perspective to the current preponderance of research focused on clinical populations. The balance of the two perspectives will give us a more complete view of the disorders we are attempting to control.

In sum, effective interventions can be developed for specific disorders even when their pathological mechanisms are not fully understood. In order to develop such interventions, however, we must set this as an explicit goal, and must have promising leads which can direct our efforts. One of the purposes of this chapter is to encourage the mental health field to set depression prevention as a goal. The following sections define key terms and describe the main elements of prevention intervention research.

DEPRESSION, PREVENTION, AND PREVENTION INTERVENTION RESEARCH

Depression

Two definitions of depression are relevant to our discussion: clinical syndromes (categorical descriptions of symptom clusters presumed to be manifestations of a single, identifiable disorder), and depressive symptomatology (usually reflected in scores on psychometric instruments).

Clinical Syndromes

The diagnostic criteria from the *Diagnostic and statistical manual of mental disorders,* (American Psychiatric Association, 1980) are widely accepted among clinicians attempting to learn about and treat psychological conditions. The disorders described there and in its revision (American Psychiatric Association, 1985) can be used by prevention practitioners and researchers to establish lines of communication with their clinical colleagues.

The principal focus throughout much of the discussion that follows will be on the "depressive disorders" (American Psychiatric Association, 1985), that is, major depression and dysthymia. Major depression is the most prevalent of the mood disorders, it has been very widely studied, and much is known about how to treat it using both psychological and pharmacological interventions (Beckham & Leber, 1985). Therefore, it is the logical first target for prevention projects. Dysthymia is less well researched, and controversy regarding whether it is best conceptualized as a specific time-limited condition or as a personality disorder still exists. Nevertheless, its similarity to major depression and its chronic course makes it also worthy of investigation from a preventive point of view.

Bipolar disorder may have many etiological connections to the depressive disorders (see chap. 15, this volume). However, they are much less prevalent, and current treatment strategies focus primarily on pharmacological interventions. Because of their relatively low incidence, and because non-pharmacological interventions have not been sufficiently developed yet, these disorders are less likely to be early targets of preventive intervention.

Other diagnostic categories that could be considered appropriate for depression prevention efforts include adjustment disorder with depressed mood and organic affective syndrome (American Psychiatric Association, 1980). The former is a likely target for prevention projects focusing on reactions to stressful life events. The latter would have great relevance to medical practice, particularly in regards to the prevention of iatrogenically produced depression.

Depressive Symptomatology

Depression levels in the general population give another important kind of information. Self-report scales are not diagnostic instruments, although they can be used to estimate the number of cases in a population. Roberts (chap. 3, this volume) presents a detailed look at this area.

Categorical definitions of clinical syndromes imply the existence of disorders that can be said to be either present or absent, and self-report scales imply a continuum model of depression. Nevertheless, the method used in current diagnostic schemes, which involves counting the number of symptoms that are present within each diagnostic category, can be construed as setting arbitrary (though clinically-informed) thresholds which, in effect, dichotomize a continuous set of observations. For example, to meet criteria for major depression, 'a person must have a certain number of symptoms. Someone having one less symptom than the number required technically does not have the disorder, although differences of one or two symptoms may be of little practical significance. Dividing people into two categorical groups means losing much information about the possible continuum of depression that exists across the entire population.

Symptom scales have a number of advantages: they generally involve continuous variables, and thus give greater statistical power (Cohen, 1977) in outcome analyses; they are not tied to the vagaries of changing criteria for diagnoses; they are considerably less expensive to administer; their psychometric properties are generally well documented; and norms across cultural and linguistic groups are easier to obtain. It is important to note that although treatment outcome studies use strict diagnostic inclusionary criteria in choosing their samples, the dependent variable most often reported is a change in symptom scales.

Some self-report depression scales which might be considered for use in prevention intervention studies include the Center for Epidemiological Studies Depression Scale (CES-D) (Radloff, 1977), the Beck Depression Inventory (BDI) (Beck, Ward, Mendelsohn, Mock, & Erbaugh, 1961), and the Zung Depression Scale (Zung, 1965). The CES-D has been used primarily in epidemiological studies, and thus has substantial normative data available (see chap. 3, this volume). The Beck Depression Inventory has been widely used in treatment outcome studies (Murphy, Simons, Wetzel, & Lustman, 1984; Rush, Beck, Kovacs, & Hollon, 1977). A review of self-report scales has been conducted by Murphy (1980).

An observer rating scale which has been frequently used in pharmacotherapy trials is the Hamilton Rating Scale for Depression (Hamilton, 1967). It is more costly, in that it is meant to be completed by a clinician. However, it does add an external perspective to the purely subjective ratings of the scales mentioned above. To obtain reliable scores with the Hamilton Rating Scale for Depression, a structured interview format should be used, such as that found in Klerman, Weisman, Rounsaville, and Chevron (1984, pp. 223–233), or in the Structured Clinical Interview for DSM-III (SCID-HAM) (Spitzer & Williams, 1985).

Prevention

The logic of prevention is compelling. Many metaphors convey the urgency that proponents of the concept put forward. For example, treatment efforts (which are clearly the predominant use of mental health resources at present) are compared to employing personnel to stand next to a river and rescue people who have fallen into the river and are calling for help. Prevention advocates would instead send someone to walk upstream and try to stop so many people from falling in. Preventive interventions might include repairing a dangerous bridge, placing caution signs along footpaths near the river, and teaching people to swim.

Another example, focusing on the relative allocation of resources for treatment versus prevention, involves questioning whether we should be spending our limited resources on doing lung transplants rather than on stepping up efforts to reduce or stop smoking.

Although the arguments are forceful, translating these good preventive intentions into effective preventive interventions is a difficult endeavor. This task is the challenge facing the prevention intervention researcher.

Prevention efforts are usually divided into three levels. Primary prevention is intended to reduce the incidence of the target disorder, that is, the number of new cases. Secondary prevention involves early identification and treatment of cases, with the intent of reducing prevalence. Tertiary prevention focuses on reduction of disability resulting from full-blown cases of the disorder, and can be properly termed rehabilitation.

Proponents of prevention have repeatedly pointed out that, strictly speaking, only primary prevention should be referred to as prevention. The other two levels are actually treatment and rehabilitation. This point, which appears minor to those new to the prevention field, is actually very important when it comes to allocation of resources. Most of the resources for mental health are presently allocated for treatment. Whenever prevention monies become available, there is a trend for treatment projects to be described as prevention projects in order to qualify for funding. By restricting the definition of prevention to primary prevention, this is less likely to happen. Following this proposed use of the term, "prevention" will refer to "primary prevention" throughout this chapter. To further define and describe the nature of prevention, some attempts at delineating its scope will be presented.

Prevention has traditionally referred to efforts aimed at "reducing the incidence of a new cases of mental disorder and disability in a population" (Caplan & Grunebaum, 1972, p.128). Cowen (1973) adds an important proviso: "Primary prevention activities are targeted impersonally to groups and communities; once individual distress is identified, intervention is other than primary" (p. 433).

Goldston (1977) has put forward the following operational definition of prevention:

> *"Primary prevention encompasses activities directed toward specifically identified vulnerable high-risk groups within the community who have not been labeled psychiatrically ill and for whom measures can be undertaken to avoid the onset of emotional disturbance and/or to enhance their level of positive mental health. Programs for the promotion of mental health are primarily educational rather than clinical in conception and operation, their ultimate goal being to increase people's capacities for dealing with crises and for taking steps to improve their own lives"* (p. 20).

Analyses of the nature and implications of prevention have been published in the series of books stemming from the annual Vermont Conference on the Primary Prevention of Psychopathology. These volumes have focused on the basic conceptual issues in prevention (Albee & Joffe, 1977), environmental influences (Forgays, 1978), social competence in children (Kent & Rolf, 1979), competence and coping in adults (Bond & Rosen, 1980), prevention through social change (Joffe & Albee, 1981), facilitation of early development (Bond & Joffe, 1982); promotion of sexual responsibility and prevention of sexual problems (Albee, Gordon, & Leitenberg, 1983); and a volume depicting progress in prevention over the ten years since the first Vermont conference (Kessler & Goldston, 1986).

A recent series of publications from the National Institute of Mental Health has addressed basic issues in primary prevention programming (Klein & Goldston, 1977), risk factor research in the major mental disorders (Regier & Allen, 1981), the prospects for preventive interventions in schizophrenia (Goldstein, 1982), prevention of the harmful consequences of severe and persistent loneliness (Peplau & Goldston, 1984), implications of stressful life event theory and research for prevention (Bloom, 1985), the prevention of stress-related psychiatric disorders (Goldman & Goldston, 1985), a guide for evaluation of prevention programs in mental health (Price & Smith, 1985), and annotated bibliographies on disasters and mental health (Ahearn & Cohen, 1984) and primary prevention in mental health (Buckner, Trickett, & Corse, 1985).

Authors addressing issues in prevention with underserved populations have discussed how to reach the underserved (Snowden, 1982), prevention among American Indians (Manson, 1982), Asians (Owan, 1985), Blacks (Hilliard, 1981; O'Gorman, 1981), Hispanics (Muñoz, 1980, 1982; Valle & Vega, 1980; Vega & Miranda, 1985), and cross cultural populations in the United States (Muñoz, Chan, & Armas, 1986).

Other presentations of prevention include a debate regarding the feasibility of prevention in mental health, with George Albee and Stephen Goldston on the affirmative, Richard Lamb and Jack Zusman on the negative, and commentary by fifteen professionals representing a diversity of opinion on primary prevention (Marlowe & Weinberg, 1985), textbooks examining various approaches to prevention (Bloom, 1975; Felner, Jason, Moritsugu, & Farber, 1983; Heller & Monahan, 1977; Iscoe, Bloom, & Spielberger, 1977; Muñoz, Snowden, & Kelly, 1979; Murrell, 1973; Myers, 1977; Price, Ketterer, Bader, & Monahan, 1980; Rappaport, 1977; Zax & Specter, 1974), and various relevant publications from influential institutions, such as the Institute of Medicine (Hamburg, Ellicott, & Parron, 1982; Osterweiss, Solomon, & Green, 1984), the Office of the Surgeon General (1979), and the American Psychiatric Association (Barter & Talbott, in press; Glasscote et al., 1980).

Prevention Intervention Research

Almost any type of research into a disorder has the potential of having preventive implications. Prevention intervention research examines specific interventions to evaluate their effectiveness in reducing incidence of the target conditions. It most closely resembles treatment outcome research.

Examples of successful prevention intervention research can be found in a special issue of the *American Journal of Community Psychology* (Cowen, 1982). Descriptions of the nature of prevention-oriented research in community contexts can be found in Muñoz, Snowden, and Kelly (1979).

ELEMENTS OF A PREVENTION INTERVENTION
RESEARCH PROJECT

At least four steps are involved in carrying out a prevention intervention research project:

1. Identifying the target of intervention. (What are you preventing?)
2. Theoretical formulation. (What mechanisms are you hypothesizing to be at work in the development of the disorder?)
3. Designing the intervention. (How do you propose to influence those mechanisms?)
4. Monitoring short- and long-term effects. (How will you know what kind of effect your intervention has had?)

For those familiar with traditional clinical research (Williams and Spitzer, 1984), it is important to note that prevention trials involve the identification of persons who are *not* clinically impaired at the beginning of the study. Thus, unlike treatment outcome studies, where participants must meet criteria for clinical disorders and severity of dysfunction, in prevention trials those participants who already meet criteria for the disorder to be prevented are screened out and referred for treatment (or to a treatment outcome study). Participants in prevention trials are at high risk, but not currently in need of treatment. The dependent variable is a lower incidence of clinical symptoms and/or of cases meeting clinical criteria in the experimental group, compared to a control group.

Identifying the Target of Intervention

The investigator must explicitly choose specific clinical diagnoses, scores on symptom scales, or both, as the dependent variable to be affected by the intervention. The prevention intervention studies which are most likely to be of interest to the clinical research community are those which focus on reducing incidence of clinical cases.

Specific clinical diagnoses should be made using such criteria as those found in the *Diagnostic and statistical manual of mental disorders* (American Psychiatric Association, 1980) or Research Diagnostic Criteria (RDC) (Spitzer, Endicott, & Robbins, 1978). The information on which diagnoses are based must itself be collected in a reliable manner, so that other investigators (as well as those who will implement the intervention in non-research settings) can identify the population to which the findings apply. Some interview protocols that might be considered include the Present Status Examination (PSE) (Wing, Cooper, & Sartorius, 1974) the Schedule for Affective Disorders and Schizophrenia (SADS) (Endicott & Spitzer, 1978), which is keyed to the Research Diagnostic Criteria; the Structured Clinical Interview for DSM-III (SCID) (Spitzer & Williams, 1985); and the NIMH Diagnostic Interview Schedule (DIS) (Robins, Helzer, Croughan, & Ratcliff, 1981), which was used in the Epidemiological Catchment Area studies (Eaton & Kessler, 1985). The latter is the only one developed explicitly to be used by trained lay interviewers, and thus may be particularly helpful for large scale studies. The other three were originally intended to be used by clinicians.

The advantages of symptom scales have been discussed above (see p. 8). The relative level of symptoms in a population being studied is of importance for a number of reasons. For example, it provides a way to compare samples which may not have similar numbers of clinical cases but may be under similar amounts of stress. The examination of symptom scales as possible predictors of later clinical cases is another source of potentially useful information. The relationship of scores on symptom scales to diagnostic criteria can also provide information on the sensitivity, specificity, positive predictive value, negative predictive value, and efficiency of these scales as screening instruments (Galen & Gambino, 1975). The availability of both types of measures can also yield information regarding which subtypes of depression appear to fit a continuous model and which do not. I strongly recommend that both diagnostic assessment and symptom scales be used in prevention studies.

The incidence of the disorder targeted must be high enough in the population being studied as to make it feasible to measure its reduction. Heller, Price, and Sher (1980) point out that in order to demonstrate a significant difference at the .05 level between experimental and control groups, one needs a very large number of participants. For example, with a very effective intervention which reduces new cases of the disorder to half of what is found in a control group, and with a disorder with a relatively high incidence of 10%, (so that the experimental group's incidence after intervention is 5%), one would need 151 participants per group. For a disorder with a much lower incidence of 1%, one would need 1611 participants per group.

These figures point out the need for identifying groups in which incidence rates are very high. If one adds to demographic screening criteria such factors as number of stressful life events (Dohrenwend & Dohrenwend, 1974), one can begin to identify a higher risk group within a high risk group. By using several of the high risk factors discussed later in this chapter, one could choose populations with predictably high incidence of depression.

A thorough review of the epidemiological literature (see chap. 3, this volume) is a first step in choosing the disorder and population to target. In many cases, there may be little or no epidemiological data on the particular group that one is interested in studying, for example, on certain minority groups.

Theoretical Formulation

There are many routes to the formulation of theoretical models for the specific disorder to be prevented. The identification of high risk groups through demographic factors may lead to hypotheses about factors which may be causing the increased risk. For example, if recent immigrants are found to have higher symptom levels, one could focus on the adaptation process as a likely source of stress, and design an intervention to facilitate adaptation.

Another source of hypotheses regarding mechanisms which may prevent the development of new disorders is effective treatment. Clinicians are in a good position to suggest mechanisms which may be involved in the development and exacerbation of particular syndromes. It is important to remember, however, that clinicians have access to a biased sample: those who go for treatment. There are many persons who do not go for treatment, but who may be willing to take part in preventive interventions which do not require them to label themselves as "mental patients." If interventions are based only on knowledge derived from clinical populations, there is a possibility that they will not be acceptable to the groups that we most need to reach: those who do not use traditional treatment services.

A possible pitfall in the development of theoretical explanations of either a correlational or a causal nature is the moderating influence of cultural factors. Relationships which hold true for mainstream groups may not hold for other groups, or may hold true with different norms. To illustrate this point, let's consider data relating beliefs to depression.

Albert Ellis (1962) has hypothesized that agreement with certain beliefs, which he has called "irrational," causes much human suffering. In a treatment-outcome study done with English-speaking, white, middle-class individuals in Eugene, Oregon (Muñoz, 1977), a measure of beliefs, labeled the "Personal Beliefs Inventory" (Muñoz & Lewinsohn, in press), was administered to depressed and nondepressed individuals. The results supported Ellis' contention: depressed individuals reported stronger agreement with these beliefs on a five-point scale. The mean for depressed participants was 2.93 (n = 64) and the mean for the nondepressed sample was 2.60 (n = 74; p < .001). In a subsequent prevention project conducted in San Francisco, the same questionnaire was administered to both English- and Spanish- speaking persons. After screening out those who met clinical criteria for depression and referring them for treatment, the remaining members of the two language groups were divided into a symptomatic and a nonsymptomatic groups using a depression symptom scale. Again, we found that symptomatic members of each group agree more with statements in the Personal Beliefs Inventory than the nonsymptomatic members. However, the baseline levels of each group are clearly different. The English-speaking sample scored as follows: nonsymptomatic group mean was 2.52 (n = 40), and the symptomatic mean was 2.78 (n = 17). The Spanish-speaking nonsymptomatic group mean score was 2.85 (n = 29), and the symptomatic group mean score was 3.03 (n = 18). Note that the nonsymptomatic Spanish-speaking mean is higher than the symptomatic English-speaking mean.

Whenever this type of finding occurs, it is imperative to consider explanations other than the possibility that these are real differences. For example, there may be translation problems, differences in mean depression levels across the groups, response styles that may be artificially affecting scores, and so on. However, for the sake of illustration, let's assume that the differences will hold up in future replications. If this is the case, the theoretical and practical implications of these findings are many. First, although there may be something maladaptive with agreeing strongly with these beliefs, the designation of the beliefs as "irrational" is questionable. In other words, culture as a mediating variable appears to "protect" Spanish-speaking people who agree with these beliefs to the same extent than depressed English-speaking people. Thus, a Spanish-speaking nonsymptomatic group can have even higher agreement scores than the English-speaking symptomatic group. Nevertheless, even within this protective cultural context, relatively higher agreement with these beliefs is still related to higher depression levels. So the theory appears to have some validity across cultures, as long as one is aware of differential base levels. The key in this case might be the value placed on interdependence. Within a fiercely individualistic culture, such as the one within which Ellis has wrought his theories, a very independent worldview may be adaptive. Latinos, on the other hand, are more likely to find social reinforcement for such beliefs as "Everyone needs the love and approval of those persons who are important to them," "Because parents or society taught acceptance of certain traditions, one must go on accepting these traditions," "What others think of you is most important," and "Depending on others is better than depending on oneself." In translating the theory to an intervention level, then, one must avoid the pitfall of attempting to change these beliefs in Latinos to match levels of mainstream U.S. norms.

The above example points out another complex issue which is very much alive in the struggles of researchers working on prevention interventions: how to intervene without causing harm. It is possible that the same cognitive, behavioral, or interpersonal patterns which make a certain group at risk for one disorder, may have little noxious effect for another group, or even protect it from another disorder. In the above instance, one can speculate that, because cultural norms encourage higher agreement with the beliefs which were measured, Latinos may be at higher risk for depression. However, these same beliefs may strengthen social bonds, thereby helping to protect Latinos from stresses that may produce other disorders.

The implications of theoretical formulations are important and must be thought through prior to the development of specific interventions. Negative effects of preventive interventions may originate in the way the problem is formulated by the mental health professional.

Designing the Intervention

This stage in the development of a prevention project involves at least four issues: 1) recruitment and retention of participants, 2) quality control over the implementation of the intervention, 3) monitoring whether the intervention produces the intended intermediate effects (usually changes in thinking, behavior, or social patterns, and 4) evaluating whether the intermediate effects influence the final goal of the intervention (for example, reducing levels of dysfunction or incidence of the disorder).

Recruitment and Retention of Participants

Recruitment issues are highlighted by reports from a depression treatment project and a depression prevention project. A recent article on media efforts to obtain participants for a treatment outcome study in Seattle (Hunt, Ward, & Bloom, 1982) reported that newspapers were the most effective medium for obtaining volunteers. In a pilot study offering depression prevention classes in San Francisco, we also used media announcements to obtain volunteers. Our study, however, was carried out in English and Spanish, and thus we were able to compare the type of media to which each of these groups responded better. Our results indicate that newspapers or bulletin boards were cited by 53% of English-speaking volunteers as their sources of information about the project. However, for Spanish-speaking volunteers, newspapers yielded only 2% of our volunteers. The overwhelming majority of Spanish-speaking participants were informed about our project via radio, television, and word of mouth. It appears, then, that recruitment efforts must take into account the communication patterns in the specific group being sought. This is not only an issue of language. In neither the Seattle nor the San Francisco samples were there any Blacks, even though the 1980 census reports show that San Francisco is 11% Black, and Seattle 9%. Obviously if one's goal is to serve the community as a whole, special efforts must be made to attract Black participants.

Retention once the sample has been recruited is another major issue. Drop out rates from treatment have generally been greater for minorities. Prevention intervention programs must attempt to retain large proportions of their participants in order to produce changes in incidence in the population being served. The nature of the attrition must be carefully examined. There is a danger of "preaching only to the converted," of reaching only those who are most likely to use other community resources, or those who are at least risk.

Specific suggestions regarding how to document recruitment and retention rates are examined in great detail in chap. 12, this volume.

Quality Control over the Implementation of the Intervention

The state of the art in treatment outcome studies is to standardize the treatment using manuals which specify the substance as well as the style in which the intervention must be carried out. Prevention intervention projects would do well to pursue a similar course. For example, in an educationally-oriented intervention, manuals or syllabi should be prepared with detailed outlines of the subject matter to be covered, examples to be used, and, if applicable, the instructional materials that are used. The persons who will implement the project should undergo a well-specified training period to standardize the intervention. And during the experimental trials, trained observers should rate the actual delivery of the intervention, to ensure that the intervention that is supposedly being evaluated is in fact being implemented. Negative results could be due merely to inadequate delivery of the intervention.

When working with groups from different cultures, the challenge of providing culturally appropriate interventions becomes of paramount importance. A "perfectly" conducted intervention done precisely "by the book" in what is perceived by the participants as a culturally awkward manner is less likely to have the expected impact.

Evaluation of Intermediate Effects

Theoretical advances in prevention will be furthered if we can document each step of the hypothesized preventive process. For example, if we hypothesize that depression is partly due to reduced activity levels, and our intervention is designed to increase activity levels in order to forestall depression, we must measure level of activity. A necessary step in evaluating such an intervention is the assessment of change in activity level. Our theory is supported if we find either that activity levels were unaffected and neither were depression levels, or that activity levels increased and depression levels decreased. If we find that activity levels increased, but depression levels were unaffected, at least we know that our intervention was successful in achieving change in activity levels, and we do not have to worry about having had a weak intervention. The focus of the intervention may need to change in future trials. If people do not become more active, but depression levels still decrease, then one must reassess one's theory. Other factors in the intervention might be producing the changes seen, such as establishing social contacts or other such unintended effects. By merely focusing on depression levels, we would miss important theoretical contributions.

The practical reasons for evaluating intermediate steps refer to future applications, funding requests, and to comparing effectiveness of the intervention across groups. If a well-specified intervention can change cognitive, behavioral, or interactional patterns valuable knowledge has been added to the mental health armamentarium *even if it does not result in the prevention of the target disorder.* Such a study would be a reasonable source of knowledge and techniques for future studies, for example, studies focused on changing modifiable high risk factors. Investigators who have shown that they can contribute something of value to the field are more likely to be seen as good risks for further funding. Comparative efficacy across groups is important in terms of effective use of interventions. If a certain intervention is very effective within a certain demographic group, but not with another, this information can be extremely helpful in deciding which groups to serve and where further development of interventions needs to be pursued.

Do Intermediate Effects Produce the Intended Final Goals?

The most important check on the intervention, from a preventive point of view, is whether it produces the intended final effect. The two-step process alluded to above is, of course, very important: are changes in the intermediate targets of the intervention related to the final preventive effects?; and, just as interesting from a pragmatic point of view, was there a measurable preventive effect? Immediate effects may have a short duration, possibly having to do with the context of the intervention itself. Perhaps the increased attention given to participants during the intervention produces a passing period of perceived well-being. However, because most prevention efforts will be focused on disorders that have a fairly low one-year incidence, immediate effects are likely to be of little consequence, unless they also have long duration. This brings us to the fourth step in the intervention-planning phase.

Monitoring Short- and Long-term Effects

Funding patterns discourage longitudinal studies. Therefore, prevention researchers must work extra hard to place themselves in a position to be able to collect longitudinal data whether or not they get continuous funding. Although there is a general skepticism regarding the duration of psychological preventive interventions, some interventions should theoretically last for a very long time. For example, an intervention focused on changing participants' feeling of control over their own lives (perhaps through changes in self-efficacy or in perceived ability to have greater control over one's emotional responses), might be expected to produce its greatest effects during crisis periods. If such periods are generally low-frequency events, the instances in which such changes in thinking style might have a protective effect would be relatively few in any one period of time. However, over a relatively long time period, the frequency of crises in the lives of a reasonably large sample might be great enough to allow for comparisons with a control group. Rates for specific disorders also point to the need to allow for long follow up periods. The point prevalence of clinical depression hovers around 6%

for the general population. Incidence rates are lower still. But lifetime prevalence rates may reach as high as 25% (Weissman & Myers, 1978). Clearly, preventive studies using effective interventions have a higher probability of showing positive effects if their followup time is of sufficient length because the probability of new cases appearing increases with time.

Short-term effects must also be evaluated, after the "glow" from active participation in a preventive project has had a chance to fade. The possibility of "sleeper" effects must also be considered. That is, although some participants may not show immediate effects, they may begin to show positive effects as they continue to practice the methods learned during the intervention phase, or as life events trigger in them the need to use these methods.

A final note regarding the necessity of longitudinal follow ups in prevention studies is that, even if preventive effects are not found, if the study is consciously structured to provide this information, the control group can serve as a prospective study sample for elucidating issues in the natural course of the target disorder *in an originally non-clinical populations* (P. Cowan, personal communication, 1982).

We turn next to a discussion of high-risk factors for depression. These factors are important both for choosing a population for prevention studies and for generating hypotheses regarding elements which affect the occurrence of depression in a population.

HIGH RISK FACTORS FOR DEPRESSION

A number of factors have been found to have a relationship to depression. None, however, has been found to be necessary nor sufficient for its appearance. The most likely interpretation of present knowledge is that the occurrence of a depressive episode is the result of the confluence of a number of contributing factors, and that the specific expression of symptoms is influenced by physiological and psychological characteristics of the individual. Therefore, it is unlikely that a single type of intervention would work to prevent depression, or to treat it.

The strategy suggested here is to examine the leads which are most likely to have the greatest impact on the greatest number of people. Our present goal should be to develop those interventions which are most practical, not necessarily those which are most elegant theoretically.

Risk factors are generally obtained from epidemiological studies. Gruenberg (1981) considers epidemiology "the study of who gets sick, and who doesn't get sick; why? (what are the risk factors?); what can we do to make the sickness less common?" (p. 8).

There are different types of risk estimates (Gruenberg, 1981), as discussed below.

Individual risk is obtained by determining the proportion of persons within a defined category (for example, age or sex) who have a certain disorder. The probability of contracting the disorder for an individual who fits the above category is assumed to be equal to the proportion of persons within the category who have the disorder in question.

Contingency risk is the increased risk that a person with a history of a risk factor has of contracting a disorder. For example, one could set up a contingency risk table for those with or without early parental loss and determine the proportion within each group who become clinically depressed. From these proportions one could determine the increase in the probability of developing depression given early parental loss.

Relative risk measures how strongly a risk factor affects incidence rates. It is the incidence of a disorder in a group exposed to a risk factor divided by the incidence of the same disorder in a nonexposed group. This estimate allows for methods to examine the total risk resulting from clusters of individual risk factors.

Attributable risk is the proportion of cases attributable to a specific risk factor. For example, if inadequate levels of pleasant activities are related to depression, what proportion of depressed cases would be prevented if one could increase a population's activity to adequate levels? These rates are best measured in preventive trials.

Prevention research could benefit much from appropriate utilization of methods to determine risk. Gruenberg's (1981) chapter is a good initial resource.

Risk factors can suggest hypotheses regarding the etiology of depression and ideas for the identification of a population at high risk. Modifiable risk factors can stimulate ideas for interventions.

Since the risk factors are not always the same for depressive symptomatology (such as that extracted from self-report symptom scales), and clinical cases of depression (which meet agreed-upon diagnostic criteria), I will be explicit as to which type has been related to each factor. The factors listed are intended to be illustrative, not exhaustive.

Demographic Characteristics

Sex

Both clinical depression and depression symptoms have been consistently found to be higher in women. Although sex is not a modifiable risk factor, if this finding is due to socially determined differences in the level of stress that men and women experience, social changes may have effects on depression rates.

Age

There are enough differences in trends found in different studies to question whether there is a reliable age effect on depressive symptoms. Cases of clinical depression in adults appear to be more prevalent at the earlier age ranges in the latest epidemiological studies (Myers et al., 1984; Robins et al., 1984). The finding that lifetime prevalence rates also drop with age has raised some questions about the validity of the ECA findings. The latter finding might be merely the result of older respondents forgetting earlier episodes. Among other alternatives is the possibility that the results reflect a true generational effect, with the present young adult group experiencing higher frequencies of clinical depression.

Social Class

There is a consistent finding of higher levels of depressive symptomatology in those with lower income (see chap. 3, this volume). However, rates of clinical depression do not appear to be consistently related to social class (Boyd and Weissman, 1982), although Brown and Harris (1978) found that working class women in London (especially those with children) are much more likely to have been in treatment than middle class women.

Race

Rates of depressive symptomatology have consistently been found to be higher for minorities in the U.S. than for whites. When socioeconomic status is controlled for, however, these differences diminish or disappear (see chap. 3, this volume). Epidemiological Catchment Area rates of clinical depression are not different for Blacks and Whites (Robins et al., 1984). The ECA study which examined Hispanic rates has not been published as of this writing.

Marital Status

Married men show the lowest rates of depressive symptoms. Divorced, widowed, and separated men and women show the highest rates. (Hirschfeld & Cross, 1981).

The Contribution of Demographic Characteristics to the Prediction of Future Depression

Although there are clear relationships between these factors and depression, taken together they account for only 7 to 13 percent of the variance (Hirschfeld and Cross, 1981). Therefore, they can only give very crude direction to prevention efforts.

Biological Characteristics Related to Depression

Genetic Contributions

A history of depression in a family increases the risk of depression for members of that family. This familial tendency could be explained on the basis of heredity, environment, or their interaction. Adoption studies strongly suggest that heredity, that is, genetic contributions, are clearly involved, especially in the more severe forms of the affective disorders (Nurnberger & Gershon, 1982). The major question for prevention is how much does heredity influence the risk of future depression. At present the answer is not known. There are likely to be different contributions of heredity for different diagnostic subgroups of depressive disorders. However, it would make sense to consider family history of depression as a risk factor in choosing a high-risk group. At the same time, it is important to recognize that genetic history only predisposes to depression. Preventive interventions could well reduce risk substantially.

Many mental health professionals shy away from, or actively express dislike of genetic explanations for behavior. In order to advance the field of depression prevention, however, it is imperative to study and assess as objectively as possible the information gathered by our fellow scientists in this area. Some refusals to consider the influences that heredity has on us, stem from uninformed overestimates of these influences. This can occur because the studies that report strong genetic effects are not carefully examined to understand their limitations, nor are their implications always thought through. Often, the implications of genetic influences are relatively limited. For example, the strongest findings in terms of increased genetic risk for depression have been reported in the most severe of the affective disorders (Nurnberger & Gershon, 1982). But the most severe of the disorders are the least prevalent (Boyd & Weissman, 1982). Thus, for most large-scale prevention programs, which would be focused on the most prevalent disorders, genetics will probably play a relatively minor role.

Neurotransmitters and Depression

Abnormalities in the transmission of nerve impulses mediated by the catecholamine system have been implicated in affective disorders (Siever & Davis, 1985; Zis & Goodwin, 1982). Pharmacologic interventions which are intended to increase available biogenic amines at the synapse produce therapeutic effects in depression. Agents which reduce their availability may precipitate depression (Whybrow, Akiskal, & McKinney, 1984). Although these observations offered tempting possibilities that depression may be related to catecholaminergic activity which was merely too high or too low, it now appears that the relationship between such activity and depressive symptomatology may be much more complex. Prange (Prange, Wilson, Lynn, Alltop, & Stikeleather, 1974) has suggested that a deficit in serotonergic transmitter levels may predispose to affective disorders, and that such a deficit permits a reduction in catecholaminergic activity to produce depression, and an increase in catecholaminergic activity to produce mania (Whybrow, Akiskal, & McKinney, 1984, pp. 135–136). More recently, Siever and Davis (1985) have suggested that persistent impairment in one or more neurotransmitter homeostatic regulatory mechanisms may confer a trait vulnerability for depression. I am aware of no proposal to correct such a vulnerability, however.

Endocrine Abnormalities

Depression has been associated with a number of pathologies in hormonal regulatory systems (Sachar, 1982). Perhaps the most studied are those related to the brain-contricosteroid axis (particularly cortisol hypersecretion), and the brain-thyroid axis (particularly a deficient thyroid stimulating hormone (TSH) response to thyrotropin-releasing hormone (TRH)) (Whybrow, Akiskal, & McKinney, 1984; Sachar, 1982). Findings in this area are replete with inconsistencies which are attributed to the heterogeneity of the depressive disorders themselves.

The Contribution of Biological Factors to the Prediction of Future Depression

At present, there are no good biological markers for identifying persons at high risk for depression. Most such markers appear to be state dependent, disappearing once the depressive episode lifts. Thus, they promise to be most helpful for diagnosis and perhaps for determining differential pharmacological therapies (Baldessarini, 1983, p. 15). Explicit attempts to delineate the preventive implications of this line of research would be potentially very influential.

The role of biological factors in depression has received so much attention and yielded so many exciting (if inconclusive) findings, that it makes sense to include these findings in the theoretical underpinnings of preventive interventions. At the very least, biological factors are part of some depressive disorders. At the same time, purely biological theories about depression seem insufficient. Theories which integrate the psychological, environmental, and biological are the most convincing (see chap. 15, this volume; Akiskal & McKinney, 1973; Whybrow, Akiskal, & McKinney, 1984, pp. 173–203).

Social Influences on Depression

Early Life Events

Early parent loss by death has been suggested as a high risk factor for depression. Paykel's (1982) review of studies concerned with this factor indicates that about half of them have shown higher frequency of early parental loss for persons with affective disorders, while the others have not.

Disruptive, hostile, and generally negative childhood home environments are reported to constitute a high risk factor by Orvaschel, Weissman, and Kidd (1980).

Current Life Events

Onset of depression following increases in stressful life events has been documented repeatedly (Paykel, 1982). Models which incorporate assumptions of additivity between events and decay of their stressful effect over time produce even more striking relationships (Surtees & Rennie, 1983). However, this triggering effect is not specific to depression, but has also been documented to affect other psychiatric disorders and medical illnesses (Bloom, 1985).

Social Support

The role of social support as a buffering element in the development of depression and other disorders has been the subject of many studies in recent years. It is likely that there are elements within the global concept of social support which could be profitably differentiated to better study hypothesized effects. These elements might include social embeddedness, perceived support, and enacted support (Barrera, 1986). The most interesting findings regarding social support are those which show that its mere absence is not sufficient to predict to onset of an episode of depression, but that once severe life events occur, the absence of social support (e.g., in the form of an intimate relationship) can greatly increase the risk of such an episode (Brown & Harris, 1978). It is this kind of interactional analysis which is most likely to yield useful information for identifying populations at current risk for depression.

Economic Factors

Common sense as well as epidemiological information (see chap. 3, this volume) points to the importance of economic factors in the development of depressive symptoms. This is an area that could well yield great preventive effects.

Unfortunately, many mental health professionals have decided that interventions focused on economic status are beyond their purview. It may be more reasonable to study economic status and its role in depression empirically. If it has a measurable effect in the onset of clinical depression, and if interventions focused on financial status have an effect on reducing the incidence of depressive episodes, then such interventions could logically become part of the mental health armamentarium. Obtaining resources for such interventions then becomes a question of feasibility.

Cultural Factors

The introduction of cultural factors into the study of depression has a major impact on the way we conceptualize our field. For some, cultural issues are mere impediments in the study of a universal phenomenon. For others, cultural issues raise basic questions about the conceptualization of depression itself, and whether it even exists (at least as we define it) in other cultures (Kleinman & Good, 1985). From a preventive perspective, the relevant questions revolve around differential rates of depression in different cultural groups; differential distribution of depression and depressive symptoms (Mezzich & Raab, 1980), even if the overall rates are similar; different high risk profiles across cultures; different terms for depression and its symptoms (Marsella, 1980); different perceived intensity of depression and subsequent impact on daily functioning; and, of course, different norms and psychometric characteristics of measurement instruments, whether or not language is an issue.

Preventive interventions in most of the U.S. should take cultural factors into account (Muñoz, Chan, & Armas, in press). In many large cities, use of non-English languages is necessary to achieve representativeness of the population in the community in research samples or in outreach projects (see chaps. 12 and 13, this volume).

Taking cultural factors into account in the prevention of depression potentially allows us to learn varied coping methods and to become familiar with the many adaptive cognitive, behavioral, and social customs that human wisdom has identified. The intent here should not be to impose "the best" cultural patterns on others, but rather to make more alternatives available for all.

Contribution of Social Influences in the Prediction of Future Depression

Empirical studies support the commonsensical notion that the socioeconomic environment and specific life events have an effect on mood and, by extension, on mood disorders. Once again, the predictive power of these factors is relatively small, but it is measurable in the aggregate. The use of these factors to choose high risk populations is reasonable.

Psychological Factors

Behavioral Factors

Lewinsohn (Libet & Lewinsohn, 1973) has found that depressed individuals demonstrate lower levels of interpersonal skills. Similarly, their level of pleasant activities is lower than for nondepressed samples (Lewinsohn & Graf, 1973), and level of unpleasant activities is higher (Grosscup & Lewinsohn, 1980; Lewinsohn & Talkington, 1979). Rehm (1977) has hypothesized that depression stems from deficiencies in self-control behaviors, such as self-monitoring, self-evaluation, and self-reward.

Cognitive Factors

Many cognitive factors have been advanced as being related to depression: a negative view of the self, the world, and the future (Beck, 1967); degree of agreement with "irrational" beliefs (Ellis, 1962); dysfunctional attitudes (Kovacs & Beck, 1978); learned helplessness (Seligman, 1975), and more specifically, global, internal, stable attributions for negative results (Abramson, Seligman, & Teasdale, 1978); increased frequency of negative thoughts and decreased frequency of positive thoughts (Muñoz, 1977); relatively high subjective probability estimates for negative events and low subjective probability estimates for positive events (Muñoz, 1977).

Personality Characteristics

A number of characteristics of depressed persons, usually derived from personality inventories, have been classified as traits associated with depression. These include neuroticism, introversion, obsessionality, dependency, and guilt (Hirschfeld & Cross, 1981). More difficult to measure are theoretical suggestions that depression involves aggression turned inward (Mendelson, 1982).

Contribution of Psychological Factors to the Prediction of Future Depression

Cognitive and behavioral factors are clearly associated with clinical depression and high depression levels. Whether these factors predispose to depression or are the result of being in a depressive episode is a much debated question (Coyne & Gotlib, 1983). A number of studies have shown that these factors dissipate once the depression lifts (Silverman, Silverman, & Eardley, 1984; Simons, Garfield, & Murphy, 1984; Zeiss, Lewinsohn, & Muñoz, 1979), and that they do not predict to later depressive episodes (Lewinsohn, Steinmetz, Larson, & Franklin, 1981). Yet, treatment outcome studies which attempt to change these factors do show credible effects (McLean & Hakstian, 1979; Murphy, Simons, Wetzel, & Lustman, 1984; Rush, Beck, Kovacs, & Hollon, 1977; Zeiss, Lewinsohn, & Muñoz, 1979). Studies which purposefully produce changes in these factors in nonclinical populations and follow these samples prospectively are very much needed.

In terms of predisposing personality characteristics, it must be remembered that associations found between depression and certain traits may be due to the development of both depression and these traits from genetic, constitutional, or learning processes, or that the experience of depression could alter personality characteristics (Hirschfeld & Cross, 1981). The same could be said of cognitive and behavioral variables which are not conceptualized as traits.

SOME CONSIDERATIONS AS WE EMBARK ON THE DEPRESSION PREVENTION ENTERPRISE

Depression prevention research has much to offer to the mental health field and to society in general. Its potential contributions include advances in theory, measurement, and description of the natural history of depression. The most direct product of such an endeavor will be interventions which reduce the rate of appearance of new cases, and which therefore avoid unnecessary human suffering. It is possible that successful preventive programs may also produce economic savings, though this is not a necessary or required outcome (Russell, 1984).

However, prevention interventions are not likely to become a priority unless they find advocates who will champion their cause. Unfortunately, our tendency is to react to dire needs and to ignore possibilities for early intervention to reduce later pain. Individuals are much more likely to pay (and to take the time) to reduce the pain of a current depression than to learn methods to forestall a possible future episode.

With few exceptions, our health system also values treatment more than prevention. The rewards at both an economic and personal level are much more easily available. A clinician who cares for a patient in whom a clinical depression is alleviated attributes the improvement to his or her work, and receives the gratitude of the patient. A prevention practitioner never knows who in a high risk group has been spared the grief of a depressive episode. The participants in such a program cannot know whether the program produced a significant effect on their lives, or if they suspect that it did, when such an effect had its impact. Thus the results are more distant, at both a subjective and temporal level.

In order to successfully pursue the prevention enterprise, it will be necessary to have a consistent public policy which recognizes that although definitive results may not appear for many years, the pursuit of preventive interventions is a long-term investment well worth making.

SUMMARY

The impact of depression on society is immense. Treatment approaches alone are unlikely to be sufficient to address the problem. Therefore, there is an urgent need to develop and evaluate preventive interventions to reduce the incidence of depression. These interventions may be successful even before etiological processes are fully understood. In fact, preventive research may help illuminate these processes, just as treatment studies have contributed to the development of productive theories and research directions.

Important elements in depression prevention research projects include defining the target of intervention, specifying the theorized mechanisms underlying the chosen approach, detailing the method of intervention to be evaluated, and measuring short- and long-term effects of the intervention on both the theorized mechanisms as well as the ultimate target.

High-risk factor research in depression can serve both to stimulate hypotheses regarding the elements which increase the chances that a depressive episode will take place, as well as to identify groups in the population that are most likely to benefit from preventive interventions. Risk factors involve demographic, biological, social, and psychological variables.

The benefits of prevention are not immediate, nor apparent at the individual level. Therefore, progress in the depression prevention area will require a long-term societal commitment. Such a commitment is possible if professional and civic leaders can share the vision of a preventively-oriented society with their communities.

REFERENCES

Abramson, L. Y., Seligman, M. E. P., & Teasdale, J. (1978). Learned helplessness in humans: Critique and reformulation. *Journal of Abnormal Psychology, 87,* 49-74.

Ahearn, F. L., Jr., & Cohen, R. E. (Eds.). (1984). *Disasters and mental health: An annotated bibliography.* (DHHS Publication No. ADM 84-1311). Washington, DC: U.S. Government Printing Office.

Akiskal, H. S., & McKinney, W. T., Jr., (1973). Depressive disorders: Toward a unified hypothesis. *Science, 182,* 20-29.

Albee, G. W., Gordon, S., & Leitenberg, H. (Eds.). (1983). *Promoting sexual responsibility and preventing sexual problems.* Hanover, NH: University Press of New England.

Albee, G. W., & Joffe, J. M. (Eds.). (1977). *Primary prevention of psychopathology: Vol. 1. The issues.* Hanover, NH: University Press of New England.

American Psychiatric Association. (1980). *Diagnostic and statistical manual of mental disorders* (3rd ed.). Washington, DC: Author.

American Psychiatric Association. (1985). *Draft: DSM-III-R in development.* Washington, DC: Author.

Baldessarini, R. J. (1983). *Biomedical aspects of depression and its treatment.* Washington, DC: American Psychiatric Press.

Barrera, M. (1986). *Distinctions between social support concepts, measures, and models. American Journal of Community Psychology, 14,* 413-445.

Barter, J. T., & Talbott, S. W. (Eds.). (in press). *Primary prevention in psychiatry: What do we know and what works?* Washington, DC: American Psychiatric Press.

Beck, A. T. (1967). *Depression: Clinical, experimental, and theoretical aspects.* New York: Hoeber. (Republished as *Depression: Causes and treatment.* Philadelphia: University of Pennsylvania Press, 1972.)

Beck, A. T., Ward, C.H., Mendelson, M., Mock, J. E., & Erbaugh, J. K. (1961). An inventory for measuring depression. *Archives of General Psychiatry, 4,* 561-571.

Beckham, E. E., & Leber, W. R. (1985). *Handbook of depression: Treatment, assessment, and research.* Homewood, IL: Dorsey.

Bloom, B. L. (1965). The medical model, miasma theory, and community mental health. *Community Mental Health Journal, 1,* 333-338.

Bloom, B. L. (1975). *Community mental health: A general introduction.* Belmont, CA: Wadsworth.

Bloom, B. L. (1985). *Stressful life event theory and research: Implications for primary prevention.* (DHHS Publication No. ADM 85-1385). Washington, DC: U.S. Government Printing Office.

Bond, L. A., & Joffe, J. M. (Eds.). (1982). *Facilitating infant and early childhood development.* Hanover, NH: University Press of New England.

Bond, L. A., & Rosen, J. C. (Eds.). (1980). *Competence and coping during adulthood.* Hanover, NH: University Press of New England.

Boyd, J. H., & Weissman, M. M. (1982). Epidemiology. In E. S. Paykel (Ed.), *Handbook of affective disorders* (pp. 109-125). New York: Guilford.

Broskowski, A., Marks, E., & Budman, S. H. (Eds.). (1981). *Linking health and mental health.* Beverly Hills: Sage.

Brown, G. W., & Harris, T. (1978). *Social origins of depression.* London: Tavistock Publications.

Buckner, J. C., Trickett, E. J., & Corse, S. J. (1985). *Primary prevention in mental health: An annotated bibliography* (DHHS Publication No. ADM 85-1405). Washington, DC: U.S. Government Printing Office.

Caplan, G. (1964). *Principles of preventive psychiatry.* New York: Basic Books.

Caplan, G., & Grunebaum, H. (1972). Perspectives on primary prevention: A review. In H. Gottesfeld (Ed.) *The critical issues of community mental health.* New York: Behavioral Publications.

Cohen, J. (1977). *Statistical power analysis for the behavioral sciences* (rev. ed.). New York: Academic Press.

Cowen, E. L. (1973). Social and community interventions. *Annual Review of Psychology, 24,* 423-472.

Cowen, E. L. (1982). Research in primary prevention in mental health [Special issue]. *American Journal of Community Psychology. 10*(3).

Coyne, J. C., & Gotlib, I. H. (1983). The role of cognition in depression: A critical appraisal. *Psychological Bulletin, 94,* 472-505.

Dohrenwend, B. S., & Dohrenwend, B. P. (1974). *Stressful life events: Their nature and effects.* New York: Wiley & Sons.

Eaton, W. W., & Kessler, L. G. (Eds.). (1985). *Epidemiologic field methods in psychiatry.* Orlando: Academic Press.

Ellis, A. (1962). *Reason and emotion in psychotherapy.* New York: Lyle Stuart.

Endicott, J., & Spitzer, R. L. (1978). A diagnostic interview: The schedule for affective disorders and schizophrenia. *Archives of General Psychiatry, 35,* 837–844.

Felner, R. D., Jason, L. A., Moritsugu, J. N., & Farber, S. S. (Eds.). (1983). *Preventive psychology: Theory, research and practice.* New York: Pergamon.

Forgays, D. G. (Ed.). (1978). *Primary prevention of psychopathology. Vol. 2. Environmental influences.* Hanover, NH: University Press of New England.

Frank, R. G., Kamlet, M. S., & Stoudemire, A. (1985, May). The social cost of depression. In A. Stoudemire (Chair), *Perspectives in the prevention of depression.* Symposium conducted at the meeting of the American Psychiatric Association, Dallas, Texas.

Galen, R. S., & Gambino, S. R. (1975). *Beyond normality: The predictive value and efficiency of medical diagnoses.* New York: Wiley & Sons.

Gershon, E. S. (1985, May). New developments in genetics of mood disorders. In R. O. Friedel (Chair), *De rerum futura: The measure of psychiatry in the 1980's and beyond.* Symposium conducted at the meeting of the American Psychiatric Association, Dallas, Texas.

Glasscote, R. M., Kohn, E., Beigel, A., Raber, M. F., Roeske, N., Cox, B. A., Raybin, J. B., & Bloom, B. L. (1980). *Preventing mental illness: Efforts and attitudes.* Washington, DC: American Psychiatric Association.

Goldman, H. H., & Goldston, S. E. (Eds.). (1985). *Preventing stress-related psychiatric disorders* (DHHS Publication No. ADM 85–1366). Washington, DC: U.S. Government Printing Office.

Goldstein, M. J. (Ed.). (1982). *Preventive intervention in schizophrenia: Are we ready?* (DHHS Publication No. ADM 82–1111). Washington, DC: U.S. Government Printing Office.

Goldston, S. E. (1977). Defining primary prevention. In G. W. Albee, & J. M. Joffe (Eds.), *Primary prevention of psychopathology: Vol. 1. The issues* (pp. 18–23). Hanover, NH: University Press of New England.

Grosscup, S. J., & Lewinsohn, P. M. (1980). Unpleasant and pleasant events, and mood. *Journal of Clinical Psychology, 36,* 252–259

Gruenberg, E. M. (1981). Risk factor research methods. In D. A. Regier & G. Allen (Eds.). *Risk factor research in the major mental disorders* (DHHS Publication No. ADM 81–1068, pp. 8–19). Washington, DC: U.S. Government Printing Office.

Hamburg, D. A., Elliott, G. R., & Parron, D. L. (Eds.). (1982). *Health and behavior: Frontiers of research in the biobehavioral sciences.* Washington, DC: National Academy Press.

Hamilton, M. (1967). Development of a rating scale for primary depressive illness. *British Journal of Social and Clinical Psychology, 6,* 278–296.

Heller, K., & Monahan, J. (1977). *Psychology and community change.* Homewood, IL: Dorsey.

Heller, K., Price, R. H., & Sher, K. J. (1980). Research and evaluation in primary prevention: Issues and guidelines. In R. H. Price, R. F. Ketterer, B. C. Bader, & J. Monahan (Eds.), *Prevention in mental health: Research, policy and practice.* (pp. 285–313). Beverly Hills, Sage.

Hilliard, T. O. (1981). Political and social action in the prevention of psychopathology of Blacks: A mental health strategy for oppressed people. In J. M. Joffe & G. W. Albee (Eds.), *Prevention through political action and social change.* (pp. 135–152). Hanover, NH: University Press of New England.

Hirschfeld, R. M. A., & Cross, C. K. (1981). Psychosocial risk factors for depression. In D. A. Regier & G. Allen (Eds.). *Risk factor research in the major mental disorders* (DHHS Publication No. ADM 81–1068, pp. 55–66). Washington, DC: U.S. Government Printing Office.

Hunt, D., Ward, N., & Bloom, V. (1982). A preliminary study of public responses to newspaper, TV, and radio presentation on depression. *Hospital and Community Psychiatry, 33,* 304–305.

Iscoe, I., Bloom, B. L., & Spielberger, C. D. (Eds.). (1977). *Community psychology in transition.* Washington, DC: Hemisphere.

Joffe, J. M., & Albee, G. W. (Eds.). (1981). *Prevention through political action and social change.* Hanover, NH: University Press of New England.

Kent, M. W., & Rolf, J. E. (Eds.). (1979). *Social competence in children.* Hanover, NH: University Press of New England.

Kessler, M., & Goldston, S. E. (Eds.). (1986). *A decade of progress in primary prevention.* Hanover, NH: University Press of New England.

Klein, D. C., & Goldston, S. E. (Eds.). (1977). *Primary prevention: An idea whose time has come* (DHHS Publication No. ADM 80–447). Washington, DC: U.S. Government Printing Office.

Kleinman, A., & Good, B. (1985). *Culture and depression: Studies in the anthropology and cross-cultural psychiatry of affect and disorder.* Berkeley: University of California Press.

Klerman, G. L., Lavori, P. W., Rice, J., Reich, T., Endicott, J., Andreasen, N. C., Keller, M. B., & Hirschfeld, R. M. A. (1985). Birth cohort trends in rates of major depressive disorder among relatives of patients with affective disorder. *Archives of General Psychiatry, 42,* 689–693.

Klerman, G. L., Weissman, M. M., Rounsaville, B. J., Chevron, E. S. (1984). *Interpersonal psychotherapy of depression.* New York: Basic Books.

Kovacs, M., & Beck, A. T. (1978). Maladaptive cognitive structures in depression. *American Journal of Psychiatry, 135,* 525–533.

Lewinsohn, P. M., & Graf, M. (1973). Pleasant activities and depression. *Journal of Consulting and Clinical Psychology, 41,*261–268.

Lewinsohn, P. M., Steinmetz, J. L., Larson, D. W., & Franklin, J. (1981). Depression-related cognitions: Antecedent or consequence? *Journal of Abnormal Psychology, 90,* 213–219.

Lewinsohn, P. M., & Talkington, J. (1979). Studies on the measurement of unpleasant events and relations with depression. *Applied Psychological measurement, 3,* 83–101.

Libet, J., & Lewinsohn, P. M. (1973). The concept of social skill with special references to the behavior of depressed persons. *Journal of Consulting and Clinical Psychology, 40,* 304–312.

MacMahon, B., & Pugh, T. F. (1970). *Epidemiology: Principles and methods.* Boston: Little, Brown.

Manson, S. M. (Ed.). (1982). *New directions in prevention among American Indian and Alaska native communities.* Portland, OR: Oregon Health Sciences University.

Marlowe, H. A., Jr., & Weinberg, R. B. (Eds.). (1985). Is mental illness preventable?: Pros and cons [Special issue]. *The Journal of Primary Prevention, 5*(4).

Marsella, A. J. (1980). Depressive experience and disorder across cultures. In J. Draguns & H. Triandis (Eds.). *Handbook of cross-cultural psychology. Vol. 6. Psychopathology* (pp. 237–289). Boston: Allyn & Bacon.

McLean, P. D., & Hakstian, A. R. (1979). Clinical depression: Comparative efficacy of outpatient treatments. *Journal of Consulting and Clinical Psychology, 47,* 818–836.

Mendelson, M. (1982). Psychodynamics of depression. In E. S. Paykel (Ed.), *Handbook of affective disorders* (pp. 164–174). New York: Guilford.

Mezzich, J. E., & Raab, E. S. (1980). Depressive symptomatology across the Americas. *Archives of General Psychiatry, 37,* 818–823.

Muñoz, R. F. (1976). The primary prevention of psychological problems: A review of the literature. *Community Mental Health Review, 1*(6), 1–15.

Muñoz, R. F. (1977). A cognitive approach to the assessment and treatment of depression. (Doctoral dissertation, University of Oregon, 1977). *Dissertation Abstracts International,* 1977, *38,* 2873B. (University Microfilms, No. 77-26, 505, 154.)

Muñoz, R. F. (1980). A strategy for the prevention of psychological problems in Latinos: Emphasizing accessibility and effectiveness. In R. Valle and W. Vega (Eds.), *Hispanic Natural Support Systems* (pp. 85–96). Sacramento: State of California Department of Mental Health.

Muñoz, R. F. (1982). The Spanish-speaking consumer and the community mental health center. In E. E. Jones, & S. J. Korchin (Eds.), *Minority mental health* (pp. 362–398). New York: Praeger.

Muñoz, R. F., Chan, F., & Armas, R. (1986). Cross-cultural perspectives on primary prevention of mental disorders. In J. T. Barter, & S. W. Talbott (Eds.), *Primary prevention in psychiatry. State of the Art.* Washington, DC: American Psychiatric Press.

Muñoz, R. F., & Kelly, J. G. (1975). *The prevention of mental disorders.* Homewood, Illinois: Richard D. Irwin.

Muñoz, R. F., & Lewinsohn, P. M. (in press). The Personal Beliefs Inventory. In M. Hersen & A. S. Bellack (Eds.), *Dictionary of behavioral assessment techniques.* New York: Pergamon.

Muñoz, R. F., Snowden, L. R., & Kelly, J. G. (Eds.). (1979). *Social and psychological research in community settings.* San Francisco: Jossey-Bass.

Murphy, G. E., Simons, A. D., Wetzel, R. D., & Lustman, P. J. (1984). Cognitive therapy and pharmacotherapy: Singly and together in the treatment of depression. *Archives of General Psychiatry, 37,* 33–41.

Murphy, J. (1980). *Psychiatric instrument development for primary care research: Patient self-report questionnaire* (Contract No. 80MO14280101D). Rockville, MD: National Institute of Mental Health.

Murrell, S. A. (1973). *Community psychology and social systems: A conceptual framework and intervention guide.* New York: Behavioral.

Myers, E. R. (1977). *The community psychology concept: Integrating theory, education and practice in psychology, social work and public administration.* Washington, DC: University Press of America.

Myers, J. K., Weissman, M. M., Tischler, G. L., Holzer, C. E., Leaf, P. J., Orvaschel, H., Anthony, J. C., Boyd, J. H., Burke, J. D., Kramer, M., & Stolzman, R. (1984). Six-month prevalence of psychiatric disorders in three communities. *Archives of General Psychiatry, 41,* 959–967.

Nurnberger, J. I., & Gershon, E. S. (1982). Genetics. In E. S. Paykel (Ed.), *Handbook of affective disorders* (pp. 126–145). New York: Guilford.

Office of the Surgeon General. (1979). *Healthy People: The Surgeon General's report on health promotion and disease prevention* (DHEW PHS Publication No. 79–55071). Washington, DC: U.S. Government Printing Office.

O'Gorman, N. (1981). The education of the oppressed child in a democracy. In J. M. Joffe & G. W. Albee (Eds.), *Prevention through political action and social change.* (pp. 275–283). Hanover, NH: University Press of New England.

Orvaschel, H., Weissman, M. M., & Kidd, K. K. (1980). Children and depression: The children of depressed parents; the childhood of depressed patients; depression in children. *Journal of Affective Disorders, 2,* 1–16.

Osterweis, M., Solomon, F., & Green, M. (Eds.). (1984). *Bereavement: Reactions, consequences, and care.* Washington, DC: National Academy Press.

Owan, T. C. (Ed.). (1985). *Southeast Asian mental health: Treatment, prevention, services, training, and research* (DHHS Publication No. ADM 85–1399). Washington, DC: U.S. Government Printing Office.

Paykel, E. S. (1982). Life events and early environment. In E. S. Paykel (Ed.), *Handbook of affective disorders* (pp. 146–161). New York: Guilford.

Peplau, L. A., & Goldston, S. E. (Eds.). (1984). *Preventing the harmful consequences of severe and persistent loneliness* (DHHS Publication No. ADM 84–1312). Washington, DC: U.S. Government Printing Office.

Perez-Stable, E. J., Muñoz, R. F., Chan, F., & Ying, Y. W. (1985). Depression in medical patients: The need for a screening test [Abstract]. *Clinical Research, 33,* 729A.

Prange, A. J., Wilson, I. C., Lynn, C. W., Alltop, L. B., & Stikeleather. R. A. (1974). L-tryptophan in mania: Contribution to the permissive hypothesis of affective disorders. *Archives of General Psychiatry, 30,* 56–62.

Price, R. H., Ketterer, R. F., Bader, B. C., & Monahan, J. (Eds.). (1980), *Prevention in mental health: Research, policy, and practice.* Beverly Hills: Sage.

Price, R. H., & Smith, S. S. (1985). *A guide to evaluating prevention programs in mental health* (DHHS Publication No. ADM 85–1365). Washington, DC: U.S. Government Printing Office.

Radloff, L. S. (1977). The CES-D scale: A self-report depression scale for research in the general population. *Applied Psychological Measurement, 1,* 385–401.

Rappaport, J. (1977). *Community psychology: Values, research, and action.* New York: Holt, Rinehart and Winston.

Regier, D. A., & Allen, G. (Eds.). (1981). *Risk factor research in the major mental disorders* (DHSS Publication No. ADM 81–1068). Washington, DC: U.S. Government Printing Office.

Rehm, L. P. (1977). A self-control model of depression. *Behavior Therapy, 8,* 787–804.

Robins, L. N., Helzer, J. E., Croughan, J., & Ratcliff, K. S. (1981). National Institute of Mental Health Diagnostic Interview Schedule: Its history, characteristics, and validity. *Archives of General Psychiatry, 38,* 381–389.

Robins, L. N., Helzer, J. E., Weissman, M. M., Orvaschel, H., Gruenberg, E., Burke, J. D., & Regier, D. A. (1984). Lifetime prevalence of specific psychiatric disorders in three sites. *Archives of General Psychiatry, 41,* 949–958.

Rush, A. J., Beck. A. T., Kovacs, M., & Hollon, S. (1977). Comparative efficacy of cognitive therapy and pharmacotherapy in the treatment of depressed outpatients. *Cognitive Therapy and Research, 1,* 17–37.

Russell, L. B. (1984). *Evaluating preventive medical care as a health strategy* (NCHSR Report No. 85–90). Washington, DC: Brookings Institution. (NTIS No. PB85-208163).

Sachar, E. J. (1982). Endocrine abnormalities in depression. In E. S. Paykel (Ed.), *Handbook of affective disorders* (pp. 191–201). New York: Guilford.

Seligman, M. E. P. (1975). *Helplessness: On depression, development, and death.* San Francisco: W. H. Freeman & Co.

Shapiro, S., Skinner, E. A., Kessler, L. G., Von Korff, M., German, P. S., Tischler, G. L., Leaf, P. J., Benham, L., Cottler, L., & Regier, D. A. (1984). Utilization of health and mental health services: Three Epidemiological Catchment Area sites. *Archives of General Psychiatry, 41,* 971–978.

Siever, L. J., & Davis, K. L. (1985). Overview: Toward a Dysregulation hypothesis of depression. *American Journal of Psychiatry, 142,* 1017–1031.

Silverman, J. S., Silverman, J. A., & Eardley, D. A. (1984). Do maladaptive attitudes cause depression? *Archives of General Psychiatry, 41,* 28–30.

Simons, A. D., Garfield, S. L., & Murphy, G. E. (1984). The process of change in cognitive therapy and pharmacotherapy for depression. *Archives of General Psychiatry, 41,* 45–51.

Snowden, L. R. (Ed.). (1982). *Reaching the underserved: Mental health needs of neglected populations.* Beverly Hills: Sage.

Spitzer, R. L., Endicott, J., & Robins, E. (1978). Research diagnostic criteria: Rationale and reliability. *Archives of General Psychiatry, 35,* 773–782.

Spitzer, R. L., & Williams, J. B. W. (1985). *Structured clinical interview for DSM-III* (SCID-HAM, 8-1-85). New York: Biometrics Research Department, New York State Psychiatric Institute.

Steinbrueck, S. M., Maxwell, S. E., & Howard, G. S. (1983). A meta-analysis of psychotherapy and drug therapy in the treatment of unipolar depression with adults. *Journal of Consulting and Clinical Psychology, 51,* 856–863.

Surtees, P. G., & Rennie, D. (1983). Adversity and the onset of psychiatric disorder in women. *Social Psychiatry, 18,* 37–44.

Teuting, P., Koslow, S. H., & Hirschfeld, R. M. A. (1981). *Special report on depression research* (DHHS Publication No. ADM 81–1085). Washington, DC: U.S. Government Printing Office.

U.S. Bureau of the Census. (1984). *Statistical abstracts of the United States* (104th ed.). Washington, DC: U.S. Government Printing Office.

Valle R., & Vega W. (Eds.). (1980). *Hispanic Natural Support Systems.* Sacramento: State of California Department of Mental Health.

Vega, W. A., & Miranda, M. R. (Eds.). (1985). *Stress & Hispanic mental health: Relating research to service delivery* (DHHS Publication No. ADM 85–1410). Washington, DC: U.S. Government Printing Office.

Weissman, M. M., & Myers, J. K. (1978). Affective disorders in a U.S. urban community: The use of Research Diagnostic Criteria in an epidemiological survey. *Archives of General Psychiatry, 35,* 1304–1311.

Whybrow, P. C., Akiskal, H. S., & McKinney, W. T., Jr. (1984). *Mood disorders: Toward a new psychobiology.* New York: Plenum Press.

Williams, J. B. W., & Spitzer, R. L. (Eds.). (1984). *Psychotherapy research: Where are we and where should we go?* New York: Guilford Press.

Wing, J. K., Cooper, J. E., & Sartorius, N. (1974). *The description and classification of psychiatric symptoms: An instruction manual for the PSE and CATEGO system.* London: Cambridge University Press.

Zax, M., & Specter, G. A. (1974). *An introduction to community psychology.* New York: John Wiley & Sons.

Zeiss, A. M., Lewinsohn, P. M., & Muñoz, R. F. (1979). Nonspecific improvement effects in depression using interpersonal skills training, pleasant activity schedules, or cognitive training. *Journal of Consulting and Clinical Psychology, 47,* 427–439.

Zis, A. P., & Goodwin, F. K. (1982). The amine hypothesis. In E. S. Paykel (Ed.), *Handbook of affective disorders* (pp. 175–190). New York: Guilford.

Zung, W. W. K. (1965). A self-rating depression scale. *Archives of General Psychiatry, 12,* 63–70.

2

Preventing Depression: The Symptom, the Syndrome, or the Disorder?

Paula J. Clayton
University of Minnesota

INTRODUCTION

The word depression can denote a mood, a symptom, a syndrome, or a disorder. As a mood it may occur in individuals as ups and downs of normal life—we have "good days" and "bad days," we get up on the wrong side of the bed, etc. As a symptom, it can be the sign of distress seen following a response to any unhappy event. Additional symptoms that we have come to associate with depression, either somatic or psychological symptoms or both, can coexist. The response is fleeting and understandable. Warheit (1979), Amenson and Lewinsohn (1981), and Andrews (1981), have clearly shown the association between stressful life events and depressive symptoms. The syndrome of depression can also appear in response to unhappy life events. The syndrome, as opposed to the symptom, is a collection of symptoms that meet the minimal criteria (e.g., either Feighner, RDC, or DSM-III) for a major depression. These symptoms are understandable given the circumstances and most of the people experiencing these symptoms do not see them as abnormal and do not seek care for them. The syndrome is less fleeting. It can last weeks or months. The perfect example of the syndrome is the response to bereavement which I will expand on later, but an equally good example would be the response to rape. The syndrome has an associated morbidity and mortality and because of this deserves critical investigation. By looking closely at the syndrome we can learn predictor and outcome variables that need to be recorded in order to strengthen intervention research. The *disorder,* depression, characteristically is what clinical investigators working with psychiatric patients (i.e., those who seek treatment for their symptoms) are interested in delineating. A disorder unlike a syndrome should have a characteristic short and long-term prognosis, family history, and laboratory tests. Investigators hope to isolate a homogeneous group or groups who then may be studied further presumably to determine a biologic etiology. In looking at patients with depressive disorder, which may resemble most closely the melancholic depression of DSM-III, there is the most controversy over the correlation between life events and the disorder. The conclusion usually reached is that the risk of developing a depression after the more stressful life events is increased six fold in the immediate six months and falls off rapidly

This research is supported, in part, by USPHS grant #MH-25430.

thereafter (Paykel, 1982). Thus, causative effects of life events are important but not overwhelming.

For the most part, people expressing the mood, the symptom, or the syndrome of depression are not seen by psychiatrists but are identified in community studies. It must be emphasized, however, because the term *major depression* refers to both the syndrome and disorder, there are people who are responding to stresses with unhappiness, demoralization, and the syndrome in clinic populations and there are patients with the disorder in the community who have not been treated. Both have affective symptoms long enough to qualify for most definitions of depression that use operational criteria. The threshold that should be used to distinguish these two is not yet clear (Wing, 1980). Certainly every episode of current or previous depression needs to be identified as occurring with or without a "significant" life stress in the preceding six months. As Bebbington et al. (1981) maintain from studying symptoms and life events in community cases and acutely ill patients, "disease theories are more likely required to explain the occurrence of the more severe affective disorders, while the less severe often have a ready explanation as understandable and unmysterious responses to adversity." Researchers must make detailed effort to describe the populations being treated in order to allow us to consider which of these populations is being treated and to help us, eventually, resolve the threshold issue. One suggested way of resolving it is to limit the disorder to recurrent depression. This would, unfortunately however, eliminate close examination of the most interesting episode of illness—the first episode.

One further issue that must be kept in mind when dealing with the concept of major depression is that this depression usually occurs in otherwise healthy individuals. A similar depression (with no distinguishing features) can result from medication, medical illness or another primary psychiatric disease. Better labeled "secondary depression" but included under the rubric of major depression preceding psychiatric symptoms, drug use (e.g., prednisone), and physical illness must be systematically inquired about and carefully recorded.

Whether identifying the syndrome or the disorder, it does not mean that interventions are not indicated. As stated there is a morbidity and mortality associated with a stress response.

DEPRESSIVE SYMPTOMS
AND THE SYNDROME OF DEPRESSION
IN BEREAVEMENT

Numerous authors, among them Freud (1957), Lindemann (1944), Marris (1958), Clayton et al. (1968, 1971), Parkes (1970, 1972), Maddison and Viola (1968), Yamamoto et al. (1969), Yamamoto (1970), Kennell et al. (1970), Levy (1976), studying the bereaved prospectively and retrospectively, have delineated the symptomatology of bereavement. It is clear that depressive symptoms dominate the picture. Just as one feels fear when confronted by an onrushing automobile, so it seems reasonable that one should feel sadness when confronted with the death of someone close. Clayton et al. (1968, 1971, 1972, 1979) have collected data on three samples of recently bereaved. The first sample was an unselected group of relatives of patients who died at a general hospital in St. Louis. The

Table 1 Frequency of depressive symptoms at 1 and 13 months

Symptom	n = 149[d]	
	1 Month % +	13 Months % +
Crying	89	33[d]
Sleep disturbance	76	48[d]
Low mood	75	42[d]
Loss of appetite	51	16[d]
Fatigue	44	30[c]
Poor memory	41	23[d]
Loss of interest	40	23[d]
Difficulty concentrating	36	16[d]
Weight loss of 2.25 kg or more	36	20[c]
Feeling guilty	31	12[d]
Restlessness (n = 89)	48	45
Reversed diurnal variation	26	22
Irritability	24	20
Feels someone to blame	22	22
Diurnal variation	17	10
Death wishes	16	12
Feeling hopeless	14	13
Hallucinations	12	9
Suicidal thoughts	5	3
Fear of losing mind	3	4
Suicide attempts	0	0
Feeling worthless	6	11
Feels angry about death	13	22[b]
Depressive syndrome	42	16[d]

[a]n varies from symptom to symptom, mostly 148
[b]Significant by McNemar's chi-square, df = 1, p ≤ 0.02
[c]Significant by McNemar's chi-square, df = 1, p ≤ 0.01
[d]Significant by McNemar's chi-square, df = 1, p ≤ 0.001

second sample was a randomly selected group of white widows and widowers chosen mostly from the death certificates, and the third was a consecutive group of young white widows and widowers chosen from a later death certificate sample. Data from the last two samples were combined since both studies were methodologically and substantially similar. In all, 171 men and women were interviewed in the first month after the deaths of their spouses and 149 were seen one year later. The average age of the 149 followed-up was 51 years. It consisted of 96 women and 53 men from all social classes. Table 1 shows the frequency of positive depression symptoms at one month and 13 months.

It is clear that the symptoms commonly seen in a typically depressed patient are also present in the first month of bereavement. By one year many of the vegetative symptoms of depression have changed significantly, although the frequency of some symptoms is still high (sleep disturbance, 48 percent; restlessness, 48 percent; low mood, 42 percent). The interesting thing is that while the somatic symptoms of depression decrease significantly, the psychological symptoms of depression, such as death wishes, hopelessness, suicidal thoughts, worthlessness and feeling angry do not decrease or may even increase by one year. This is in keeping

Table 2   Frequency of depressive symptoms at any time in the first
year of bereavement and in controls

Symptom	Probands % n = 149[a]	Controls % n = 131[a]
Crying	90	14[e]
Sleep disturbance	79	35[e]
Low mood	80	18[e]
Loss of appetite	53	4[e]
Fatigue	55	23[e]
Poor memory	50	22[e]
Loss of interest	48	11[e]
Difficulty concentrating	40	13[e]
Weight loss of 2.25 kg or more	47	24[e]
Feeling guilty	38	11[e]
Restlessness	63	27[e]
Irritability	35	21[b]
Diurnal variation	22	14
Death wishes	22	5[e]
Feeling hopeless	19	4[d]
Hallucinations	17	2[e]
Suicidal thoughts	8	1[c]
Fear of losing mind	7	5
Suicide attempts	0	0
Worthlessness	14	15
Depressive syndrome	47	8[d]

[a]n varies from symptom to symptom
[b]Significant by chi-square, df = 1, p < .05
[c]Significant by chi-square, df = 1, p < .01
[d]Significant by chi-square, df = 1, p < .0005
[e]Significant by chi-square, df = 1, p < .0001

with similar findings of Blanchard et al. (1976), from a retrospective study of widows. Their conclusion was that early in bereavement the physiological symptoms of depression predominate, but as the bereaved turns to looking toward the future and reorganizing her life, the psychological symptoms become predominant. Parkes (1972) discusses the physiological response of an animal to stress. He speaks of sympathetic stimulation and parasympathetic inhibition and three distinct components of the overall response—level of arousal, autonomic disturbance, and emotional reaction. Our findings are reminiscent of this. It seems the level of arousal and the autonomic disturbance are prominent early in bereavement and that the emotional reaction surfaces in the later stage.

Table 2 compares the frequency of depressive symptoms occurring at any time during the first year in the 149 bereaved and a group of 131 married community controls matched for age (average age 52.6), sex, and neighborhood. Most symptoms are more common in the bereaved. Hallucinations are reported by the bereaved, a finding confirmed by Rees (1971). The hallucinations pertain to the deceased.

Several further comments should be made. There are several depressive symptoms that are rare in bereavement or are qualitatively different. Suicidal thoughts are uncommon. They occur normally in younger male bereaved in the first month, but under any other circumstances they can be considered pathological. Retardation is also rare and probably pathological. We have never observed a "retarded" depression in bereavement, a finding similar to Lindemann (1944) and Parkes (1970). Although guilt is frequently noted, it usually is guilt of "omission," chiefly things that were or were not done during the terminal illness or at the death. Pervasive guilt and rumination are not seen. Nor is there morbid cultivation of the deceased, referred to as "mummification," and reported further by Gardner and Pritchard (1977). In this abnormal state, the living preserve the dead's environment unchanged for months or years after. The usual example is Queen Victoria's behavior after Prince Albert's death. She extended from past to present by having his clothes and shaving water brought to their dressing room daily for several years. Finally, although hallucinations are present as noted, delusions are never recorded. These symptoms may indicate true psychiatric disability. By one year most of the bereaved can discuss the dead person with relative equanimity. A "severe" (Bornstein & Clayton, 1972) anniversary reaction is rare and indicates a poor outcome.

Although sleep remains disturbed for one year, by four months most bereaved have regained their appetites and begun to gain weight. Parkes (1970) reports, "Nineteen (86 percent) widows claimed that they lost their appetites during the first month of bereavement, and in 15 this brought about recognized loss of weight. Six widows lost 6 kg or more in the course of the first month, and only one gained weight during this period. After the end of the first month, however, anorexia and weight loss were much less common, and from the third month onward it was weight gain that was more likely to be regarded as a 'problem.'" In the book, by Glick et al. (1974), *The First Year of Bereavement,* Glick confirms this without giving frequencies. He says, "In time some found the weight loss to be not altogether displeasing—our one year interviews suggest that they rather like the improvement in their figures, and there was not at any point fear that anorexia might be entrenched as there was in relation to insomnia." Sexual interests also return by four months although this is more variable. Low mood is still reported by many at one year, but it is not a sustained low mood and most of the bereaved report that they can easily be distracted from it. The mood is always noticeably disturbed on holidays, anniversaries, the anniversary of the death and other personal meaningful events. Since the bereaved continue their normal functioning, this should not be considered pathological.

The pertinent question then is since bereaved suffer from and report significant depressive symptoms, how many have enough symptoms to be "labeled" as having the syndrome of depression? Using criteria of Feighner et al. (1972) in our first study of widowhood (Maddison & Viola, 1968; Bornstein et al., 1973; Clayton et al., 1974), (sample's average age: 62), 35 percent at one month, 25 percent at four months and 17 percent at one year could be classified as depressed. Forty-five percent were depressed at some point during the year and 13 percent were depressed for the entire year. Adding in the younger sample (see Table 1), 42 percent at one month and 16 percent at one year met the criteria. Forty-seven percent of the sample were depressed at one of the two points and 11 percent were depressed for the entire year. In the controls, who were excluded if they lost a first degree relative in the preceding year, eight percent reported a depressive syndrome, a one year incidence figure that can be compared to the 47 percent in the widowed population (see Table 2). This emphasizes the necessity of taking the bereavement reaction into account in any study of the population prevalence of depression, as Weissman and Myers (1978) have recently done. They reported a lifetime prevalence for grief reactions of 10.4 percent, defining a grief reaction as "symptoms that met the criteria for major depression by the SADS (Spitzer et al., 1978) if they began within three months of the death of a close relative and lasted up to one year." Such reactions were more often reported in women and in those from the lower classes. The DSM-III (1980) likewise acknowledges this syndrome in its category "uncomplicated bereavement." Unfortunately, this is the only stress that is so acknowledged, unless one considers post traumatic stress syndrome.

MORBIDITY AND MORTALITY OF BEREAVEMENT

There is still a good deal of controversy over the physical symptoms associated with normal bereavement and the physical morbidity of bereavement. In reviewing all the prospective studies of bereavement, Clayton (1982) concluded there is less physical distress than has previously been emphasized. There is a hint from the literature that young widowed have more anxiety symptoms and perhaps more hospitalizations. Except for those already ill, older men and women have very few changes in their physical health, physician visits and hospitalizations. The startling outcome is that all studies show an increase in cigarette smoking, alcohol consumption and either tranquilizer or hypnotic use or both. The serious morbidity then is the potential abuse of substances.

Depressive symptoms and a persistent depressive reaction also constitutes a morbidity. The relationship between recent death and psychiatric consultation is unclear. Psychiatric hospitalization after a bereavement is rare and probably occurs so infrequently that bereavement need not be considered as a cause of serious mental illness (Clayton, 1982). Our data from the collaborative study of depressive disorder (Hirschfeld et al., 1983) shows that four percent of depressed patients had a recent death of a first degree relative or spouse one to 12 months before *onset* and 6% had such a death in the last 12 months (ignores onset). In the community controls for the bereavement study, 6% were excluded because they had lost a spouse or a first degree relative in the year before the interview. Thus, bereavement alone cannot account for a depressive *disorder*. In the introduction we discussed life events and depressive disorder, and even with pooling of events there is still only a modest association.

Careful re-reading of the mortality data (Clayton, 1982), along with a fine recent set of papers (Helsing & Szklo, 1981; Helsing et al., 1981, 1982), shows there is no increase in mortality in the first year of bereavement for women. There definitely is an increase in mortality for older men and probably for younger men also.

Suicide deserves special mention. Shepherd and Barraclough (1974) have shown that spouses of suicides have no increased mortality in the first year of bereavement. Over a longer period, 58 months, there were 10 deaths in 44 spouses showing a trend that indicates survivors of suicide have a greater risk of death than survivors of other deaths. Compared to mortality rates of married rather than widowed, there probably was a statistically significant excess mortality. Five of 10 spouses who died were mortally ill before the spouse committed suicide and the authors felt the consequences of these illnesses seemed to have increased the risk of suicide in the spouse. This sheds light on the complicated interactions in studying mortality in bereavement and is consistent with similar findings about poor health and mortality in the Ward data (1974, 1976) and poor health and increased physician visits in the Wiener et al. data (1975). Numerous studies from vital statistics records and survey data (Bock & Webber, 1972) have documented an increased number of suicides in the widowed (never as high, though, as single, divorced and separated) compared to an age and sex matched married population. This is particularly striking for elderly men. Three studies have attempted to examine entry into widowhood and suicide. McMahon and Pugh (1965) reviewed the death certificates of all widowed over a five year period in Massachusetts. They selected widowed who had died by suicide and an appropriate comparison group of widowed deaths from other causes. Then they searched the death certificates prior to these deaths for spouses' death certificates, to ascertain the length of widowhood in both the deaths by suicide and from other causes. They found the spouses' death certificates in 80 percent of the cases. The final group consisted of 320 widowed suicides and 320 widowed comparison deaths. Compared with deaths from other causes, deaths from suicide clustered in the first four years of widowhood and particularly in the first year. It appeared that most of this difference could be accounted for by widowed males, 60 and over, in the first year. The relative risk of suicide was estimated to be 2.5 times higher in the first year of bereavement and 1.5 times higher in the second, third and fourth years. They had excluded in their original study design all homicide-suicide combinations. There were no suicides on the anniversary of spouses' deaths.

Bunch (1972) looked at the relationship between recent bereavement and suicide in 75 individuals. She found, compared to appropriate living controls, there was an excess of parental and spouse deaths in the suiciders in the five years before. Comparing the 27 bereaved suicides to 19 living controls who had experienced a similar bereavement, she found that there were no differences in the number and geographical distribution of first degree relative, but the suicides were seeing less of their relations. This could be because of their depressive illnesses, which she documented. Significantly more of the suicides had had psychiatric treatment and/or made a suicide attempt before they were bereaved. Thus, previous psychiatric history may predict a bereavement outcome of suicide in individuals so disposed.

Helsing et al. (1982) reported deaths from infectious diseases, accidents, and suicide were significantly higher than expected among widowed males and from cirrhosis of the liver in widowed females.

PREDICTOR AND OUTCOME VARIABLES TO A STRESS-LIKE BEREAVEMENT

Against a background of realizing that "outcome" variables differ from study to study, it seems clear that the best predictor of poor outcome is poor prior physical or mental health. Those who are physically ill before the bereavement will be most likely to be ill after the bereavement, with more physician visits and perhaps even the greater risk of death in the first year. And those with a previous psychiatric disorder, especially misuse of drugs or alcohol, will be the most vulnerable psychiatrically. This observation is in keeping with all studies that looked at these variables in bereavement as well as many other reported studies dealing with the effects of different stresses, such as floods, being a sudden refugee, hysterectomy, rape, etc.

Alcoholism is a condition that illustrates this point. In all bereavement studies, it has been shown that alcohol consumption increases following bereavement and that the alcoholic is more likely to be doing poorly at one year. If psychiatric hospitalization occurs, the diagnosis is likely to be one of alcoholism (Frost & Clayton, 1977). In addition, it has been shown that among suicides (Murphy & Robins, 1967; Frost & Clayton, 1977), alcoholics are particularly likely to commit suicide within six weeks of a loss.

Thus, those who are physically or mentally ill, or have a propensity toward such, appear to be more vulnerable to various stressful life experiences.

Other variables which are less firmly associated with poor outcome in that they have been reported in one study, but not necessarily replicated in another, are lack of social supports, being in an environment that has a high level of perceived non-support, low socioeconomic status, young age, sex, no previous experience with death, presence of concurrent life crises and short duration of illness. Raphael (1977) has shown that perceived non-support in recently widowed women is associated with poor outcome. It is unclear, however, whether there really were unsupportive people in the environment and therefore, it might have been a variant of the first of these listed variables (lack of social support) or whether this was a symptom of a particular kind of bereaved, that is, one who misinterprets the attitude of others. She did not find that additional stresses produced poorer outcome. Vachon et al. (1982) also showed that social support, poor health and financial problems correlated with enduring distress.

Listing these predictor variables should draw attention again to definitions. For instance, listing "sex" as a predictor clearly has certain implications. If the outcome measure is remarriage, men will have a better outcome. If the outcome measure is death, women will have a better outcome. If the outcome measure is general life satisfaction, since many men remarry and/or die, those who remain widowed in some studies have poorer scores on this item than widowed women. The same problem of definition applies to short duration of illness, sudden death, unanticipated or untimely death. In each study, the definition varies.

There have been several studies of interventions in the recently bereaved picking high risk populations based on factors like lack of social supports, previously discussed. They usually show a tendency or a very modest significant improvement in those who had the interventions (Raphael, 1977; Singh & Raphael, 1981; Parkes, 1981). Colin Murray Parkes (1980) recently reviewed such interventions and felt that on the whole they showed some modest improvement.

Frank and Stewart (1983) looked at the response to rape and recorded the frequency of depressive symptoms and the syndrome variables that might predict a depressive outcome and even included a noncontrolled psychotherapeutic intervention. They found in assessing consecutive rape victims from two rape crisis centers (50% agreed to participate) that 24% had a score of 6 or above on the Beck Depression Inventory and 53% of these met RDC criteria for major depressive disorder. They looked at the factors that might correlate with depression and they found that factors within the rape situation did not account for the differences among the victims, but a past history of psychiatric problems and a nonsupportive or a hostile social network after the stress represented two categories of predictors of depressive symptoms in the aftermath of rape. The time course of this depressive reaction is yet to be documented.

INTERVENTION

Since we know so little about treatment, intervention should be tested separately for the syndrome and the disorder. This is not to say that both will not respond to a variety of nonsomatic therapies (just as many medical illnesses do), but that the target symptoms, length of treatment, or intensity of treatment may be different. Since the syndrome probably clears more spontaneously than the disorder, it may be that under these circumstances, no intervention is as effective and/or less costly than even a brief intervention. The discussion will focus on factors that need to be considered when planning an intervention study of the syndrome. The intervention could be for any stress-related depression, but most of the considerations are based on outcome data from the bereavement literature. Presumably with the disorder, depression, which is probably more lethal, different strategies are necessary.

Preventive intervention and/or early intervention is indicated in those acute stresses that are known to produce a depressive syndrome in a significant minority of subjects as long as it includes a control group with no intervention. As reviewed, stress also produces physical morbidity and has an increased mortality. From the time course of bereavement, since many people with depressive symptoms and/or a depressive syndrome improve, the intervention should be started or planned to occur at a point after which the majority have shown improvement. If not many will improve and the treatment effects will be minimized or buried in the overall improvement. Thus, a bereavement intervention should probably be started 4–6 months after the stress. As an alternative, it is possible to identify patients with "high risk" for developing a continuous depressive response and earlier intervention is indicated. An outline of risk factors is presented below:

1. Definite risk factors for increased morbidity after stress
   Poor previous physical health
   Poor previous mental health
   Use or misuse of substances such as alcohol or drugs or cigarettes
2. Less definite risk factors for morbidity after stress
   Lack of social supports
   Sex—males
   Low income
   No previous experience with death (in bereavement)
   Individual symptoms such as psychomotor retardation, suicidal thoughts, morbid guilt
3. Probable factors for low risk of morbidity after stress
   Employment, job satisfaction
   Individual symptom—*No* insomnia immediately following the stress

Since most studies indicate that those who have had psychological problems (alcohol or drug abuse, suicide attempts, known psychiatric disorders) or poor physical health do less well, these variables need to be included as past history on any individual who is participating in a program. In addition, a careful drug and alcohol history as well as smoking habits should be included.

Most stress researchers believe that personality attributes probably account for some of the outcome differences. Although none of the studies in bereavement have included personality assessment, in new research some personality assessment prior to the intervention also should be done. Since many psychiatric disorders run in families, careful family histories need to be taken. It may be that a subject from a family with a heavy loading of alcoholism or affective disorder or antisocial personality is at more risk for developing a depressive syndrome than one without such a family history. Thus, by including this it may be possible to identify another high risk group.

A good intervention study should also include a careful psychiatric diagnostic interview with each of the participants. Since the epidemiologic branch of the NIMH is conducting a large-scale study using the DIS (Robins et al., 1981) (Diagnostic Interview Schedule) to ascertain the prevalence of psychiatric disorders in the community, the best psychiatric diagnostic interview at this point probably is the DIS. Although these interviews are lengthy, the data gathered is essential. Thus, the researcher could tell whether his/her population contains more of a particular group of psychiatric patients than would be expected from a community sample. For example, in looking at the survivors of the younger deaths, we had the impression that a certain group of families led rather chaotic lives which contributed to the death of one of the spouses and a more deleterious bereavement in the survivor. Even the children seemed more disturbed (Van Eerdewegh et al., 1982). This seemed particularly true of those deaths which were either accidental or due to alcoholism or suicide. The same factors did not seem to be operating in those spouses who died of natural causes like cancer, myocardial infarct, cerebral vascular accidents, etc.

As many reports of depressive syndrome and disorder (Flaherty et al., 1983) discuss social supports as a modifier of outcome, a social support inventory is important. Several should be reviewed and the one most appropriate to the study population should be chosen (Corney et al., 1982).

Control groups are essential. In the bereavement intervention studies usually the technique was to identify a high risk group and intervene and then compare the outcome to a low risk group. A stronger design would be to use a random assignment in the high risk group as well as to follow a low risk group.

Lastly, it is important to decide the outcome variables before the study is started. These should include scores on a well-accepted depression rating scale, such as the Hamilton or the Beck Depression Inventory, scores on a more global health questionnaire like the Goldberg Health Questionnaire, numbers of doctors' visits and reasons for care, numbers of hospitalizations and reasons for hospitalizations, a quantitative score on drug use, alcohol use, smoking, and some simple measure of concurrent life events such as Paykel's (1971) modified Holmes Rahe Scale. Consider other outcomes; for instance in bereavement, remarriage for men is possible, dating or making new friends for both sexes, moving, change of income (more or less), and death.

The methodologic advances of psychiatric research have been so tremendous in the past two decades that the time seems right for well-controlled, well-done prevention intervention studies of a stress-induced depression.

REFERENCES

Amenson, C. S., and Lewinsohn, P. M. (1981). An investigation into the observed sex difference in prevalence of unipolar depression. *Journal of Abnormal Psychology 90:*1–13.

Andrews, G. (1981). A prospective study of life events and psychological symptoms. *Psychological Medicine 11:*795–801.

Bebbington, P. E., Tenant, C., and Hurry, J. (1981). Adversity and the nature of psychiatric disorder in the community. *Journal of Affective Disorders 3:*345–366.

Blanchard, C. G., Blanchard, E. G., and Becker, J. V. (1976). The young widow: Depressive symptomatology throughout the grief process. *Psychiatry 39:*394–399.

Bock, E. W., and Webber, J. L. (1972). Suicide among the elderly: Isolating widowhood and mitigating alternatives. *Journal of Marriage and the Family 34:*24–31.

Bornstein, P. E., and Clayton, P. J. (1972). The anniversary reaction. *Diseases of the Nervous System 33:*470–471.

Bornstein, P. E., Clayton, P. J., Halikas, J. A., Maurice, W. L., and Robins, E. (1973). The depression of widowhood after thirteen months. *British Journal of Psychiatry 122:*561–566.

Bunch, J. (1972). Recent bereavement in relation to suicide. *Journal of Psychosomatic Research 16:*361–366.

Clayton, P. J., Desmarais, L., and Winokur, G. (1968). A study of normal bereavement. *American Journal of Psychiatry 125:*168–178.

Clayton, P. J., Halikas, J. A., and Maurice, W. L. (1971). The bereavement of the widowed. *Diseases of the Nervous System 32:*597–604.

Clayton, P. J., Halikas, J. A., and Maurice, W. L. (1972). The depression of widowhood. *British Journal of Psychiatry 120:*71–78.

Clayton, P. J., Herjanic, M., Murphy, G. E., and Woodruff, R., Jr. (1974). Mourning and depression: Their similarities and differences. *Canadian Psychiatric Association Journal 19:*309–312.

Clayton, P. J., and Darvish, H. S. (1979). Course of depressive symptoms following the stress of bereavement. In J. D. Barrett (Ed.), *Stress and Mental Disorder.* New York: Raven Press.

Clayton, P. J. (1982). Bereavement. In E. S. Paykel (Ed.), *Handbook of Affective Disorders.* London: Churchill Livingstone.

Corney, R. H., Clare, A. W., and Fry, J. (1982). The development of a self-report questionnaire to identify social problems—a pilot study. *Psychological Medicine 12*(4):903–909.

Diagnostic and Statistical Manual of Mental Disorders—DSM III (1980). Third Edition. Washington, D.C.: American Psychiatric Association.

Feighner, J. P., Robins, E., Guze, S. B., Woodruff, R. A., Jr., Winokur, G., and Muñoz, R. (1972). Diagnostic criteria for use in psychiatric research. *Archives of General Psychiatry 26:*57–63.

Flaherty, J. A., Gaviria, F. M., Black, E. M., Atlman, E., and Mitchell, T. (1983). The role of social support in the functioning of patients with unipolar depression. *American Journal of Psychiatry 140:*473–476.

Frank, E., and Stewart, B. D. (1983). Treatment of Depressed Rape Victims: An Approach to Stress-Induced Symptomatology. In P. J. Clayton and J. E. Barrett (Eds.), *Treatment of Depression: Old Controversies and New Approaches.* New York: Raven Press.

Freud S. (1957). Mourning and Melancholia. In *The Complete Work of Sigmund Freud,* Vol. 14, pp. 243–258. London: Hogarth Press.

Frost, N. R., and Clayton, P. J. (1977). Bereavement and psychiatric hospitalization. *Archives of General Psychiatry 34:*1172–1175.

Gardner, A., and Pritchard, M. (1977). Mourning, mummification, and living with the dead. *British Journal of Psychiatry 130:*23–28.

Glick, I. O., Weiss, R. S., and Parkes, C. M. (1974). *The First Year of Bereavement.* New York: John Wiley & Sons.

Helsing, K. J., and Szklo, M. (1981). Mortality after bereavement. *American Journal of Epidemiology 114:*41–52.

Helsing, K. J., Szklo, M., and Comstock, G. W. (1981). Factors associated with mortality after widowhood. *American Journal of Public Health 71:*802–809.

Helsing, K. J., Comstock, G. W., and Szklo, M. (1982). Causes of death in a widowed population. *American Journal of Epidemiology 116:*524–532.

Hirschfeld, R. M. A., Klerman, G. L., Clayton, P. J., and Keller, M. G. (1983). Personality and Depression: Empirical Findings. *Archives of General Psychiatry, 40:*993–998.

Kennell, J. H., Slyter, H., and Klaus, M. H. (1970). The mourning response of parents to the death of a newborn infant. *New England Journal of Medicine 283:*344–349.

Levy, B. (1976). A study of bereavement in general practice. *Journal of the Royal College of General Practitioners 26:*329–336.

Lindemann, E. (1944). Symptomatology and management of acute grief. *American Journal of Psychiatry 101:*141–148.

MacMahon, B., and Pugh, T. F. (1965). Suicide in the widowed. *American Journal of Epidemiology 81:*23–31.

Maddison, D., and Viola, A. (1968). The health of widows in the year following bereavement. *Journal of Psychosomatic Research 12:*297–306.

Marris, P. (1958). *Widows and Their Families.* London: Routledge and Kegan Paul.

Murphy, G. E., and Robins, E. (1967). Social factors in suicide. *Journal of the American Medical Association 199:*303–308.

Murphy, G. E., Armstrong, J. W., Hermele, S. L., Fischer, J. R., and Clendenin, W. W. (1979). Suicide and alcoholism. Interpersonal loss confirmed as a predictor. *Archives of General Psychiatry 36:*65–69.

Parkes, C. M. (1970). The first year of bereavement: A longitudinal study of the reaction of London widows to the deaths of their husbands. *Psychiatry 33:*444–467.

Parkes, C. M. (1972). *Bereavement: Studies of Grief in Adult Life.* New York: International Universities Press.

Parkes, C. M., and Brown, R. J. (1972). Health after bereavement: A controlled study of young Boston widows and widowers. *Psychosomatic Medicine 34:*449-469.

Parkes, C. M. (1980). Bereavement counselling. Does it work? *British Medical Journal 281:*3–6.

Parkes, C. M. (1981). Evaluation of a bereavement service. *Journal of Preventive Psychiatry 1:*179–188.

Paykel, E. S. (1982). Life events and early environment. In E. S. Paykel (Ed.), *Handbook of Affective Disorders.* London: Churchill Livingstone.

Paykel, E. S., Prusoff, B. A., Uhlenhuth, E. H. (1971). Scaling of life events. *Archives of General Psychiatry 25:*340-347.

Raphael, B. (1977). Preventive intervention with the recently bereaved. *Archives of General Psychiatry 34:*1450-1454.

Rees, W. D. (1971). The hallucinations of widowhood. *British Medical Journal 4:*37–41.

Robins, L. N., Helzer, J. E., Croughan, J., and Ratcliff, K. S. (1981). National Institute of Mental Health Diagnostic Interview Schedule. *Archives of General Psychiatry 38:*381–389.

Shepherd, D., and Barraclough, B. M. (1974). The aftermath of suicide. *British Medical Journal 2:*600–603.

Singh, B., and Raphael, B. (1981). Postdisaster morbidity of the bereaved. A possible role for preventive psychiatry? *Journal of Nervous and Mental Disease 169:*203–212.

Spitzer, R. L., Endicott, J., and Robins, E. (1978). *Research Diagnostic Criteria* (3rd Edition), Biometrics Research, New York State Department of Mental Hygiene, New York.

Vachon, M. L. S., Sheldon, A. R., Lancee, W. J., Lyall, W. A., Rogers, J., and Freeman, S. J. J. (1982). Correlates of enduring distress patterns following bereavement. Social network, life situation, and personality. *Psychological Medicine 12:*783–788.

Van Eerdewegh, M. M., Biere, M. D., Parrilla, R. H., and Clayton, P. J. (1982). The bereaved child. *British Journal of Psychiatry 140:*23–29.

Ward, A. W. M. (1974). Terminal care in malignant disease. *Social Science and Medicine 8:*413–420.

Ward, A. W. M. (1976). Mortality of bereavement. *British Medical Journal 1:*700–702.

Warheit, G. J. (1979). Life events, coping, stress and depressive symptomatology. *American Journal of Psychiatry 136:*502–507.

Weissman, M. M., and Myers, J. (1978). Affective disorders in a U. S. urban community: The use of research diagnostic criteria in an epidemiological survey. *Archives of General Psychiatry 35:*1304–1311.

Wiener, A., Gerber, I., Battin, D., and Arkin, A. M. (1975). The process and phenomenology of bereavement. In B. Schoenberg, I. Gerber, A. Wiener, A. H. Kutscher, D. Peretz and A. C. Carr (Eds.), *Bereavement: Its Psychological Aspects.* New York: Columbia University Press.

Wing, J. K. (1980). Methodological issues in psychiatric case-identification. Editorial in *Psychological Medicine 10*:5–10.

Yamamoto, J., Okonogi, K., Iwasaki, T., and Yoshimura, S. (1969). Mourning in Japan. *American Journal of Psychiatry 125*:1660–1665.

Yamamoto, I. J. (1970). American and Japan—Two ways of mourning. Annual meeting of American Psychiatric Association, San Francisco.

3

Epidemiological Issues in Measuring Preventive Effects

Robert E. Roberts
The University of Texas Health Science Center, Houston

INTRODUCTION

Depression, considered in all its myriad forms, is ubiquitous. Since antiquity depressive phenomena have been among humanity's most common afflictions. Yet in spite of their common-place occurrence and deleterious effects on the human condition, we still know very little about the etiology of the wide spectrum of depressive disorders. This is not to say that we know nothing about depression. We know a good deal, much more than we did even a decade ago. But our knowledge is still fragmented and incomplete. It may be accurate to say that our current state of knowledge permits us, perhaps for the first time, to feel some confidence that we are beginning to understand depressive disorders.

In this regard, it may be instructive to review what we know, or at least what we think we know, about the epidemiology of depression. I will focus my discussion on incidence and prevalence of depression, risk factors and high risk populations, and issues in assessing incidence and prevalence and changes in these over time or in response to intervention programs.

INCIDENCE AND PREVALENCE

Prevalence in epidemiologic research refers to *all* cases of a disorder existing in a population for a defined time period, such as now, the past week, the past month, or past year. Incidence on the other hand, refers to *new* cases of this disorder occurring during a given time period (Fox, Hall & Elveback, 1970; Mausner & Bahn, 1974). In general, prevalence data are available much more frequently than incidence data, largely because measurement of incidence involves the difficult problems of establishing date of onset and assessing change over time. Data on the incidence and prevalence of psychopathology, including depression, historically have come from two sources: (1) statistics on admission to and discharge from varied types of treat-

This research was supported in part by a Research Scientist Development Award (MH 00047) and by Grant No. MH 36960 from the National Institute of Mental Health. Appreciation is expressed to Catherine Ramsay Roberts for her assistance and comments, and to Kenneth Reed who also provided an insightful review.

ment facilities or sources of help for human problems, and (2) statistics derived from studies conducted with individuals or groups regardless of their treatment status. Case-ascertainment in psychiatric epidemiology has relied on two different measurement approaches: (1) Clinical diagnosis, based on either structured or unstructured interviews, and (2) impairment estimates based on symptom checklists or rating scales which yield impairment scores that typically are not diagnosis specific. Such checklists or scales are widely used, primarily because of their economy and feasibility (Seiler, 1973).

A number of authors (Akiskal & McKinney, 1975; Friedman, 1974; Robins & Guze, 1972; Whybrow & Palatore, 1973) have pointed out that a source of confusion in depression research is the heterogeneity of depressive phenomena. Researchers frequently do not specify what type of depressive phenomena they are studying. A consequence of this lack of precision is reduced comparability and a subsequent attentuation of our ability to generalize the results of our research. Akiskal (1979) has distinguished four types of depressive phenomena: (1) Normal depression, (2) situational or reactive depression, (3) secondary depression, and (4) primary depression or melancholia. The first two phenomena are subclinical mood disturbances, differing from each other in terms of severity and duration. Normal depression is seen as a universal adaptive response to stress, frustration, or loss, ordinarily lasting a few hours to a few days. Situational or reactive depression is more severe, usually lasting from several weeks to several months. Grief in response to loss of a love object or pronounced nostalgia are examples of this type of depressive phenomena. Primary and secondary depressions are examples of clinical depression. Secondary depressions are analogous to situational depressions, except that they are more severe and are sequelae of other serious medical or psychiatric disorders. The dysphoria usually parallels the course of the primary disorder (Guze, Woodruff, & Clayton, 1971; Woodruff, Murphy, & Herjanic, 1967) and rarely reaches melancholic proportions (Winokur, 1972). Contrasted with situational and secondary depressions, primary depressions or melancholias either arise without pre-existing or concurrent nonaffective disorders or seem out of proportion to life changes preceding them. Akiskal points out that primary depression is where one finds the development of the full syndrome which has many attributes of a disease state, such as disruption of psychomotor and vegetative functions, considerable morbidity and mortality, autonomous course, and favorable response to specific pharmacologic agents (see also Prange, 1973).

In terms of a discussion of incidence and prevalence of depressive phenomena, Akiskal's (1979) fourfold classification can be reduced to a dichotomy, i.e., clinical depression and nonclinical depression. The rationale for this bit of reductionism is twofold. First, if we are interested in the descriptive epidemiology of depression, we are concerned primarily with issues of magnitude (incidence and prevalence) and distribution rather than with issues of origin (etiology). Put another way, our interest is primarily in whether disease is present, its severity, and duration. Several of the distinctions made by Akiskal (normal/situational, primary/secondary) involve at least partially notions of etiology, in addition to phenomenology, severity, and duration. Second, classifying depressive phenomena as clinical or nonclinical gives us the advantage of having a disease classification which closely mirrors measurement approaches extant in psychiatric epidemiology, i.e., clinical and psychometric (Dohrenwend & Dohrenwend, 1982). Making the most of this fortuitous circumstance, let us turn to a review of the available evidence on the incidence and prevalence of clinical and nonclinical depression. I might note that other authors (Boyd & Weissman, 1981; Hirshfeld & Cross, 1982) use the terms depressive syndrome and depressive symptoms to refer respectively to clinically diagnosed depression and depression assessed using symptom checklists.

Clinical Depression

Several problems confront us when we attempt to estimate the incidence and prevalence of clinical depression from the published research literature. First, treatment data are not very instructive. There have been numerous studies of persons in treatment for depression (treatment prevalence), and about the most we can say at this point is that prevalence estimates based on treatment data greatly underestimate true prevalence, and that we seldom know the nature and extent of the bias involved. By way of illustration, studies by Weissman, Myers, and Thompson (1981) and by Roberts and Vernon (1982) indicate that only about one out of five persons with a clinical diagnosis of depression have seen a mental health professional in the past year. These findings are consistent with the results of 11 studies reviewed by Link and Dohrenwend (1980), in which a variety of case-finding techniques were used. Second, when we turn to studies of untreated or true incidence and prevalence, it turns out that there have been very few community-based epidemiologic studies of clinical depression in the United States. Furthermore, there have been no incidence studies of clinical depression in American communities published to date. Third, when we examine studies of the true prevalence of psychiatric disorder we find little comparability among them in terms of research methodology employed, particularly in terms of diagnostic procedures.

To illustrate the problem, let us refer to one of the most systematic attempts to date to estimate the prevalence of psychiatric disorder in the U.S. adult population. Neugebauer, Dohrenwend, and Dohrenwend (1980) reviewed studies of functional disorders among adults published since 1950, and found only three which presented data separately for affective psychoses and which also satisfied their criteria for methodologic rigor. The prevalence rates varied from none to 0.41 percent. Based on their analyses, they estimated the true prevalence of affective psychosis to be 0.3 percent. They also reviewed six studies which presented data separately for the neuroses. The prevalence rates varied from less than one percent to 40 percent. Their estimate of the true prevalence of the neuroses ranged from 8 to 15 percent. The variability was equally great for other disorders. In fact, the prevalence rate for all disorders ranged from less than one percent to nearly 70 percent, with a median of nearly 23 percent. Clearly the estimates from this body of research are not very instructive concerning the true prevalence of clinical depression in the United States.

In a more recent assessment, Boyd and Weissman (1982) review 14 studies (only one conducted in the U.S.) of the full range of non-bipolar clinical depression and report that the point prevalence in industrialized countries was between 1.8 and 2.2 percent for men and between 2.0 and 9.3 percent for women. The overall prevalence ranged from 1 to 11 percent. These were all community studies using clinical diagnosis to ascertain caseness. These results present a somewhat more coherent view than the survey by Neugebauer, Dohrenwend, and Dohrenwend (1980).

Fortunately, there is some good news. Two lines of investigation have emerged in the past several years which are providing more concordant estimates of the prevalence of clinical depression using diagnostic criteria extant in contemporary Ameri-

Table 1 Six month prevalence of affective disorders for three ECA sites

Affective disorder	Baltimore	New Haven	St. Louis
Major depressive episode	2.2%	3.5%	3.2%
Manic episode	0.4	0.8	0.7
Dysthymia	2.1	3.2	3.8

can psychiatry and, in one case, which will provide community-based incidence data as well.

The first set of investigations consists of two community-based surveys, one in New Haven, Connecticut, and the other in Alameda County, California, which collected data using the Schedule for Affective Disorders and Schizophrenia (SADS) and made diagnoses using the Research Diagnostic Criteria (RDC). The SADS-RDC represents a categorical approach to psychiatric diagnosis in which a series of operational definitions are used to classify respondents into discrete nosologic groups (Endicott & Spitzer, 1978; Spitzer, Endicott, & Robins, 1978). Weissman and Myers (1978) report that the current point prevalence of major depression in New Haven was 4.3 percent and minor depression was 2.5 percent, for a total of 6.8 percent. Lifetime prevalence was 20 percent for major and 9.2 percent for minor depression. The lifetime rate for major and/or minor depression was 26.7 percent. Roberts and Vernon (1982), in a partial replication of the New Haven study, report that the current point prevalence rates in Alameda County were 2.1 percent for major depression and 1.3 percent for minor depression (3.4 percent overall). The lifetime rates of major and minor depression were 15.7 and 8.5 percent, respectively.

The second line of investigation is represented by the National Institute of Mental Health's Epidemiologic Catchment Area (ECA) research program. The ECA effort consists of a series of five epidemiologic research studies performed by independent research teams in New Haven, Connecticut, Baltimore, Maryland, St. Louis, Missouri, Los Angeles, California, and Durham, North Carolina (Eaton, Regier, Locke, & Taube, 1981). The basic objective is to obtain population-based data on the incidence and prevalence of clinical psychiatric disorders as well as data on utilization of health services. All the sites are employing the same research design and core set of data collection instruments, including a structured clinical interview, the Diagnostic Interview Schedule (DIS). The DIS, designed to be used by trained lay interviewers in community settings, elicits data to permit most of the DSM III adult diagnoses to be made, as well as those using Feighner and Research Diagnostic Criteria (Robins, Helzer, Croughan, & Ratcliff, 1981). Although two of these studies have not been completed yet, three of the projects (New Haven, Baltimore and St. Louis) reported results from the prevalence surveys recently (Myers et al., 1984) and the results are quite interesting. Thus far only six-month prevalence figures have been reported. Table 1 summarizes the results for affective disorders using six-month prevalence rates.

As you can see, there is comparatively close agreement among the sites. Using DSM III criteria, about 2.2–3.5 percent of adults in three urban areas reported a major depressive episode in the six-month period prior to the study; the six-month prevalence for all disorders ranged from 16.8 to 23.4 percent. Interestingly, these preliminary data are extremely similar to data in two papers in which the authors used DSM III criteria to reanalyze data collected some years ago. Blazer and Williams (1980) reanalyzed data from a community survey of elderly residents of Durham, North Carolina, conducted in 1972, and report that the point prevalence of DSM III major depression among the population 65 or older was 3.7 percent. Murphy (1980), in an attempt to determine comparability of prevalence rates across time and studies, applied DSM III criteria to the original Stirling County survey data and reports the prevalence of depression so defined is 4.1 percent of the population.

By contrast, the lifetime prevalence rates for the three ECA sites ranged from 3.7 to 6.7 percent for a major depressive episode, 0.6 to 1.1 percent for a manic episode, and 2.1 to 3.8 percent for dysthymia. Clearly these lifetime rates for major depression are significantly lower than those reported by Weissman and Myers (1978) or by Roberts and Vernon (1982) using the RDC. Lifetime prevalence for all disorders combined was 28.8 percent in New Haven, 38.0 percent in Baltimore and 31.0 percent in St. Louis (Robins et al., 1984).

Nonclinical Depression

What does the research literature tell us about the incidence and prevalence of nonclinical depression? Several things.

First, it is not clear exactly what the prevalence of nonclinical depressive phenomena is in the United States. A variety of measures of nonclinical psychopathology have been developed over the years by mental health researchers (see Boyd & Weissman, 1981; Dohrenwend, Oksenberg, Shrout, Dohrenwend, & Cook, 1981; Link & Dohrenwend, 1980). Although there seems to be a common universe of content to which the items in these various symptom checklists refer, there is still substantial diversity in actual item content. Furthermore, there is considerable conceptual confusion concerning what exactly is being measured. Constructs used to describe the phenomenon being measured have included mental illness, psychological impairment, psychophysiological distress, psychological distress, nonspecific psychological distress, minor psychiatric morbidity, expressed distress, psychological well-being, psychiatric symptoms, and other variations of these themes (see Seiler, 1973, for example). Some measures have been developed specifically to measure depressive symptoms, and are so labelled. Perhaps two of the better known examples are the 20-item Zung Self-Rating Depression Scale (Zung, 1965) and the 20-item Center for Epidemiologic Studies Depression (CES-D) Scale (Radloff, 1977), although there are others.

In addition to suffering from the problems of content variability and conceptual diversity, these symptom checklists also are related only indirectly to clinical psychiatric disorder (Dohrenwend, 1973). For example, Wheaton (1982) examined the ability of the Langner 22-item index (Langner, 1962) to identify subjects who also had a diagnosed psychiatric disorder. Only 52-56 percent of those individuals with the highest symptom scores on the Langner index also had some current diagnosis. While the majority of those scoring high were clinically depressed, a substantial proportion had a wide range of other diagnoses. Clearly the Langner index, the most widely used symptom checklist in the past 20 years, measures something other than clinical psychopathology. Another example is the CES-D. Two studies have examined concordance in community surveys between the CES-D and clinical diagnoses of depression suing the RDC (Myers & Weissman, 1980; Roberts & Vernon, 1983). In both of these studies, the CES-D correctly identified about 60 percent of those subjects with clinical depression. The CES-D also picks up other psychiatric diagnoses. In both studies about 1 in 5 of the CES-D "cases" had a clinical diagnosis other than depression. However, about half of the CES-D "cases" had no RDC diagnosis. Both studies suggest that the CES-D is reasonably good at screening out the nondepressed (true negatives), but is not very efficient in identifying true positives. Part of the explanation for this lack of concordance is methodological, in particular the inclusive nature of the symptom checklist and the exclusive nature of the clinical criteria (Roberts & Vernon, 1983). A central problem is that the checklists, due to their brevity and nonspecificity, do not permit differential diagnoses. However, there is another hypothesis, and a highly plausible explanation.

Dohrenwend and his colleagues (Dohrenwend, Shrout, Egri, & Mendelsohn, 1980; Link & Dohrenwend, 1980) argue that what these instruments measure is best defined using Frank's (1973) concept of "demoralization." The central features of this phenomenon are low self-esteem, helplessness-hopelessness, sadness and anxiety. Frank posits that this condition is a major factor leading people to seek help and is also the condition that psychotherapy attempts to relieve (p. 278). Dohrenwend and his coworkers argue that demoralization is a condition that is likely ". . . to be experienced in association with a variety of problems, including severe physical illness, particularly chronic illness, stressful life events, psychiatric disorders, and perhaps conditions of social marginality as experienced by minority groups and persons such as housewives and the poor whose social positions block them from mainstream strivings (Link & Dohrenwend, 1980, p. 115)." A measure of demoralization even has been developed (Dohrenwend et al., 1980) incorporating the central features of Frank's concept.

Second, symptoms of demoralization ostensibly indicative of depressive phenomena are quite prevalent in American society (and, indeed, probably in all societies). Weissman and Myers (1978) reviewed five community surveys conducted in the years around 1970 and reported that the estimated prevalence rates varied from 16 to 20 percent. In a recent update of this review of community studies, Boyd and Weissman (1981) examined 11 studies (including many of the earlier ones reviewed) and report that the prevalence rates varied from 9 percent to 20 percent. All of the studies reviewed were carried out in local communities. Link and Dohrenwend (1980) included in their review 14 local community studies conducted since 1950 in the United States in different regions of the county in varying urban and rural contexts, and using different measures. The median estimated prevalence for these studies was 24.5 percent. Link and Dohrenwend also included two nationwide studies for comparison. The prevalence rates for these two studies were 25.9 and 31.8 percent. Based on their review, Link and Dohrenwend estimate that the prevalence of depressive symptoms in the United States approaches one-quarter of the population. A national study not included in their review (Sayetta and Johnson, 1980) estimates the prevalence of depressive symptomatology to be 17.3 percent of the U.S. population, aged 25–74 years of age. This study was based on the 1974–75 Health and Nutrition Examination Survey (HANES) and used the CES-D to estimate prevalence. This national estimate is within the range suggested by Weissman and Myers (1978) in their review.

One of the problems in attempting to generalize from the plethora of local community studies using symptom checklists is that different measures are used and, more importantly, the criterion for caseness varies widely. It might be instructive to examine studies which have used the same instrument and the same caseness criterion and for which both national and local community data are available.

Table 2 Prevalence of demoralization based on population surveys in the U.S. employing the CES-D for case ascertainment

Study	Location	Prevalence (%)*	
Sayetta & Johnson (1980)	National Survey	Total	17.3
Eaton & Kessler (1981)	National Survey	Whites	15.3
		Blacks	28.5
Comstock & Helsing (1976)	St. Louis, MO	Total	21.5
		Whites	19.8
		Blacks	26.4
	Washington County, MD	Total	17.0
Husaini, Neff, & Stone (1979)	Rural Tennessee	Total	11.9
Boyd & Weissman (1981)	New Haven, Conn.	Total	9.0
Frerichs, Aneshensel, & Clark (1981)	Los Angeles, Calif.	Total	19.1
		Whites	15.6
		Blacks	21.8
		Hispanics	27.4
Vernon & Roberts (1982)	Alameda County, Calif.	Total	19.6
		Anglos	14.6
		Blacks	18.1
		Chicanos	28.9

*A score ≥ 16.

Fortunately such data exist. Table 2 presents the results of community surveys using the CES-D which also used the caseness criterion of a score of 16 or greater. The HANES results published by Sayetta and Johnson (1980) provide national baseline data for comparative purposes. The national prevalence was 17.3 percent. Four of the six local community studies report rates between 17 and 21 percent. The two exceptions are rural Tennessee and New Haven. Compared to other urban surveys, and even the national survey, the New Haven prevalence (9 percent) is quite low. Reasons why this might be so are not readily apparent, although the data emanate from the third and final wave of a seven-year prospective study, and the CES-D was given after the SADS interview. The Tennessee sample is rural, which may partially account for the low rate. Washington County is a largely rural area, and it had a prevalence lower than many other areas. As Dohrenwend and Dohrenwend (1974) have pointed out, available data (such as there are) suggest that psychiatric disorders may be less prevalent in rural areas.

The incidence of demoralization in community populations is largely unknown. There are several reasons for the dearth of data on incidence. First, as noted earlier, estimation of incidence requires longitudinal data, permitting the partition of the sample into noncases, old (prevalent) cases, and new (incident) cases. Although an increasing number of longitudinal or prospective studies are being done, the focus is usually analytic rather than descriptive, and little or no attempt is made to measure incidence per se. Second, most symptom checklists inquire about symptoms experienced over a very brief span of time, such as "currently," "the past week," or "the past month." To estimate incidence, studies must employ a design in which intervals between assessments reflect the time referents of the instruments. Clearly not many studies attempt to assess symptoms as frequently as monthly, much less weekly. A notable exception is the study of stress and illness among air traffic controllers (Barrett, Hurst, DiScala, & Rose, 1978). In this study, subjects were assessed each month using the Zung Self-Rating Depression

Scale (Zung, 1965). About 91 percent of the subjects did not experience any significant depressive symptoms during a given month. Only about 7 percent reported mild depressive symptoms and about 2 percent moderate to severe symptomatology. During the 12-month follow-up period, 71 percent of the subjects reported no significant depressive symptoms at any time, 19 percent reported mild symptoms and 10 percent reported moderate to severe symptoms at some time during the year. Mild depression was experienced an average of 3 months and moderate to severe depression was experienced an average of about 1 month. Two patterns seemed to emerge, acute episodic disorder in which more pronounced depressive symptoms occurred relatively rarely and lasted 1-3 months, and a more chronic condition, in which symptoms fluctuated and the duration of time with more depressive symptoms was longer. Thus, for this group of men selected for physical and psychologic health, the point prevalence of demoralization (mild–severe) was about 9 percent and the 12-month period prevalence was about 29 percent. However, the researchers did not report monthly incidence data, i.e., new cases each month who did not report depressive symptoms or demoralization in the previous month.

Before leaving this discussion, there is one other issue worth noting. We have some data on the relationship of demoralization to clinical depression, but only from the perspective of assessing the efficacy of symptom checklists in identifying those with clinical depression. In terms of measurement issues and descriptive epidemiology, this is of course important. But in terms of etiology and, therefore, primary prevention, there is an equally important question regarding the relationship between demoralization and clinical or depressive syndrome depression (or psychiatric disorder more generally). This question addresses the extent to which demoralized individuals become clinically depressed, and the extent to which the clinically depressed remain demoralized once the major depressive episode has remitted. Several authors (Akiskal, 1979; Klein, 1974), for example, have noted that a state of demoralization is commonly observed in lifelong psychiatric disorder, presumably stemming from the episodic and unpredictable exacerbations of the disease, ambiguities about etiology and outcome, as well as the social and interpersonal costs incurred. Link and Dohrenwend (1980) suggest that about half of those who are demoralized also are impaired clinically. Other data (Myers & Weissman, 1980; Roberts & Vernon, 1983) suggest a majority of these individuals are suffering from clinical depression. However, we do not know the role of demoralization in the etiology and course of depressive disorders. Does demoralization increase the risk of clinical depression and, if so, in whom and under what circumstances? Given the high prevalence of demoralization, demonstration of the extent and nature of an etiologic role in the development of more severe and chronic manifestations of depressive disorders might assist in identification of a large population-at-risk for primary and secondary prevention activities.

RISK FACTORS IN DEPRESSION

Although in epidemiology we are interested ultimately in establishing the primary or specific cause of a disease (Lilienfeld & Lilienfeld, 1980; MacMahon & Pugh, 1970), most chronic diseases prevalent in contemporary urban industrial societies do not have a known etiologic agent. Indeed, the unicausal model used in early research on infectious diseases has given way to a model which views disease as the product of multiple factors (Susser, 1973) whose interactions contribute an increased risk of disease in individuals or groups (Fox, Hall, & Elveback, 1970; Lilienfeld & Lilienfeld, 1980).

Psychiatric disorders in general and depressive phenomena in particular are among the most prevalent of the chronic diseases. The primary cause or causes of depressive phenomena are unknown. However, we do know something about factors that seem to increase the risk of depression. Given our current state of knowledge, what are these risk factors for depression? As in our earlier discussions, we will dichotomize our discussion of risk factors in terms of clinical depression and nonclinical depression or demoralization where data permit.

Some of the better discussions of risk factors in clinical depression have been by Akiskal (Akiskal, 1979; Akiskal & McKinney, 1973). He argues that our understanding of clinical depression (more specifically melancholia) will require consideration of genetic and developmental factors as well as interpersonal and acquired psychological causes. To summarize his argument, he sees melancholia as a psychobiologic state representing a final common pathway involving ". . . (a) life events or chemical stressors that so overwhelm the adaptive skills of the affectively ill that they see themselves as losing control over their destiny; (b) escalating levels of subjective turmoil; (c) heightened neuronal excitability and arousal with interplay of genetically or developmentally vulnerable neuronal circuits in the diencephalon; (d) impaired monoaminergic transmission; (e) derangement of the neurochemical substrates of reinforcement; (f) further breakdown in coping mechanisms; and (g) a vicious cycle of more turmoil, arousal and hopelessness . . ." (Akiskal, 1979, p. 431). According to this model of the etiology of melancholia, depression is the result of various factors that converge in areas of the diencephalon that modulate arousal, mood, motivation, and psychomotor functions. Briefly stated, melancholia is a final common pathway in which alterations in functional levels of biogenic amines, production of faulty neurotransmitters, and accumulation of intraneuronal sodium are generated by the interaction of four classes of factors: physiological stressors, genetic predisposition, psychosocial stressors, and developmental predispositions. Among the biologic factors (physiological and genetic), Akiskal discusses reserpine, hypothyroidism, viral infections, leaky presynaptic membranes, and decreases in postsynaptic receptor sensitivity. While the model posed by Akiskal is parsimonious and coherent, the biological components offer little promise, at least in the foreseeable future, for intervention in terms of primary prevention. First, our knowledge of the role of biologic factors is still rudimentary, albeit the implications of this knowledge are provocative and profound. Second, our knowledge of clinical depression or melancholia is based entirely on the study of cases treated in tertiary care psychiatric facilities, generally university teaching hospitals and public mental hospitals. The extent to which the biological risk factors for depression identified in treated cases are operant in the full spectrum of melancholia, treated and untreated in the general population, is not known. As noted earlier, as many as 80 percent of the individuals with clinical depression have not sought nor recieved professional treatment. Third, early identification of those at biologic risk generally would require some type of community screening using biological and chemical tests which are too cumbersome and expensive to implement on a broad scale, even if we knew which factors to screen for (which we at present do not) and had tests with acceptable sensitivity and specificity.

There is a potential exception to the argument against biologic risk factors as a focus in the primary prevention of clinical depression. There is considerable evidence indicating that depressive disorders are familial in nature and that part of this familiality is genetic in nature (Clayton, 1981; Gershon, Bunney, Leckman, vanErdewegh, & deBauche, 1976; Nurnberger & Gershon, 1982; Weissman, et al., 1984; Winokur, 1978). Ostensibly the offspring of parents with depressive disorders represent a group at increased risk of developing depressive disorders at sometime during their life, and consequently may constitute a likely target for preventive interventions. In particular, individuals with first degree relatives who have alcoholism, sociopathy, or depression, singly or in combination, appear to be at much greater risk of developing unipolar clinical depression (Winokur, 1979; Andreasen & Winokur, 1979). However, implementing such interventions poses problems, for several reasons. First, we do not know the true prevalence of familial clustering of depressive disorders in the population, nor the nature and extent of such clustering. Again, virtually all our data on familial linkage have emanated from studies of patients. Second, since primary prevention of familial disorders requires identification of affected parents in order to identify offspring at risk, efforts in the foreseeable future of necessity must focus almost exclusively on treated populations. Third, prospective studies of the risk of depressive disorders and factors increasing risk of these disorders in offspring are for the most part still in progress and at this point provide few guides for specific preventive efforts. Fourth, since there are no unequivocal genetic or biological markers for depression, we must rely on a proxy measure—family history—to estimate genetic vulnerability. The problem with this is that a family history of depressive disorder is neither a necessary nor sufficient cause of depression. Even if depression were strictly a genetically transmitted disease, some individuals with a family history would not develop depression and some without a family history would (Erlenmeyer-Kimling, 1979), for reasons which have been elaborated by Akiskal (1979) as well as Depue, Monroe, and Shackman (1979).

In spite of these problems, family history does appear to increase substantially the risk for various manifestations of depressive phenomena (at least in treated populations), its presence can be ascertained with acceptable reliability and validity (Andreasen, Endicott, Spitzer & Winokur, 1977; Merikangas & Spiker, 1982; Thompson, Orvaschel, Prusoff, & Kidd, 1982; Winokur, Tsuang, & Crowe 1982), and it does identify a clearly-defined population-at-risk before the disease manifests itself, often long before. Given these considerations, plus the fact that a large portion of the variance in depression, even when there is a positive family history, is attributable to psychosocial risk factors, suggests that this high risk population should be considered of primary importance in prevention efforts.

Given the preceding discussion, it seems to me that the primary prevention of clinical depression must of necessity focus on the identification of population groups in the community which have higher incidence and prevalence of depressive disease and those population subgroups which, because of their exposure to or risk of exposure to stressful factors in the psychosocial environment, are believed to be at greater risk of developing clinical depression. Here again, however, we are still somewhat at a disadvantage because of limitations of the knowledge base. Studies of risk factors in clinical depression also have been limited to patients, by and large, the body of literature on psychosocial stressors is not yet extensive, and the findings often (in fact, much too often) are equivocal. Still, the research literature provides some insight into possible target groups for intervention programs to reduce the incidence and prevalence of clinical depression.

Four general classes of psychosocial risk factors in depression now will be discussed: social status, life stress, personal resources, and family history. An outline of these risk factors is presented below:

1. Status Attributes
   age
   sex
   social class
   marital status
2. Personal Resources
   personality
   coping behaviors
   social networks/social support
3. Life Stress
   object loss
      predisposing (distal)
      precipitating (proximal)
   illness
      somatic (heart disease, stroke, etc.)
      psychological (alcoholism, anxiety disorders, etc.)
   childbirth
   other events of an undesirable or threatening nature
   life strains
4. Family History
   first degree relatives with depression, alcoholism, or sociopathy, singly or in combination.

The various factors listed in the outline are described as "putative risk factors" for several reasons. There is a presumption of increased risk attributable to factors, and some evidence for the associations, but, in general, the data are not conclusive. Furthermore, even in those instances where there is reasonable evidence for a statistical association, the evidence for the most part comes from prevalence studies, so that the etiologic role of the factors is not demonstrated.

Social Status

The social statuses or positions that individuals occupy locate them in the social structure and are important determinants of the life experience, including illness experience. Such status attributes as age, sex, marital status, social class, and ethnicity long have been associated with differential risks of disease, including psychiatric disease (Dohrenwend & Dohrenwend, 1969, 1974). Events that alter the life experience, particularly in a negative or undesirable manner, likewise long have been considered to increase the risk of untoward health effects, including psychiatric disorder (Dohrenwend & Dohrenwend, 1974, 1981a). Attributes which increase or decrease the individual's vulnerability to noxious stimuli, such as social support, social skills, coping styles, and personality also have been considered important in the etiology of psychiatric disorders. (See Akiskal, 1979; Depue, Monroe, & Shackman, 1979; Hirschfeld & Cross, 1982, for general discussions of these issues.) Rather than review in detail specific studies of risk factors in these three categories, I will refer whenever possible to recent reviews of the epidemiology of clinical depression and demoralization. In addition, to make comparisons easier, whenever possible the data for each class of risk factors will be presented for both clinical depression and demoralization in the same discussion.

Hirschfeld and Cross (1982) in their recent review conclude that the risk of clinical depression (or depressive syndrome, to use their terminology) is greater for women than men (see also Weissman & Klerman, 1977), for younger rather than older adults, for the separated and divorced (see also Roberts & Roberts, 1982), and for the socioeconomically disadvantaged (see also Dohrenwend & Dohrenwend, 1981a). They found no evidence of differential risk for clinical depression based on race or religion.

The relationships between various status attributes and risk of demoralization are somewhat better documented than is the case for clinical depression. This is partly because the data emanate from community surveys and partly because status attributes are frequently the primary explanatory and/or control vairables in such surveys. Recent reviews (Eaton, 1980; Hirschfeld & Cross, 1982; Link & Dohrenwend, 1980; Roberts, Roberts, & Stevenson, 1982) point out that the risk of demoralization is consistently greater for women, for younger adults, for the poor, and for the separated and divorced. I should note, however, that the evidence for greater risk of demoralization among women is not as monolithic as much of the literature would have us believe. There have been a number of studies in a variety of contexts which report no significant gender differences in demoralization (Berkman, 1971; Comstock & Helsing, 1976; Hammen & Padesky, 1977; Neff & Husaini, 1980; Parker, 1979; Roberts & Roberts, 1982; Roberts, Stevenson, & Breslow, 1981; Schwab, McGinnis, & Warheit, 1973). I suspect that if one were to examine more data sets, carefully controlling for correlated socioeconomic and deographic factors, there would be even less evidence for gender differences (see Cleary & Mechanic, 1983). Such counter evidence raises questions concerning the ubiquity of gender differences in demoralization suggested in recent reviews of this topic (see Dohrenwend & Dohrenwend, 1976; Weissman & Klerman, 1977). Clearly, the use of symptom checklists has not resolved this issue. In an interesting paper bearing on this issue, Newmann (1984) reports data suggesting that the female excess reported in studies using summated demoralization scores may be largely a function of excess levels of commonly occurring, but clinically trivial, feelings of distress among women, rather than excess levels of more severe, clinically relevant symptoms.

The role of race and ethnicity as risk factors for demoralization is interesting as well. The majority of these studies compare rates of demoralization among black and whites (see Comstock & Helsing, 1976; Neff & Husaini, 1980; Roberts, Stevenson, & Breslow, 1981; Warheit, Holzer, & Arey, 1975) although a few studies have included Hispanics (Dohrenwend & Dohrenwend, 1969; Frerichs, Aneshensel, & Clark, 1981; R. E. Roberts, 1980). These studies implicitly or explicitly examine two competing hypotheses, one which argues that ethnic differences are due solely to social class and the other that there are ethnic effects in addition to social class effects. At this point, the evidence in general is much more supportive of the social class argument. While the crude prevalence rates of demoralization for disadvantaged minorities are higher than for the majority population (see the data in Table 2, for illustration) most studies report few or no ethnic differences when controls are implemented for age, sex, and socioeconomic factors.

I might note also, before leaving this subject, that the relationship of age to depression really is not clear. Boyd and Weissman (1982) report that rates are higher for younger women and for older men, although the overall rate is higher for the total population under 45. For clinical depression, the highest rates seem to be for women aged 35–45. The pattern for men is much less clear, although data suggest again that it is somewhat higher for older men (Boyd & Weissman, 1982). In a more recent discussion of this issue, Feinson (1984) examined 27 studies of both clinical depression and demoralization and reported that 10 of these studies found no age difference, 8 found higher rates among younger adults, 3 found mixed results, and only 6 found higher rates among older adults.

Life Stress

From an historical perspective, one of the more pervasive themes in the scientific health literature has been that disease can be precipitated by environmental stress (see, for example, Wolff, Wolf, & Hare, 1950; Selye, 1956). This theme is particularly pronounced in psychosocial epidemiology. For example, the major focus of two books on stressful life events which have appeared in the last 10 years, both edited by the Dohrenwends (Dohrenwend & Dohrenwend, 1974, 1981b), is on psychological disorder. There seems little question at this point that there is an association between life stress and risk of psychological impairment in general. There are questions, as we shall see, about the meaning of this relationship, from both a methodological and a theoretical perspective (but more on this later).

First, let me review the evidence on life stress as a risk factor for depression. Two recent reviews (Hirschfeld & Cross, 1982; Mueller, 1980) summarize the results of about a dozen community studies in which stressful life events are moderately correlated with elevated scores on self-report symptom checklists of the type that I have suggested measure demoralization. Several recent reviews which focus specifically on life events as risk factors for clinical depression (Lloyd, 1980a, 1980b; Hirschfeld & Cross, 1982; Paykel, 1982) also report that a majority of studies report a positive association.

The review by Lloyd, one of the more comprehensive assessments of life events as risk factors in depressive disorder published to date, is presented in a two-part discussion (Lloyd, 1980a, 1980b). I will summarize her findings briefly. She divided life events into predisposing factors and precipitating factors, and included in her assessment only studies of clinical depression. The predisposing factor examined was childhood bereavement or other childhood loss events (1980a). Of the studies of early object loss as a predisposing factor in adult depressive disorder, the majority (8 of 11 studies) found an increased prevalence of loss among the depressives compared to controls. Among the studies reporting an association, Lloyd calculated that childhood loss of a parent by death generally increased the relative risk of adult depression by a factor of 2 or 3. In addition, early loss events also seem to be related to severity of subsequent depression and to attempted suicide. Even so, Lloyd estimates that between 60 and 80 percent of adults with clinical depression have not experienced an early loss event. A more recent review by Paykel (1982), however, is not as encouraging. He notes that about half the studies of parental death have found it more common among depressives than controls, which suggests a real effect, but not conclusively.

Turning her attention to studies examining the hypothesis that life events may precipitate a depressive episode, Lloyd (1980b) concludes that although some contradictory results exist, the majority of studies indicate that depressed patients experience more stressful events preceding their disorder than do normal controls or schizophrenics. The relative risk of depression in the six months after an event occurs appears to be on the order of 5 to 6 (Paykel, 1978). In the studies reviewed, certain events, such as undesirable loss or severely threatening events, were particularly likely to precede a depression. Lloyd concludes that life events are associated with increased risk for depression, but that most of the evidence supporting this conclusion has come from retrospective studies, and corroborating prospective studies are needed. She also notes that not all depressives report precipitating events, so that other factors are clearly operant. Paykel (1982) also finds that the majority of studies of life events as precipitants of depression support the conclusions of Lloyd.

A good deal of research has been done on object loss in adulthood and its relationship to depression and other psychiatric disorder, physical morbidity and mortality. Clayton, who has been a major contributor to this literature, recently reviewed the evidence on bereavement (Clayton, 1982). She reports that many of the symptoms commonly seen in depressed patients are also present in bereavement, particularly during the first month. But after a year, their frequency is substantially reduced. Still, her own studies (Bornstein, Clayton, Halikas, Maurice, & Robins, 1973; Clayton, Halikas, & Maurice, 1972; Clayton, Herjanic Murphy, & Woodruff, 1974) suggest that the prevalence of clinical depression is about 42 percent at one month and 16 percent at one year using Feighner criteria. Weissman and Meyers (1978) report a lifetime prevalence of 10 percent for grief reactions in a community sample, defining a grief reaction using the RDC, criteria for major depression as grief beginning within three months of the death of a close relative and lasting up to a year.

It also should be noted that an increased risk of depression has been found to be associated with the presence of a variety of other medical and psychiatric disorders, such as alcoholism, anxiety, cancer, myocardial infarction, stroke, and childbirth (see, for example, Boyd & Weissman, 1982; Hirschfeld & Cross, 1982). There is overwhelming evidence that the post-partum period (up to six months) carries an excess risk for more serious disorders (Paffenberger & McCabe, 1966; Pugh, Jerath, Schmidt, & Reed, 1963; Weissman & Klerman, 1977), and most of this excess is depression. Pitt (1982) reviews a number of studies, almost all based on patients, and reports that the prevalence of moderate to severe depression is about 10 percent in these studies, and that of nonclinical depression (or the "blues") about 50 percent. He also expresses doubt that there are clinical features which distinguish depression associated with childbirth from that occurring at other times. Although there is not a clear consensus on the relationship between anxiety and depression (see Downing & Rickels, 1974; Gersh & Fowles, 1979), there have been at least three recent papers which suggest that the prevalence of secondary depression in persons suffering from anxiety disorders may be in the range of 30–40 percent (Clancy, Noyes, Hoenk, & Slymen, 1978; Dealy, Ishiki, Avery, Wilson, & Dunner, 1981; Noyes, Clancy, Hoenk, & Slymen, 1980). Petty and Nasrallah (1981) review clinical studies of the association between alcoholism and depression and conclude that the relationship appears to be unidirectional, i.e., alcoholism predisposes to depression but not the reverse. Another disease in which researchers have studied secondary depression is cancer. Petty and Noyes (1981), based on an extensive review of the literature, estimated that 17–25 percent of patients hospitalized with neoplastic disease suffer from depression severe enough to warrant psychiatric intervention. Petty and Noyes also point out a number of methodologic problems which compromise much of the research on the psycholog-ical impact of cancer, as do Freidenbergs, et al. (1981–82). Still, the consensus seems to be that cancer patients, compared to the general population, are at in-creased risk of both clinical depression and demoralization. There is also evidence for a relationship between cardiovascular disease and depression. For example, there is a higher prevalence of both demoralization (Huapaya & Onanth, 1980) and clinical depression (Rabkin, Charles, & Kass, 1983) among hypertensives than among nonhypertensives, although an etiological explanation for this association is not yet available. A high prevalence of depression also has been reported among stroke patients (Post, 1982; Storey, 1967), although Robins (1976) has argued that depression in stroke patients is a non-specific affective response to the complex physical and psychological stresses imposed by severe illness. This interpretation doubtless is applicable to the psychological impact of severe illnesses generally. To further illustrate this point, a number of investigators (Cassem & Hackett, 1971; Wishnie, Hackett, & Cassem, 1971; Wynn, 1967) have reported that symptoms of anxiety and depression are quite common among patients who have experienced a myocardial infarction. Cassem and Hackett report prevalences of 32 percent for anxiety and 30 percent for depression.

Andreasen and Winokur (1979) point out that the clinical and research signifi-cance of secondary depression is not a trivial issue. Secondary depression is a very common diagnosis in both inpatient services and ambulatory clinics. They note that research results suggest that depression secondary to other psychiatric disor-ders is potentially more severe and familial than primary depression, tending to be more colorful and florid, with patients making more suicide attempts, showing more psychotic symptoms, and complaining more of phobias, anger, difficulty falling asleep, and somatic problems. They also suggest that primary and second-ary depression appear to be identical from the perspective of clinical care.

There is considerable debate in the life events literature on the question of what types of events are most stressful or what aspects of events are most stressful. In the case of depression, there is substantial evidence that losses or exits from the social field are the events of most importance (Paykel, 1982). Mueller (1980) notes that this category of events, more so than others, clearly involves substantial disruptions in personal networks. For depression in particular it appears that the stressfulness of events is closely tied to the degree of disruption they create in the social network. In view of this, Mueller argues that one productive research strat-egy in studying the stressful events-depression relationship may be to measure the magnitude of life stress in terms of the level of disruption of network relationships. He suggests that the disruptiveness of any particular event is dependent on the centrality of the network members it affects, the intensity of the relationships involved, and the availability of alternative sources of support within the network.

A number of authors (Antonovsky, 1974; Brown, 1974; Dohrenwend & Dohrenwend, 1974, 1981b; Paykel, 1982; Rabkin & Struening, 1976) have identified a number of conceptual and methodological issues in life event research, which I will not recapitulate here. Rather, I will note a number of issues which render the results of research on life events and depression problematic.

For the most part, studies of life events and clinical depression have been studies of patients. While the results from these studies seem plausible and may accurately reflect the stress process involved, we do not know whether the findings generalize to the spectrum of clinical depression which exists in the general population. Second, both community studies and studies of patients to date have relied overwhelmingly on cross-sectional or case-control study designs in which the relationship between life events and depression is assessed retrospectively. Lloyd (1980a, 1980b), Mueller (1980), and Paykel (1982) have pointed out the difficulties inherent in this approach. A critical issue is the difficulty in causal attribution, since the association could be due to the etiologic role of life events or to the fact that depressives experience more events because of their disorder. In studies of patients there is even a third possibility, that life events may increase the probability of help-seeking for an already existing depressive disorder. A longitudinal study by Aneshensel and Stone (1982) which examines the relationship between stress, support and depression, using the CES-D, indicates that there is a reciprocal relationship between life events and depression. That is, recent stress was found to be related to an increase in current depression, but depression was also related to subsequent experience of stressful life events. Third, the data reported in different studies have been collected using a wide variety of techniques ranging from simple self-administered checklists (Holmes & Rahe, 1967) to detailed and lengthy interviews (Brown & Harris, 1978). For most of these measures we have little or no information on their reliability and validity. Fourth, the problem of how and under what circumstances life events engender depressive phenomena has been conceptualized rather simplistically in most studies (Dohrenwend & Dohrenwend, 1981a; Gore, 1981).

All things considered, however, I fear the field of life events research does not yet provide much opportunity for intervention from the perspective of primary prevention. In their recent review of research issues in this field, the Dohrenwends (Dohrenwend & Dohrenwend, 1981b) point out that while we know that life stress sometimes plays a part in the onset of a variety of psychological and somatic disorders, we do not yet understand the life-stress process well enough to predict and control its pathological effect. Day (1981) is even more explicit, asserting that from a public health perspective the accumulated results of life event research provide very little information that can be used to design primary, secondary or even tertiary intervention programs.

Stressors can be viewed as acute or chronic. Acute stressors refer to events or processes with a delimited time referent, i.e., they are discreet, typically brief in duration, with an observable beginning and end. The archetypal definition of acute stressor is embodied in the contents of most life event inventories that have been developed over the past several decades. The proliferation of such inventories and investigations in which they are employed reflects a distinct bias in the life stress literature; virtually all research on this topic has emphasized the effects of acute stress. Chronic stressors are persistently difficult life conditions or enduring life strains. By definition they are longer-lived, repetitive (either continuous or inter-mittent), and do not necessarily have well-defined origins or end-points. The idea of chronic stressors and their role in depression is preeminently associated with the work of Pearlin and his co-workers. Beginning in the mid-seventies they began publishing a series of papers in which they examined the relationship between social statuses, life strains, coping, and nonclinical depression (Pearlin, 1980; Pearlin & Johnson, 1977; Pearlin & Lieberman, 1979; Pearlin, Lieberman, Menaghan, & Mullan, 1981; Pearlin & Schooler, 1978). In this series of papers they found that life strains increase symptoms of depression, and that coping and social support mediate the effects of life strain. More recently, Wheaton (1983) has presented a more formal discussion of the concept of chronic stressors. He notes that five themes underlie the idea of chronic stress (Wheaton, 1983, pp. 213–214): (1) the perception of barriers to the achievement of life goals or lack of improve-ment in life conditions (Merton, 1968); (2) a perception that rewards in various roles are not commensurate with effort or qualifications (Pearlin & Schooler, 1978; Walster, Berscheid, & Walster, 1973); (3) excessive or inadequate demand in the environment compared to the response capacity of the individual (French, Rodgers, & Cobb, 1974; LaRocco, House, & French, 1980); (4) frustration of role expectations (Pearlin & Schooler, 1978); and (5) the absence of basic and necessary resources for adequate existence. His approach to measurement involves both subjective and objective indicators; the former measuring perceived life strain (Pearlin & Schooler, 1978) and the latter measuring chronic stressors in terms of actual problematic stimuli, e.g., low occupational status or marital disruption (di-vorce or separation). Wheaton presents some interesting data which suggest that while both acute and chronic stressors are related to increased nonclinical depres-sion, their effects are somewhat different and these effects are influenced differen-tially by selected personal coping resources. In view of this, it would appear useful for future studies of risk factors in depression to focus on both acute and chronic stressors and their interaction with each other as well as with various types of personal resources and social statuses. Such an approach would appear particularly important in view of the unpromising results obtained thus far from traditional approaches to life event research (Tennant, 1983).

Personal Resources

In an interesting paper on the structure of coping, Pearlin and Schooler (1978) suggest that individuals use various coping repertoires and that in developing them they rely on three types of personal resources: social resources, psychological resources, and specific coping responses. Social resources are represented by the interpersonal networks of which people are part and which are a potential source of support: family, friends, fellow workers, neighbors, and voluntary associations. General psychological resources of people, on the other hand, are the personality characteristics that people draw upon to help them withstand threats in the environ-ment. In particular, Pearlin and Schooler note self-esteem, self-denigration, and mastery are important. In distinction to general psychological resources are spe-cific coping responses: the behaviors, cognitions, and perceptions in which people engage when actually contending with their life problems. What does the available research tell us about personality, social support, and coping behaviors vis-á-vis depression?

Personality as a risk factor for depression has been a subject of considerable interest in the mental health field (see Chodoff, 1972, and vonZerssen, 1982, for reviews of this literature). However, two recent reviews of the epidemiology of depression do not cite a single study in which the focus was on the relationship between personality characteristics and nonclinical depression or demoralization (Boyd & Weissman, 1982; Hirschfeld & Cross, 1982). In fact, the former cite only one study of personality factors in clinical depression, the latter cite only four (Hirschfeld & Klerman, 1979; Kendall & Discipio, 1976, 1979; Standman, 1978). Hirschfeld and Cross conclude that the traits that have been found to be associated with depression (i.e., neuroticism, introversion, obsessionality, guilt, and dependency) suggest that depressives are more worrisome, less socially adept, more insecure, more sensitive, and more likely to break down under stress than persons who display such traits to a lesser degree. However, it should be noted that these findings are retrospective or crossectional, and are based on patients. Furthermore, as Hirschfeld and Cross note, an association between depression and certain personality characteristics does not necessarily imply these characteristics predispose to depression. The experience of depression, particularly severe melancholia, could alter personality characteristics, or the two could be the result of a third factor such as the same underlying genetic or constitutional processes. In his review, vonZerssen also raises this possibility, suggesting that the "melancholic personality" may be a habitual manifestation of a constitutional predisposition to episodic loss of balance in a system for the regulation of general activity, mood, self-esteem and, partially, sleep and other autonomic functions.

Although there is an extensive literature on coping and stress (see, for example, Coelho, Hamburg, & Adams, 1974; Cohen & Lazarus, 1979; Monat & Lazarus, 1977), there has been little systematic research on specific coping responses and their relationship to clinical depression or demoralization. A notable exception is the paper by Pearlin and Schooler (1978) cited above. These investigators report that the style and content of coping do make a difference for the psychological well-being of people, and that the greater scope and variety of the individual's coping repertoire, the more protection coping affords. The data suggest as well that coping efficacy depends not only on what people do, but on the context in which it is done, for the same kinds of coping mechanisms were not equally effective in different role areas. Their measure of impairment was an index of life stress analogous to demoralization and among the specific coping behaviors assessed were self-reliance versus help-seeking, negotiation, selective ignoring, positive comparison, self-assertion versus passive forbearance, and controlled reflectiveness versus emotional discharge. Pearlin and Schooler also report that the effectiveness of coping varied systematically across subgroups. In particular, there was a tendency for women and those disadvantaged by virtue of less education or lower income to employ coping behaviors that were less effective in ameliorating stress. What is intriguing about these results is that they are consistent with the data suggesting that the prevalence of demoralization and clinical depression is higher among lower status populations. Certainly strategies such as those used by Pearlin and Schooler seem useful for helping us to better understand depressive phenomena. There is a clear need to replicate their results, in particular the role of specific coping behaviors in relationship to both demoralization and clinical depression. In addition, future research on this subject would benefit from the conceptual and methodological strategies developed by Lazarus and his colleagues (Folkman & Lazarus, 1980; Lazarus, 1981; Lazarus, Kanner, & Folkman, 1980). This approach, termed "cognitive-phenomenological," is a more formal and precise strategy than that of Pearlin and Schooler although the central ideas of the two approaches are similar. The Lazarus model is more situation-oriented, emphasizing how people actually cope in specific stressful situations, and transactional in that person and environment are seen in an on-going reciprocal relationship mediated by two processes: appraisal and coping. A questionnaire and scoring procedure have been developed which operationalizes these notions (see Folkman & Lazarus, 1980).

There seems little doubt at this point that social support is inversely related to risk of psychiatric disorder in general. Extensive reviews by Cassel (1976), Cobb (1976), and Caplan (1981) document numerous studies indicating that social support is negatively related to impairment in the presence of such stressors as life events, natural disasters, and war experiences. Mueller (1980), in one of the most extensive reviews to date, concludes that there is considerable evidence for a link between lack of social support and psychiatric morbidity. The evidence is of several kinds. For example, there is a long tradition in the behavioral sciences (particularly sociology) of examining the relationship between psychopathology in communities and a wide range of socioenvironmental conditions such as social isolation, social marginality, and social disorganization. Studies commonly find higher rates of disorder under such conditions, which Mueller argues is consistent with the notion that reduced or impaired social support increases the risk of psychopathology. There is evidence from clinical studies that persons with psychiatric disorders have personal networks that are smaller in size than non-psychiatrically ill persons (Henderson, Duncan-Jones, McAuley, & Ritchie, 1978; Pattison, Defrancisco, Wood, Frazier, & Crowder, 1975; Sokolovsky, Cohen, Berger, & Geiger, 1978). There is also evidence that social support, particularly in the form of close, confiding relationships, is inversely related to risk of depression, especially among women (Brown & Harris, 1978; Henderson, Byrne, et al., 1978; Henderson, Duncan-Jones, McAuley, & Ritchie, 1978; Miller, Ingham, & Davidson, 1976; Roy, 1978). Whether social support is differentially implicated in clinical and nonclinical depression is not known. Researchers have examined social support in relation to both, and seem to obtain the same general findings, i.e., lower morbidity in the presence of greater support.

At this point there seem to be three central, unresolved issues in regard to social support and depression: (1) The nature of the social support effect; (2) conceptualization and measurement of support; and (3) the specificity of social support effects in depression.

From the available studies, there is some question as to whether the effects of social support on psychiatric impairment are limited to moderating the impact of life stress (the buffering hypothesis), or whether social support has an effect independent of the presence of life stress (direct effect hypothesis) (see, for example, Mueller, 1980; Thoits, 1982; Turner & Noh, 1982; Williams, Ware, & Donald, 1981). A serious shortcoming of previous research has been the lack of attention to the conceptual and methodologic properties of measures of social support (McQueen & Celentano, 1982; Thoits, 1982). There is no clear consensus regarding definition of the concept. There appears to be an emerging consensus that the concept is multi-dimensional (McQueen & Celentano, 1982; Thoits, 1982; Wellman, 1981), although there is not yet agreement as to what these dimensions are.

Only a few investigators (Donald & Ware, 1982; Duncan-Jones, 1981a, 1981b; Lin, Dean, & Ensel, 1981; McFarlane, Neale, Norman, Roy, & Streiner, 1981) have made systematic attempts to develop social support scales. Scales often are constructed in an ad hoc manner, or proxy measures such as marital status or employment status are used as indicators of social support. As Mueller (1980) notes, research thus far does not indicate the kind and quality of support that is protective against, or lowers the risk of, psychiatric disorder. Until more systematic efforts are made to specify the dimensions of social support, the questions of how and under what circumstances support reduces the risk of disorder will remain unanswered.

Although there is substantial evidence to suggest that social support is related to the occurrence of psychiatric disorder, there is little evidence to suggest that there are social support effects specific to depression, or that the effects are different for clinical and nonclinical depression. In view of this, Mueller (1980) urges that future investigations of the relationship of social support to onset of psychiatric disorder focus on specific effects. This will require studies involving comparison of depressives with other psychiatric disorders, ideally with nonpsychiatric controls drawn from either treatment facilities or the general population. The question of differential social support effects among depressives would require further differentiation, say between clinical and nonclinical depression, or between primary and secondary depression.

ASSESSING THE IMPACT OF INTERVENTIONS

Assessing the impact of interventions to reduce the incidence and prevalence of depressive phenomena is an integral, as well as critical, part of any prevention effort. The discussions of prescriptions and proscriptions regarding collection, analysis, and interpretation of data from experimental and quasiexperimental interventions are myriad. I will not attempt to review these here (interested readers are referred to Breckinridge's discussion of statistical issues presented at this workshop, or to such books as Attkisson, Hargreaves, Horowitz, & Sorenson, 1982; Cook & Campbell, 1979; Kirk, 1968; Underwood, 1957; Winer, 1971). Instead, I will suggest and discuss some possible outcome variables and issues in their measurement from an epidemiologic perspective.

Outcomes for assessing the impact of interventions in the community should be broadly conceived. In the case of a specific disease or disorder, the measures of outcome should reflect as accurately as possible the spectrum of the disease's manifestation. In the case of depressive phenomena, outcomes can be considered in terms of at least the two broad classes discussed earlier: (1) depression; (2) demoralization.

Depression, in the context of this discussion, again refers to the clinical syndrome, whether primary or secondary in nature. Likewise, demoralization refers to a broad range of symptoms reflecting low self-esteem, helplessness-hopelessness, sadness, and anxiety (Frank, 1973). We have already noted a number of facets of the epidemiology of these two types of depressive phenomena, including the fact that indicators of social status such as age, sex, marital status and social class as well as indicators of psychosocial risk factors such as life change and personal resources seem to operate in a similar fashion in regard to both. Consequently, I suggest that intervention efforts which have as their objective the primary prevention of depressive phenomena must include both of these manifestations as outcome measures. I suggest this for several reasons. First, clinical depression is fairly prevalent, is a serious behavioral disorder with life-threatening implications (e.g., suicide), and in the case of melancholia, a chronic disease with considerable illness burden. Failure to include an assessment of clinical depression and changes in its incidence and prevalence in response to intervention efforts ignores the more serious form of the disease. Second, demoralization is extremely prevalent in our society, is also the source of considerable suffering, and is related to clinical depression, although at this juncture we are not sure how. Link and Dohrenwend (1980) have suggested that a population may be partitioned into four groups: (1) those persons manifesting clinical disorder and demoralization; (2) those having only clinical disorders; (3) those having only demoralization; and (4) those having neither. I suggest this scheme could be a useful strategy for designing and assessing intervention programs using these two outcomes.

The assessment of outcomes obviously requires the existence of reliable and valid indicators. In psychiatric epidemiology our measures are still far from perfect, but we are better off now that at any time in the past. Historically, one of the limitations in conducting large-scale community studies of clinical psychiatric disorder was that procedures for eliciting symptoms and making clinical decisions were not standardized so that they could be used to generate comparable results across studies. In recent years several structured clinical interview instruments have been developed which employ explicit criteria for making psychiatric diagnoses. Three of these are being used increasingly in both clinical and community studies: the Present State Examination (PSE) developed at the Institute of Psychiatry in London (Wing, Cooper, & Sartorius, 1974); the SADS-RDC, developed primarily at the New York State Psychiatric Institute (Endicott & Spitzer, 1978); and the DIS developed by Robins and her colleagues at Washington University (Robins, Helzer, Croughan, & Ratcliff, 1981). All of these procedures have facilitated greatly our ability to generate more valid and reliable estimates of the incidence and prevalence of psychiatric disorder in both treatment and community settings, and should be strongly considered by researchers interested in clinical disorder as an outcome. Likewise, at this point we have sufficient evidence on the psychometric properties of most symptom checklists to suggest that they all have good reliability and that they seem to tap a common underlying dimension. The CES-D has much to recommend it: it is brief (20 items), is easily scored, has been used in cross-cultural contexts (R. E. Roberts, 1980; Vernon & Roberts, 1982), and has been used in a variety of clinical and community studies, including a national survey. However, if we agree that what such inventories assess is most likely demoralization, then another useful instrument is the Psychiatric Epidemiology Research Interview (PERI) subscales which Dohrenwend and his colleagues (Dohrenwend, Shrout, Egri, & Mendelsohn, 1980) have combined into a measure of demoralization. The PERI is brief, is suitable for use in clinical or community settings, has been used in cross-cultural contexts (Vernon & Roberts, 1981) and is composed of distinct subscales measuring the central dimensions of Frank's construct (1973).

CONCLUDING REMARKS

We have seen that depressive phenomena are relatively common afflictions of the human condition. Although we do not know the incidence of clinical or non-clinical depression, based on the best available data, it appears that 3–4 percent of the adult population may be suffering from a major depressive episode at any given time, and as many as 15–20 percent report having experienced a major depressive episode at some time in their life. Demoralization is more prevalent, with most studies suggesting that the point prevalence of demoralization in the general population is in the 20–25 percent range. We do not know the lifetime prevalence of demoralization. In terms of sheer numbers of people affected, clearly we are not dealing with a trivial issue. It seems equally apparent that reduction of this illness burden would effect enormous societal benefit in both humanitarian and economic terms.

From an epidemiologic perspective, what are some key issues to consider if we wish to effect such a reduction? I will discuss two of these issues: morbidity measurement and risk factors.

In terms of measurement, there is a critical need for incidence data. If we are talking about primary prevention, our objective is to prevent the occurrence of *new* or *first* episodes of depressive phenomena. A reduction in prevalence does not necessarily tell us anything about success of primary prevention efforts, since a reduction in duration of episodes can reduce prevalence without any change occurring in incidence. Diminution of duration effects are important, of course, in terms of secondary prevention. If we are interested in factors involved in the etiology of initial episodes of depression phenomena, then again we need incidence data. Factors related to increased prevalence may actually be related to duration effects and not to etiologic effects. That is, the factors sustain the illness rather than cause it. The only way out of this dilemma is at some point to assess the relative contributions of factors such as those listed in Table 3 on incident cases as contrasted with prevalent cases. In terms of research design, this ultimately means large-scale prospective investigations over as long a time interval as possible.

There seems little doubt, given our current state of knowledge, that depressive phenomena are multifactorial in origin, almost certainly resulting from the lifelong interaction of biological, psychological, and socioenvironmental factors (see Akiskal, 1979, for example). It seems equally apparent that there is a broad array of psychosocial factors implicated in depression. I have summarized the factors for which there seems to be both consensus and some supporting data in Table 3. However, there are a number of problems which limit the usefulness of this set of risk factors for primary prevention. First, the correlation of these factors, singly and in varying combinations, with depression are quite modest. Second, since there are individuals identified as being at risk on such factors who never have depression and there are depressives who are not at risk in terms of these factors, they clearly are neither necessary nor sufficient causes of depression. At most, psychosocial factors may increase the probability of depression occurring, given other factors.

Third, although some of these factors are strongly implicated in the etiology of depression, we still know very little about how or under what circumstances they are operant. This problem could be reduced if studies were designed to systematically examine more of these putative risk factors within the same design, thereby permitting multivariate comparisons of a broad range of alternate risk factors and the relative contributions of each. Fourth, the specificity of these psychosocial risk factors is unknown. Most probably can be viewed as having nonspecific effects. However, unless comparative designs are used involving multiple diagnostic categories, the extent and nature of their specificity cannot be assessed. In fact, since some classes of these factors (such as status attributes and perhaps even life stress and family history) cannot be manipulated, their use is limited largely to identifying target populations, rather than as variables to be modified by intervention programs. The most likely class of factors in terms of potential for modification vis-á-vis primary prevention is personal resources, particularly coping behaviors and social networks/social support. In fact, much of the prevention intervention in mental health has emphasized strengthening personal resources, as Heller, Price, and Sher (1980), have pointed out.

I am suggesting that the fields of primary prevention and epidemiology would be advanced considerably if preventive interventions were done using standard measures of psychopathology and if the interventions and the measures of outcome focused on the full spectrum of depressive phenomena, including measures of both clinical and subclinical manifestations of depression. As I indicated in my earlier remarks, depressive phenomena are heterogeneous, and intervention efforts should acknowledge this. First, any given intervention, or set of interventions, may impact multiple depressive phenomena, and may do so differentially. Unless the intervention design explicitly recognizes this, our ability to assess its effectiveness will be attenuated. Second, I suggest that programs to prevent depression should focus both on more prevalent/less severe and less prevalent/more severe illness, the former because it is more tractable and the latter because it involves greater illness burden. Furthermore, an intervention that prevents a broad range of depressive phenomena is much more robust than one that does not. The use of standard assessment procedures would address a major limitation of most intervention efforts to date, i.e., noncomparability of results across studies. When studies of ostensibly the same factors produce divergent results, which unhappily occurs all too often, it is difficult to interpret the findings because research designs usually are not replicates. This problem obviously is not limited to intervention research. For example, reviewers of epidemiologic studies almost invariably comment on the wide variability of results and the problem of noncomparable procedures. As I noted in the discussion of incidence and prevalence, however, when comparisons are made controlling for type of assessment procedures, a remarkable degree of concordance emerges. At this point there are several alternative procedures for assessing both clinical depression and demoralization suitable for use with general populations, and for which we have some evidence of reliability and validity. I refer specifically to the SADS-RDC and the DIS-DSM III for clinical diagnosis and the Zung SDS, the CES-D, and the PERI-D for assessing demoralization. I submit that if these procedures for assessing outcomes were systematically and widely used in primary prevention efforts our ability to generalize, and consequently to understand depression, would be enhanced considerably.

There are good reasons, in fact, to include multiple measures of psychopathology in our research. Shrout and Fleiss (1981) have demonstrated that multimethod procedures are virtually mandatory if accurate case ascertainment is to be achieved. Moreover, there is considerable evidence for the construct validity of multi-method approaches in psychological measurement (Campbell & Fiske,

1959). In a recent discourse on this topic, Dohrenwend and Dohrenwend (1982) discuss the application of the multi-method approach to multi-stage screening programs in community populations. In this instance, they propose using symptom checklists (with their strong psychometric properties and economy of administration) as initial assessments, followed by assessments using clinical diagnostic procedures. However, the model can be generalized to multiple assessments within stages as well, as is discussed in the chapter by Breckinridge in this volume, particularly in reference to the use of LISREL analytic procedures.

But more can be done to advance the field of primary prevention than what I have discussed thus far. What I have reference to specifically is the research model being used. Most research in mental health, whether in prevention or epidemiology, is carried out by independent investigators in local community settings employing ideosyncratic research designs. This cottage industry approach is neither parsimonious nor productive, given the scope of the problem. I say this because there is another research model which has a much greater potential for scientific and, ultimately, programmatic yield. This model has been widely used in other public health sectors, sometimes with spectacular results. I am referring to the large-scale clinical trial or multi-site collaborative research study. These joint ventures have a long history in somatic disease studies, for example, those of polio, heart disease and stroke. The advantage is that a common conceptual model can be assessed simultaneously across multiple community settings using a standard research design and uniform assessment procedures. Because comparability across studies is maximized, and the overall sample is large and more representative of the larger society than any single study sample, the results have the potential for much greater impact. The usefulness of this model is becoming more widely recognized in mental health. Two notable examples are the NIMH collaborative studies of the psychobiology of depression (Katz & Klerman, 1979) and the ECA collaborative community survey (Eaton, Regier, Locke, & Taube, 1981). I suggest that this model may be equally applicable to the field of primary prevention and that reductions in the incidence and prevalence of depressive phenomena ultimately will require large-scale demonstration projects that identify classes of risk factors and strategies that modify them. The extent to which preventive efforts are able to employ this research model will go a long way toward determining the viability of the concept of primary prevention of depression.

REFERENCES

Andreasen, N.C., Endicott, J. Spitzer, R. L., & Winokur G. (1977). The family history method using diagnostic criteria. *Archives of General Psychiatry, 34,* 1229–1235.

Andreasen, N. C., & Winokur, G. (1979). Secondary depression: Familial, clinical, and research perspectives. *American Journal of Psychiatry, 136,* 62–66.

Aneshensel, C. S., & Stone, I. D. (1982). Stress and depression: A test of the buffering model of social support. *Archives of General Psychiatry, 39,* 1392–1396.

Antonovsky, A. (1974). Conceptual and methodological problems in the study of resistance resources and stressful life events. In B. S. Dohrenwend, & B. P. Dohrenwend (Eds.), *Stressful life events: Their nature and effects* (pp. 245–258). New York: John Wiley and Sons.

Akiskal, H. S. (1979). A biobehavioral approach to depression. In R. A. Depue (Ed.), *The psychobiology of the depressive disorders: Implications for the effects of stress* (pp. 409–438). New York: Academic Press.

Akiskal, H. S., & McKiney, W. T. (1973). Depressive disorders: Toward a unified hypothesis. *Science, 182,* 20–29.

Akiskal, H. S., & McKinney, W. T. (1975). Overview of recent research in depression: Integration of ten conceptual models into a comprehensive clinical frame. *Archives of General Psychiatry, 32,* 285–305.

Attkisson, C. C., Hargreaves, W. A., Horowitz, M. J., & Sorenson, J. E. (1982). *Evaluation of human service programs.* New York: Academic Press.

Barrett, I., Hurst, M. W., DiScala, C., & Rose, R. M. (1978). Prevalence of depression over a 12-month period in a nonpatient population. *Archives of General Psychiatry, 35,* 741–744.

Berkman, P. L. (1971). Measurement of mental health in a general population survey. *American Journal of Epidemiology, 94,* 105–111.

Blazer, D., & Williams, C. D. (1980). Epidemiology of dysphoria and depression in an elderly population. *American Journal of Psychiatry, 137,* 439–444.

Bornstein, P. E., Clayton, P. J., Halikas, J. A., Maurice, W. L., & Robins, E. (1973). The depression of widowhood after thirteen months. *British Journal of Psychiatry, 122,* 561–566.

Boyd, J. H., & Weissman, M. M. (1981). Epidemiology of affective disorders: A reexamination and future directions. *Archives of General Psychiatry, 38,* 1039–1046.

Boyd, J. H., & Weissman, M. M. (1982). Epidemiology. In E. S. Paykel (Ed.), *Handbook of affective disorders* (pp. 109–125). New York:Guilford Press.

Brown, G. W. (1974). Meaning, measurement, and stress of life events. In B. S. Dohrenwend & B. P. Dohrenwend (Eds.), *Stressful life events: Their nature and effects* (pp. 217–244). New York: John Wiley & Sons.

Brown, G. W., & Harris, T. (1978). *Social origins of depression: A study of psychiatric disorder in women.* London: Tavistock.

Campbell, D. T., & Fiske, D. W. (1959). Convergent and discriminant validation by the multi-trait-multi-method matrix. *Psychological Bulletin, 56,* 81–105.

Caplan, G. (1981). Mastery of stress: Psychosocial aspects. *American Journal of Psychiatry, 138,* 413–420.

Cassel, J. (1976). The contribution of the social environment to host resistance. *American Journal of Epidemiology, 104,* 107–123.

Cassem, N. H., & Hackett, T. P. (1971). Psychiatric consultation in a coronary care unit. *Annals of Internal Medicine, 75,* 9–14.

Chodoff, P. (1972). The depressive personality. *Archives of General Psychiatry. 27,* 666–673.

Clancy, J., Noyes, R., Hoenk, R. P., & Slymen, D. J. (1978). Secondary depression in anxiety neurosis. *Journal of Nervous and Mental Disease, 166,* 846–850.

Clayton, P. J. (1981). The epidemiology of bipolar affective disorder. *Comprehensive Psychiatry, 22,* 31–43.

Clayton, P. J. (1982). Bereavement. In E. S. Paykel (Ed.), *Handbook of affective disorders* (pp. 403–415). New York: Guilford Press.

Clayton, P. J., Halikas, J. A., & Maurice, W. L. (1972). The depression of widowhood. *British Journal of Psychiatry, 120,* 71–78.

Clayton, P. J., Herjanic, M., Murphy, G. E., & Woodruff, R., Jr. (1974). Mourning and depression: Their similarities and differences. *Canadian Psychiatric Association Journal, 19,* 309–312.

Cleary, P. D., & Mechanic, D. (1983). Sex differences in psychological distress among married people. *Journal of Health and Social Behavior, 24,* 111–121.

Cobb, S. (1976). Social support as a moderator of life stress. *Psychosomatic Medicine, 38,* 300–314.

Coelho, G. V., Hamburg, D. A., & Adams, J. E. (Eds.). (1974). *Coping and adaptation.* New York: Basic Books.

Cohen, F., & Lazarus, R. S. (1979). Coping with the stress of illness. In G. C. Stone & N. E. Adler (Eds.), *Health psychology,* (pp. 217–254). San Francisco: Jossey-Bass.

Comstock, G. W., & Helsing, K. J. (1976). Symptoms of depression in two communities. *Psychological Medicine, 6,* 551–563.

Cook, T. D., & Campbell, D. T. (1979). *Quasi-Experimentation.* Boston: Houghton Mifflin.

Day, R. (1981). Afterword: Recent directions in life stress research from a public health perspective. In B. S. Dohrenwend & B. P. Dohrenwend (Eds.), *Stressful life events and their contexts* (pp. 279–283). New York: Neale Watson Academic Publications.

Dealy, R. S., Ishiki, D. M., Avery, D. H., Wilson, L. G., & Dunner, D. L. (1981). Secondary depression in anxiety disorders. *Comprehensive Psychiatry, 22,* 612–618.

Depue, R. A., Monroe, S. M., & Shackman, S. L. (1979). The psychobiology of human disease:

Implications for conceptualizing the depressive disorders. In R. A. Depue (Ed.), *The Psychobiology of the depressive disorders: Implications for the effects of stress* (pp. 3–20). New York: Academic Press.

Dohrenwend, B. P. (1973). Some issues in the definition and measurement of psychiatric disorders in general populations. In *Proceedings of the 14th National Meetings of the Public Health Conference on Records and Statistics* (DHEW Publication No. 74-1214, pp. 480–489). Washington, D. C.: U.S. Government Printing Office.

Dohrenwend, B. P., & Dohrenwend, B. S. (1969). Social status and psychological disorder. New York: John Wiley & Sons.

Dohrenwend, B. P., & Dohrenwend, B. S. (1974). Social and cultural influences on psychopathology. *Annual Review of Psychology, 25,* 417–452.

Dohrenwend, B. P., & Dohrenwend, B. S. (1976). Sex differences in psychiatric disorder. *American Journal of Sociology, 81,* 1447–1454.

Dohrenwend, B. P., & Dohrenwend, B. S. (1981a). Socioenvironmental factors, stress, and psychopathology (Part 1). Quasi-experimental evidence on the social causation-social selection issue posed by class differences. *American Journal of Community Psychology, 9,* 128–159.

Dohrenwend, B. S., & Dohrenwend, B. P. (1981b). Life stress and illness: Formulation of the issues. In B. S. Dohrenwend & B. P. Dohrenwend (Eds.), *Stressful life events and their contexts* (pp. 1–27). New York: Neal Watson Academic Publications.

Dohrenwend, B. P., & Dohrenwend, B. S. (1982). Perspectives on the past and future of psychiatric epidemiology. *American Journal of Public Health, 72,* 1271–1279.

Dohrenwend, B. P., Oksenberg, L., Shrout, P. E., Dohrenwend, B. S., & Cook, D. (1981). What brief psychiatric screening scales measure. In Sudman, S. (Ed.), *Health survey research methods: Third Biennial Conference* (pp. 188–189). Washington, D.C.: National Center for Health Services Research.

Dohrenwend, B. P., Shrout, P. E., Egri, G., & Mendelsohn, F. S. (1980). Nonspecific psychological distress and other dimensions of psychopathology. *Archives of General Psychiatry, 37,* 1229–1236.

Donald, C. A., & Ware, J. E. (1982). *The quantification of social contacts and resources.* Santa Monica: The Rand Corporation.

Downing, R. W., & Rickels, K. (1974). Mixed anxiety—depression: Fact or myth? *Archives of General Psychiatry, 30,* 312–317.

Duncan-Jones, P. (1981a). The structure of social relationships: Analysis of a survey instrument (Part 1). *Social Psychiatry, 16,* 55–61.

Duncan-Jones, P. (1981b). The structure of social relationships: Analysis of a survey instrument (Part 2). *Social Psychiatry, 16,* 143–149.

Eaton, W. W. (1980). *The sociology of mental disorders.* New York: Praeger.

Eaton, W. W., & Kessler, L. G. (1981). Rates of symptoms of depression in a national sample. *American Journal of Epidemiology, 114,* 528–538.

Eaton, W. W., Regier, D. A., Locke, B. Z., & Taube, C. A. (1981). The epidemiologic catchment area program of the NIMH. *Public Health Reports, 96,* 319–325.

Endicott, J., & Spitzer, R. L. (1978). A diagnostic interview: The schedule for affective disorders and schizophrenia. *Archives of General Psychiatry, 35,* 837–844.

Erlenmeyer-Kimling, L. (1979). Advantages of a behavior-genetic approach to investigating stress in the depressive disorders. In R. A. Depue (Ed.), *The psychobiology of the depressive disorders: Implications for the effects of stress* (pp. 391–407). New York: Academic Press.

Feinson, M. C. (1984). Aging and mental health: Challenging a scientific myth. Paper presented at the annual meeting of the American Sociological Association, San Antonio, Texas.

Folkman, S., & Lazarus, R. S. (1980). An analysis of coping in a middle-aged community sample. *Journal of Health and Social Behavior, 21,* 219–239.

Fox, J. P., Hall, C. E., & Elveback, L. R. (1970). *Epidemiology: Man and disease.* Toronto: McMillan Company.

Frank, J. D. (1973). *Persuasion and healing.* New York: Schocken Books.

Freidenbergs, I., Gordon, W., Hibbard, M., Levine, L., Wolf, C., & Diller, L. (1981–82). Psychosocial aspects of living with cancer: A review of the literature. *International Journal of Psychiatry in Medicine, 11,* 303–329.

French, J. R. P., Rodgers, W., & Cobb, S. (1974). Adjustment as person-environment fit. In G. V. Coelho, D. A. Hamburg, & J. E. Adams (Eds.) *Coping and adaptation* (pp. 316–333). New York: Basic Books.

Frerichs, R. R., Aneshensel, C., & Clark, V. (1981). Prevalence of depression in Los Angeles County. *American Journal of Epidemiology, 113,* 691–699.

Friedman, R. J. (1974). The psychology of depression: An overview. In R. J. Friedman, & M. M. Katz (Eds.), *The psychology of depression: Contemporary theory and research* (pp. 281-298). Washington, D.C.: U.S. Government Printing Office.

Gersh, F. S., & Fowles, D. L. (1979). Neurotic depression: The concept of anxious depression. In R. A. Depue, (Ed.), *The psychobiology of the depressive disorders: Implications for the effects of stress* (pp. 81-104). New York: Academic Press.

Gershon, E. S., Bunney, W. E., Leckman, J. F., vanErdewegh, M., & deBauche, B. A. (1976). The inheritance of affective disorders: A review of data and of hypotheses. *Behavioral Genetics, 6,* 227-261.

Gore, S. (1981). Stress-buffering functions of social supports: An appraisal and clarification of research models. In B. S. Dohrenwend, & B. R. Dohrenwend (Eds.), *Stressful life events and their contexts* (pp. 202-222). New York: Neale Watson Academic Publications.

Guze, S. B., Woodruff, R. A., & Clayton, P. J. (1971). "Secondary" affective disorder: A study of 95 cases. *Psychological Medicine, 1,* 426-428.

Hammen, C. L., & Padesky, C. A. (1977). Sex differences in the expression of depressive responses on the Beck Depression Inventory. *Journal of Abnormal Psychology, 86,* 609-614.

Heller, K., Price, R. H., & Sher, K. J. (1980). Research and evaluation in primary prevention: Issues and guidelines. In R. H. Price and Associates (Eds.), *Prevention in mental health: Research, policy and practice* (pp. 285-313). Beverly Hills: Sage.

Henderson, S., Duncan-Jones, P., McAuley, H., & Ritchie, K. (1978). The patient's primary group. *British Journal of Psychiatry, 132,* 74-86.

Hirschfeld, R. M. A., & Cross, L. K. (1982). Epidemiology of affective disorders. *Archives of General Psychiatry, 39,* 35-46.

Hirschfeld, R. M. A., & Klerman, G. L. (1979). Personality attributes and affective disorders. *American Journal of Psychiatry, 136,* 67-70.

Holmes, T. H., & Rahe, R. H. (1967). The social readjustment rating scale. *Journal of Psychosomatic Research, 11,* 213-218.

Huapaya, L., & Onanth, J. (1980). Depression associated with hypertension: A review. *Psychiatric Journal of the University of Ottawa, 5,* 58-62.

Husaini, B. A., Neff, J. A., & Stone, R. H. (1979). Psychiatric impairment in rural communities. *Journal of Community Psychology, 7,* 137-146.

Katz, M. M., & Klerman, G. L. (1979). Introduction: Overview of the clinical studies program of the National Institute of Mental Health—Clinical Research Branch Collaborative Program on the Psychobiology of Depression. *American Journal of Psychiatry, 136,* 49-51.

Kendall, R. E., & Discipio, W. J. (1976). Eysenck personality inventory scores of patients with depressive illness. *British Journal of Psychiatry, 114,* 767-770.

Kendall, R. E., & Discipio, W. J. (1979). Obsessional symptoms and obsessional personality traits in patients with depressive illness. *Psychological Medicine, 1,* 65-72.

Kirk, R. E. (1968). Experimental design procedures for the behavioral sciences. Belmont, CA: Brooks/Cole.

LaRocco, J. M., House, J. S., & French, J. R. P. (1980). social support, occupational stress, and health. *Journal of Health and Social Behavior, 21,* 202-218.

Langner, T. S. (1962). A twenty-two item screening score for psychiatric symptoms indicating impairment. *Journal of Health and Social Behavior, 3,* 269-276.

Lazarus, R. S. (1981). The stress and coping paradigm. In C. Eisdorfer, D. Cohen, A. Kleinman, & P. Maxim (Eds.), *Theoretical bases of psychopathology* (pp. 177-214). New York: Spectrum.

Lazarus, R. S., Kanner, A., & Folkman, S. (1980). Emotions: A cognitive-phenomenological analysis. In R. Plutchik, & H. Kellerman (Eds.), *Theories of emotion* (pp. 189-217). New York: Academic Press.

Lilienfeld, A. M., & Lilienfeld, D. E. (1980). *Foundations of epidemiology.* (2nd ed.). New York: Oxford.

Lin, N., Dean, A., & Ensel, W. M. (1981). Social support scales: A methodological note. *Schizophrenia Bulletin, 7,* 73-89.

Link, B., & Dohrenwend, B. P. (1980). Formulation of hypotheses about the true prevalence of demoralization in the United States. In B. P. Dohrenwend, B. S. Dohrenwend, M. S. Gould, B. Link, R. Neugebauer, & R. Wunsch-Hitzig (Eds.), *Mental illness in the United states: Epidemiological estimates* (pp. 133-149). New York: Praeger.

Lloyd, C. (1980a). Life events and depressive disorder reviewed—I: Events as predisposing factors. *Archives of General Psychiatry, 37,* 529-535.

Lloyd, C. (1980b). Life events and depressive disorder reviewed—II: Events as precipitating factors. *Archives of General Psychiatry, 37,* 541–549.

MacMahon, B., & Pugh, T. F. (1970). *Epidemiology—principles and methods.* Boston: Little Brown & Company.

Mausner, J. S., & Bahn, A. K. (1974). *Epidemiology: An introductory text.* Philadelphia: W. B. Saunders Co.

McFarlane, A. H., Neale, K. A., Norman, G. R., Roy, R. G., & Streiner, D. L. (1981). Methodological issues in developing a scale to measure social support. *Schizophrenia Bulletin, 7,* 90–100.

McQueen, D. V., & Celentano, D. D. (1982). Social factors in the etiology of multiple outcomes: The case of blood pressure and alcohol consumption patterns. *Social Science and Medicine, 16,* 397–418.

Merikangas, K. R., & Spiker, D. G. (1982). Assortative mating among inpatients with primary affective disorder. *Psychological Medicine, 12,* 753–764.

Merton, R. K. (1968). *Social Theory and Social Structure.* New York: Free Press.

Miller, P.M., Ingham, J. C., & Davidson, S. (1976). Life events, symptoms and social support. *Journal of Psychosomatic Research, 20,* 515–522.

Monat, A., & Lazarus, R. S. (Eds.), (1977). *Stress and coping: An anthology.* New York: Columbia University Press.

Mueller, D. P. (1980). Social networks: A promising direction for research on the relationship of the social environment to psychiatric disorder. *Social Science and Medicine, 14,* 147–161.

Murphy, J. M. (1980). Continuities in community-based psychiatric epidemiology. *Archives of General Psychiatry, 32,* 1215–1223.

Myers, J. K., & Weissman, M. M. (1980). Use of a self-report symptom scale to detect depression in a community sample. American Journal of Psychiatry, 137, 1081–1084.

Myers, J. K., Weissman, M. M., Tischler, G. L., Holzer, C. E., Leaf, P. J., Orvaschel, H., Anthony, J. C., Boyd, J. H., Burke, J. D., Kramer, M., & Stoltzman, R. (1984). Six-month prevalence of psychiatric disorders in three communities: 1980 to 1982. *Archives of General Psychiatry, 41,* 959–967.

Neff, J. A., & Husaini, B. A. (1980). Race, socioeconomic status, and psychiatric impairment: A research note. *Journal of Community Psychology, 8,* 16–19.

Neugebauer, R., Dohrenwend, B. P., & Dohrenwend, B. S. (1980). Formulation of hypotheses about the true prevalence of functional psychiatric disorders among adults in the United States. In B. P. Dohrenwend, B. S. Dohrenwend, M. S. Gould, B. Link, R. Neugebauer, & R. Wunsch-Hitzig (Eds.), *Mental illness in the United States* (pp. 45–94). New York: Praeger.

Newman, J. P. (1984). Sex differences in symptoms of depression: Clinical disorder or normal distress? *Journal of Health and Social Behavior, 25,* 136–159.

Noyes, R., Clancy, J. Hoenk, P. R., & Slymen, D. J. (1980). The prognosis of anxiety neurosis. *Archives of General Psychiatry, 37,* 173–178.

Nurnberger, J. I., & Gershon, E. S. (1982). Genetics. In E. S. Paykel (Ed.), *Handbook of affective disorders* (pp. 126–145). New York: The Guilford Press.

Paffenberger, R. S., & McCabe, L. J. (1966). The effect of obstetric and perinatal events on risk of mental illness in women of childbearing age. *American Journal of Public Health, 56,* 400–407.

Parker, G. (1979). Sex differences in non-clinical depression. *Austrialia and New Zealand Journal of Psychiatry, 13,* 127–132.

Pattison, E. M., Defrancisco, D., Wood, P., Frazier, H., & Crowder, J. (1975). A psychosocial kinship model for family therapy. *American Journal of Psychiatry, 132,* 1246–1251.

Paykel, E. S. (1978). Contribution of life events to causation of psychiatric illness. *Psychological Medicine, 8,* 245–253.

Paykel, E. S. (1982). Life events and early environment. In E. S. Paykel (Ed.), *Handbook of affective disorders* (pp. 146–161). New York: Guilford Press.

Pearlin, L. I., & Johnson, J. S. (1977). Marital status, life-strains, and depression. *American Sociological Review, 42,* 704–715.

Pearlin, L. I., & Lieberman, M. A. (1979). Social sources of emotional distress. In R. Simmons (Ed.), *Research in community and mental health* (Vol. 1, pp. 217–248). Greenwich, CT.: JAI Press.

Pearlin, L. I., Lieberman, M. A., Menaghan, E. G., & Mullan, J. T. (1981). The stress process. *Journal of Health and Social Behavior, 22,* 337–356.

Pearlin, L. I., & Schooler, C. (1978). The structure of coping. *Journal of Health and Social Behavior, 19,* 2–21.

Petty, F., & Nasrallah, H. A. (1981). Secondary depression in alcoholism: Implications for future research. *Comprehensive Psychiatry, 22,* 587–595.

Petty, F., & Noyes, R., Jr. (1981). Depression secondary to cancer. *Biological Psychiatry, 16,* 1203–1220.

Pitt, B. (1982). Depression and childbirth. In E. S. Paykel (Ed.), *Handbook of affective disorders* (pp. 361–378). New York: Guilford Press.

Post, F. (1962). The significance of affective symptoms in old age. (Maudsley Monographs, No. 10). London: Oxford University Press.

Prange, A. (1973). The use of drugs in depression: Its theoretical and practical basis. *Psychiatric Annuals, 3,* 55–75.

Pugh, T. F., Jerath, B. K., Schmidt, W. M., & Reed, R. B. (1963). Rates of mental disease related to childbearing. *New England Journal of Medicine, 268,* 1224–1228.

Rabkin, J. G., & Struening, E. L. (1976). Life events, stress and illness. *Science, 194,* 1013–1020.

Rabkin, J. G., Charles, E., & Kass, F. (1983). Hypertension and DSM-III depression in psychiatric outpatients. *American Journal of Psychiatry, 140,* 1072–1074.

Radloff, L. S. (1977). The CES-D Scale: A self-report depression scale for research in the general population. *Applied Psychological Measurement, 1,* 385–401.

Roberts, C. R. (1980). *Predicting perceived health status: The role of psychological well-being.* Unpublished master's thesis, The University of Texas School of Public Health, Houston, TX.

Roberts, C. R., Roberts, R. E., & Stevenson, J. M. (1982). Women, work, social support and psychiatric morbidity. *Social Psychiatry, 17,* 167–173.

Roberts, R. E. (1980). Prevalence of psychological distress among Mexican Americans. *Journal of Health and Social Behavior, 21,* 134–145.

Roberts, R. E. (1981). Prevalence of depressive symptoms among Mexican Americans. *Journal of Nervous and Mental Disease, 169,* 213–219.

Roberts, R. E., Stevenson, J. S., & Breslow, L. (1981). Symptoms of depression among Blacks and Whites in an urban community. *Journal of Nervous and Mental Disease, 169,* 213–219.

Roberts, R. E., & Roberts, C. R. (1982). Marriage, work and depressive symptoms among Mexican Americans. *Hispanic Journal of Behavioral Sciences, 4,* 199–221.

Roberts, R. E., & Vernon, S. W. (1982). Depression in the community: Prevalence and treatment. *Archives of General Psychiatry, 39,* 1407–1409.

Roberts, R. E., & Vernon, S. W. (1983). The center for epidemiologic studies depression scale: Its use in a community sample. *American Journal of Psychiatry, 140,* 41–46.

Robins, A. H. (1976). Are stroke patients more depressed than other disabled subjects? *Journal of Chronic Disease, 29,* 479–482.

Robins, E., & Guze, S. (1972). Classification of affective disorders: The primary-secondary, the endogenous-reactive, and the neurotic-psychotic concepts. In T. A. Williams, M. M. Katz & J. A. Shields (Eds.), *Recent advances in the psychobiology of the depressive illness* (pp. 283–293). Washington, D.C.: U.S. Government Printing Office.

Robins, L. N., Helzer, J. E., Croughan, J., & Ratcliff, K. S. (1981). National Institute of Mental Health Diagnostic Interview Schedule: Its history, characteristics, and validity. *Archives of General Psychiatry, 38,* 381–389.

Robins, L. N., Helzer, J. E., Weissman, M. M., Orvaschel, H., Gruenberg, E., Burke, J. D., & Regier, D. A. (1984). Lifetime prevalence of specific psychiatric disorders in three sites. *Archives of General Psychiatry, 41,* 949–958.

Roy, A. (1978). Vulnerability factors and depression in women. *British Journal of Psychiatry, 3,* 106–110.

Sayetta, R. B., & Johnson, D. P. (1980). *Basic data on depressive symptomatology: United States, 1974–1975: Data from the National Health Survey* (Series 11, No. 216., DHEW Pub. No. 80-1666). National Center for Health Statistics.

Schwab, J. J., McGinnis, N. H., & Warheit, G. J. (1973). Social psychiatric impairment: Racial comparisons. *American Journal of Psychiatry, 130,* 183–187.

Seiler, L. H. (1973). The 22-item scale used in field studies of mental illness: A question of method, a question of substance and a question of theory. *Journal of Health and Social Behavior, 14,* 252–264.

Selye, H. (1956). *Stress of life.* New York: McGraw-Hill.

Shrout, P. E., & Fleiss, J. L. (1981). Reliability and case detection. In J. K. Wing, & P. Bebbington (Eds.) What is a case: The problem of definition in psychiatric community surveys (pp. 117–128). London: Grant & McIntyre.

Sokolovsky, J., Cohen, C., Berger, D., & Geiger, J. M. (1978). Personal networks of ex-mental patients in a Manhattan sro hotel. *Human Organization, 37,* 5–10.

Spitzer, R. L., Endicott, J., & Robins, E. (1978). Research diagnostic criteria: Rationale and reliability. *Archives of General Psychiatry. 35*, 773–782.

Standman, E. (1978). Psychogenic needs in patients with affective disorders. *Acta Psychiatrica Scandinavia, 58*, 16–29.

Storey, P. B. (1967). Psychiatric sequelae of subarachnoid haemorrhage. *British Medical Journal, 3*, 261–266.

Susser, M. (1973). Causal thinking in the health sciences: Concepts and strategies of epidemiology. New York: Oxford University Press.

Tennant, C. (1983). Life events and psychological morbidity: The evidence from prospective studies. *Psychological Medicine, 13*, 483–486.

Thoits, P. A. (1982). Conceptual, methodological and theoretical problems in studying social support as a buffer against life stress. *Journal of Health and Social Behavior, 23*, 145–159.

Thompson, W. D., Orvaschel, H., Prusoff, B. A., & Kidd, K. K. (1982). An evaluation of the family history method for ascertaining psychiatric disorders. *Archives of General Psychiatry, 39*, 53–58.

Turner, R. J., & Noh, S. (1982). *Social support, life events and psychological distress: A three wave panel analysis.* Paper presented at the annual meeting of the American Sociological Association, San Francisco.

Underwood, B. J. (1957). *Psychological Research.* Englewood Cliffs, New Jersey: Prentice-Hall.

Vernon, S. W., & Roberts, R. E. (1981). Further observations on the problem of measuring nonspecific psychological distress and other dimensions of psychopathology. *Archives of General Psychiatry, 38*, 1239–1247.

Vernon, S. W., & Roberts, R. W. (1982). Prevalence of treated and untreated psychiatric disorders in three ethnic groups. *Social Science and Medicine, 16*, 1575–1582.

vonZerssen, D. (1982). Personality and affective disorder. In E. S. Paykel (Ed.), *Handbook of affective disorders.* New York: Guilford Press.

Walster, E., Berscheid, E., & Walster, G. W. (1973). New directions in equity research. *Journal of Personality and Social Psychology, 25*, 151–176.

Warheit, G. J., Holzer, C. E., & Arey, S. A. (1975). Race and mental illness: An epidemiologic update. *Journal of Health and Social Behavior, 16*, 243–256.

Weissman, M. M., Gershon, E. S., Kidd, K. K., Prusoff, B. A., Leckman, J. F., Dibble, E., Hamovit, J., Thompson, W. D., Pauls, D. L., & Guroff, J. J. (1984). Psychiatric disorders in the relatives of probands with affective disorders. *Archives of General Psychiatry, 41*, 13–21.

Weissman, M. M., & Klerman, G. L. (1977). Sex differences and the epidemiology of depression. *Archives of General Psychiatry, 34*, 98–111.

Weissman, M. M., & Myers, J. K. (1978). Rates and risks of depressive symptoms in a United States urban community. Acta Psychiatrica Scandinavia, 57, 219–231.

Weissman, M. M., Myers, J. K., & Thompson, W. D. (1981). Depression and its treatment in a United States urban community 1975–1976. *Archives of General Psychiatry, 38*, 417–421.

Wellman, B. (1981). Applying network analysis to the study of support. In B. H. Gottlieb (Ed.), *Social Networks and Social Support* (Vol. 4, pp. 171–200). Sage Studies in Community Mental Health. Beverly Hills, CA.: Sage Publications.

Wheaton, B. (1982). Uses and abuses of the Langner Index: A reexamination of findings on psychological and psychophysiological distress. In D. Mechanic (Ed.), *Symptoms, illness behavior, and help-seeking* (pp. 25–54). New York: Prodist.

Wheaton, B. (1983). Stress, personal coping resources, and psychiatric symptoms: An investigation of interactive models. *Journal of Health and Social Behaviors, 24*, 208–229.

Whybrow, P., & Palatore, A. (1973). Melancholia, a model in madness: A discussion of recent psychobiologic research into depressive illness. *International Journal of Psychiatry in Medicine, 4*, 351–378.

Williams, A. W., Ware, J. E., & Donald, C. A. (1981). A model of mental health, life events, and social supports applicable to general populations. *Journal of Health and Social Behavior, 22*, 324–336.

Winer, B. J. (1971). Statistical principles in experimental design (2nd ed.) New York: McGraw-Hill.

Wing, J. K., Cooper, J. E., & Sartorius, H. (1974). *The measurement and classification of psychiatric symptoms.* London: Cambridge University Press.

Winokur, G. (1972). Family history studies VIII. *Diseases of the Nervous System, 33*, 94–99.

Winokur, G. (1978). Mania and depression: Family studies and genetics in relation to treatment. In M. A. Lipton, A. SiMascio, K. F. Killan (Eds.), *Psychopharmacology: A generation of progress* (pp. 1213–1221). New York: Raven.

Winokur, G. (1979). Unipolar depression: Is it divisible into autonomous subtypes? *Archives of General Psychiatry, 24*, 135–155.

Winokur, G., Tsuang, M. T., & Crowe, R. R. (1982). The Iowa 500: Affective disorder in relatives of manic and depressed patients. *American Journal of Psychiatry, 139*, 209–212.

Wishnie, H. A., Hackett, T. P., & Cassem, N. H. (1971). Psychological hazards of convalescence following myocardial infarction. *Journal of American Medical Association, 215*, 1292–1296.

Wolff, H. G., Wolf, S. G., & Hare, L. L. (1950). *Life stress and bodily disease.* Baltimore: Williams and Wilkins.

Woodruff, R. A., Murphy, G. E., & Herjanic, M. (1967). The natural history of affective disorders—I: Symptoms of 72 patients at the time of index hospital admission. *Journal of Psychiatric Research, 5*, 255–263.

Wynn, A. (1967). Unwarranted emotional distress in men with ischaemic heart disease. *The Medical Journal of Australia and New Zealand, 2*, 847–851.

Zung, W. W. K. (1965). A self-rating depression scale. *Archives of General Psychiatry, 12*, 63–70.

II

TOWARD THE PREVENTION OF DEPRESSION: LIFE CYCLE PERSPECTIVES

Depression is not a static, time-bound condition. It is a process which is the combined result of influences experienced throughout a person's life. Its expression is greatly influenced by the developmental stage during which it occurs. Preventive interventions must take this variability into account. It is very likely that different approaches will be effective with different age groups.

At another level, preventive thinking naturally leads one to consider early interventions. Anyone working on preventive interventions with adults will soon find himself or herself speculating on whether interventions earlier in life, say, during high school, or even earlier, might have had powerful effects in reducing the probability of depression in later life.

For both of the above reasons, it seemed important to include in this volume contributions explicitly related to different stages in the life cycle. The authors in this section share with us theoretical concepts, empirical information, reviews of the literature, as well as specific research studies addressing depression at different ages.

Lynn Rehm extends his well-known contributions to the treatment of depression in adults to the realm of childhood. The self-control mechanisms which he has studied extensively must have developed throughout life. His present line of research addresses the types of self-control processes identifiable during the early school years, and examines their relationship to depression. The literature on child depression is reviewed by Ginsburg and Twentyman. Their chapter emphasizes the limitations of present research and theory as they apply to depression prevention efforts. It is clear from this chapter that prevention researchers must chart new territory if they hope to develop effective programs.

An interesting preventively-oriented project carried out in a high school serves as the source of theoretical and practical advice for future prevention researchers in the chapter by Klein and colleagues. It is this kind of creative attempt to carry out and study preventive interventions in a natural setting which will ultimately develop practical prevention programs. Klein and colleagues also highlight the need to consider the possibly deleterious effects of preventive interventions which require excessive self-control, especially in adolescents.

The role of exercise in the prevention of depression is covered by Wesley Sime. His work in alleviating symptoms of depression in a college population is used to suggest possible applications of physical exercise to the prevention of depression. Sime also reviews treatment studies of depression using exercise as one of the interventions.

The life cycle approach is perhaps most clearly brought to mind by the chapter on postpartum depression by Cynthia Telles. It is during the post-birth period that the emotional state of an adult has the strongest effects on the experiences of a new human being. Telles focuses primarily on depression in the mother. Nevertheless, it is reasonable to consider the possible effects that preventing depression in this population might have on their babies. Telles also addresses explicitly the need to take into account characteristics of special population subgroups, in this case, a group that differs socioeconomically and culturally from the mainstream, namely low-income Hispanic women.

Peter Lewinsohn, one of the pioneers in the behavioral treatment of depression, illustrates the way in which treatment approaches, especially those which are of an educational nature, can be applied to prevention. His work in developing a course that will be effective in the treatment of nonpsychotic, nonbipolar depression leads directly into preventive applications.

Unlike all of the other contributors to the book, Betty Tableman does her work outside of a university context. She is the Director of Prevention and Demonstration Projects in the State of Michigan Department of Mental Health. Her chapter, focused on adult women on public assistance, foreshadows the type of development that will be needed to make the knowledge gathered in academic settings available to the general public. The future of the prevention movement in mental health will ultimately be determined outside of academia. Tableman's work should remind others in the public sector that they do not have to wait for researchers to provide all the answers. It is at least as likely that practitioners in applied settings will provide leadership for this new field.

An intervention for the elderly is described by Steinmetz Breckenridge, Zeiss, and Thompson. Their careful analysis of the elements which are related to the greatest amount of impact of their intervention is a model for prevention researchers who are interested in studying the manner in which their intervention has its effect.

As a group, the eight chapters in this section provide a number of different approaches to consider as possible preventive interventions. At the same time, their focus on different populations and on different stages in the life cycle remind us that any approach will have to be carefully adapted to its intended audience.

4

Approaches to the Prevention
of Depression with Children:
A Self-Management Perspective

Lynn P. Rehm
University of Houston

INTRODUCTION

My purpose in this paper is to discuss the applicability of psychological concepts of self-control or self-management to depression in children as a means of preventing depression in adulthood. I plan to outline the nature of models of self-management, their applicability to depression and their advantages in developing preventive strategies in children. I will briefly describe our model of self-management and then summarize some research findings from a series of psychopathology studies of childhood depression. Based on these ideas and a small amount of data, I want to suggest some strategies for preventions of depression. Finally I want to suggest some directions for future research.

SELF–MANAGEMENT

Definition

There are probably as many definitions of self-management as there are theorists and researchers in the area, but the following definitions will serve the purpose of this paper. Self-management refers to those processes and strategies by which individuals organize and direct their behavior toward long range goals in the relative absence of, or in opposition to, immediate environmental controls. The goal of self-management is to maximize long range reinforcement. Models of self-management postulate processes descriptive of the manner in which control may be exerted with implications of individual differences. People vary in the nature, style, skillfulness, and effectiveness of their repertoire of self-control strategies. Self-management implies organization, direction, and planning of behavior. Prediction and evaluation of outcomes and estimations of value and of control are all involved. Self-control is attributed to persons when their goal directed behavior is not easily attributable to external agents. However, self-managed behavior may be *acquired* from experience with external environmental control, and external reinforcers may well be the goal toward which self-managed behavior is directed. Self-management behavior supplements or modulates response to external sources of control. The goals of self-managed behavior are delayed. Time-binding or choosing between immediate and delayed reinforcement is indicated with the implied goal of maximizing obtained reinforcement over time. Most models of self-management involve a feedback process whereby behavior is adjusted according to its effects or to changes in the environment.

Models of Self-Management

Many different models have been proposed which more or less correspond to this overall definition of self-management. Within a strict behavioral paradigm Skinner (1957) suggested a number of strategies whereby individuals manipulate their environment in order to influence their own future behavior. Bandura has contributed in several ways to research and theory in self-management, most recently, in his self-efficacy model (1977). Kanfer (1970; Kanfer & Karoly, 1972a, b) developed a three stage feedback-loop model and has recently proposed a more elaborate flow chart for modeling self-control behavior (Kanfer & Hagerman, 1981). Information processing models have been applied to problems of self-control by Carver and Scheier (1982). A cognitive self-instructional strategy for self-control in children and adults has been developed by Meichenbaum & Cameron (1974), and Eric Klinger (1982) has proposed a model involving the cognitive structuring of plans and concerns. Richard Lazarus' (1981) work on stress coping strategies and homeostatic feedback models (e.g., Schwartz, 1977) for biological self-regulation as applied to biofeedback might also be included. Each of these models has been applied in one way or another to the phenomena of depression. For the purpose of this paper, the Kanfer three stage model with some additional considerations will serve as an organizing framework.

Characteristics of Models
of Self-Management

Models of self-management have generally had sufficient breadth of applicability to bridge between areas of clinical interest and topics of interest in basic research in psychology. For example, studies of self-monitoring blend with and draw from basic areas in cognitive psychology such as selective attention and memory. Self-evaluation studies deal with some basic issues in social psychology such as social cognition and social comparison processes. Self-management overlaps with social skill research areas and with studies of interpersonal systems. The acquisition of self-management behavior is becoming an important area, and developmental theory has influenced thinking about self-management. Models of self-management also provide a bridge between treatment approaches for such diverse problems as depression, anxiety, and addiction.

There are a number of characteristics of models of self-control which make them particularly suited to application to depression. First, self-management models tend to posit multiple factors to account for self-managed behavior. These factors, processes, stages, or constructs are interrelated within the models. Depression is a complex and multifaceted phenomenon which may require a multiple factor model to account for its various component phenomena. A multifactor model may be able to address and differentiate the various forms and patterns which depression takes. A number of authorities have recently argued the desirability of multifactor models of depression to replace earlier single factor models (e.g., Craighead, 1980).

Self-managed behavior is behavior that has a long range goal. A delayed external reinforcement is worked toward despite immediate reinforcement for alternative behavior (e.g., resisting temptation or persisting in a difficult endeavor). The assumption is that this "time binding" ability is accomplished by internal manipulation of stimuli and consequences related to component behaviors. The behavior of depressed persons is characterized by deficiencies in behaviors aimed at long range goals. Depressed persons may ruminate about desired delayed goals, but behavior aimed toward these goals deteriorates first in depression while behavior under the control of immediate consequences is maintained. Depressed persons lack persistence and initiative and are often self-indulgent. These are patently self-management deficits.

Self-management models also deal with adjustment to change. For example, Kanfer argues that behavioral self-regulation is engaged primarily under conditions when the person perceives a change or deficiency in the outcome produced by current behavior (e.g., lack of success in social relationship). A major loss of a source of reinforcement (e.g., loss of job or of a loved one) involves reactive depressive behavior which diminishes as the person adjusts to the loss. Failure to readjust signifies a clinically significant depression. Self-management is concerned with effective and ineffective styles of coping with change. The models are active, process models as opposed to many more passive, static models of depressive deficits. As models or readjustment, self-management can be thought of as a way of thinking about the interaction between individual differences in coping styles and stress. Vulnerability to depression may exist in the form of maladaptive coping styles whereas the full blown disorder is not apparent until an environmental stressor necessitates coping behavior. Predictions of susceptibility to depression should be derivable from self-management models.

A Self-Management Model of Depression

A number of models have been proposed for applying self-management concepts to the phenomena of depression. For the purposes of this paper, Rehm's (1977) self-control model of depression will be employed as an organizing framework for discussion. This model is based on an adaptation of Kanfer's (1970) three stage model. According to Kanfer's model, when individuals perceive that some form of behavior is not functioning or will not be able to function to achieve desired outcomes, a self-monitoring, self-evaluation, self-reinforcement feedback sequence is engaged. Self-monitoring involves observation of one's own performance including its antecedents, consequences and concomitants. Information gathered regarding performance is then compared to an internal standard. Evaluative success-failure decisions are made on the basis of this comparison. In a 1977 paper, I amended this model by adding in a self-attribution process which acts as a modifier on self-evaluation (Rehm, 1977). That is, in order to make an evaluative judgement one must attribute the performance to internal causes such as skill or effort. Actions perceived as externally caused are personally neither praiseworthy nor blame-worthy. Finally, in Kanfer's model self-evaluation is the cue for self-administered reward or punishment. These rewards or punishments may be covert or overt and are assumed to influence behavior in the same manner that externally administered contingent reinforcement influences behavior. Self-administered reinforcement supplements external reinforcement in guiding behavior toward long range external goals. Individuals vary in their self-management skills or style. Good self-management means that the person organizes, initiates, and maintains behavior aimed at desired long term goals. Poor self-management would imply lack of organization of goals and standards, control by immediate external factors and lack of persistence. In the original model, I postulated six factors within the model which typified a depressive self-management style. These factors were: self-monitoring characterized by (1) selective attention to negative events, and (2) selective attention to immediate as opposed to delayed consequences of events; self-evaluation characterized by (3) stringent self-evaluative standards; self-attribution characterized by (4) a negative attributional style; and self-reinforcement characterized by (5) insufficient contingent self-reward, and (6) excessive self-punishment. Each of these factors is reflected in depressive behavior (e.g., pessimism, low self-esteem, guilt) and the aggregate results in a low rate of behavior, lack of initiation of behavior, and lack of persistence.

APPLICATIONS TO CHILDREN

My intent is to discuss the possibilities of intervening in self-management with children to prevent depression in adulthood. I do so well aware that a number of controversial assumptions are implied. Such an approach assumes that depression or a psychological prodrome of depression can be identified in children. It assumes that there may be some form of continuity in psychological vulnerability to depression across stages of development from childhood to adulthood. In addition, it assumes that modifying a psychological risk factor at one stage of development will reduce susceptibility to depression at a later stage.

A number of risk factors for depression have been identified or could be postulated in considering depression proneness in children. Familial depression has been identified as a risk factor. Parental depression with particular emphasis on maternal depression has also been noted. In considering depression in children maternal depression may be a risk factor as a concurrent influence, as a prior influence at a vulnerable stage of development, or as merely a strong indicator of genetic predisposition. The mode of transmission might be genetic, modeling, deficient stimulation or contingent reinforcement of depressive behavior. It should be noted that other forms of parental psychopathology have also been linked to depression. Parental loss has also been linked to later adult depression.

Adult depression may be associated with various factors identifiable in the childhood of the patient. Childhood depression would appear to be a prime candidate as a factor but childhood psychopathology in general may also place the individual at risk for depression. Specificity of risk factors for a variety of adult disorders. Finally, it may be possible to identify psychological factors in the child which may or may not be associated with depression in the child, yet which may constitute vulnerability factors for depression later in adulthood. Self-management deficits are a possible set of candidates for this form of risk factor.

RESEARCH ON DEPRESSION
IN CHILDREN

Rationale

I would now like to shift my focus to some of the results of our studies of childhood depression. These data will then be related back to assumptions about children at risk for adult depression.

Let me say from the outset that our research has been directed at studying depressive psychopathology in children. It has not attempted to intervene in childhood depression nor to prevent later depression. It is seen as basic research on which intervention or prevention programs might be constructed.

The overall strategy of our program involves a number of elements. First, we essentially bypassed the controversy about the existence of depression in children by simply adopting current "state-of-the-art" methods of identifying cases and then examined the correlates of this classification. Mindful of the assessment issues involved, we have been, however, very interested in the reliability of our assessment methods. Second, our primary interests were in the correlates of depression. We have been interested in both concomitant symptoms of psychopathology and in those self-management factors which have been related to depression in adulthood. Current theoretical models of depression postulate a number of social-cognitive factors as central to depression (e.g., attributional style, cognitive distortion, self-control deficits). Research with adults has demonstrated their association with depressed behavior. We have used the self-control model of depression as a heuristic for organizing and studying these factors as they related to depression in children. Third, we have taken a developmental perspective in our approach to depressive phenomena in children. We assume that although there may be some continuity in psychological risk factors across childhood, nevertheless, it is important to take into account the child's stage of psychological development and organization, and also the environmental challenges that children face at different stages of development. Fourth, we have been interested in assessing parental factors and their relationship to depression in children. Specifically, we have been interested in parental depression and parental self-management as they relate to child depression and child self-management.

These studies have been conducted as part of a program of research developed by me, Nadine Kaslow, and Alex Siegel (a developmental psychologist) in cooperation with Stephen Pollack (a child psychologist). Most of these studies have been funded by the Hogg Foundation in Texas. Our research group has included a number of graduate students who conducted specific studies in the general program. I will review data collected by Harriet Schultz and Nadine Kaslow.

Specific studies assessed (1) normal children in first, fourth and eight grades (Kaslow, 1981), (2) depressed and non-depressed children in a clinic and their mothers (Schultz, 1981), and (3) depressed and non-depressed clinic children, a sample of normal children, and both parents of each child (Kaslow, 1983).

Table 1 Intercorrelations among depression measures (Schultz, 1981)

Variable	CHILD			MOTHER	
	BID–CHILD	BID–MOTHER	DSM–III	BECK	SADS
CDI	.65	.30	.41	.01	.14
	p = .001	p = .009	p = 001	NS	NS
BID–CHILD		.38	.56	.18	.24
		p = .001	p = .001	NS	p = .03
BID–MOTHER			.53	.42	.23
			p = .001	p = .001	p = .04
DSM–III				.17	.24
				NS	p = .03
BECK–MOTHER					.65
					p = .001

Results of the Studies

Diagnostic Reliability

Our studies have used several instruments for assessing depression. These include the Children's Depression Inventory (CDI; Kovacs & Beck, 1977), a self report instrument; the Bellevue Index of Depression (BID; Petti, 1978), a structured clinical interview with an adult informant; and the KIDDIE–SADS (Puig-Antich & Chambers, 1978), a structured clinical interview for child or adult informant. While interrater reliability has been fairly good for the same interview and test-retest reliability for the CDI is adequate, the consensual reliabilities among instruments, and agreements among informants have been considerably lower than those found with adults. An example of this can be seen in Table 1. Intercorrelations among depression measures were calculated for a sample of 62 children and their mothers in a child guidance clinic (Schultz, 1981). In this sample, the CDI correlated fairly well with the Bellevue interview given to the child but considerable disparity occurs when data are derived from two different informants (e.g., child and mother Bellevues). Interestingly, parental interviews concerning the child are influenced by parents' level of depression.

In our most recent study (Kaslow, 1983), three independent KIDDIE–SADS interviews were conducted and then cases were identified by a conferenced protocol agreed on by the interviewers. Again, informant (child, mother or father) was a major source of variance. Reliable assessment and identification of cases remains a major impediment to high quality research on depression in children.

Correlates of Depression

Many additional symptoms correlate with depression in normal and clinic children. These include a variety of age appropriate manifestation of psychopathology and child perceptions of family maladjustment (Kaslow, 1981; 1983; Schultz, 1981). We began by exploring the relationship of depression to so-called "masking symptoms" but have recently developed the concern that measures of depression may merely measure severity of psychopathology, i.e., children with many complaints are identified as depressed but are high on virtually any symptom scale.

Again research is hampered by a lack of discriminant validity in the assessment instruments.

With regard to social-cognitive (self-management) factors as correlates of depression the results are less strong and less consistent. This may be due in part to the fact that these measures are much more experimental. For instance, Kaslow (1981) assessed a number of specific dimensions of self-control in the context of behavioral task (e.g., figure copying) with a sample of 108 normal children drawn from first, fourth and eighth grades. Subjects respond to questions about the task before and after attempting it. Overall, Table 2 illustrates that there is moderate evidence that depressed children expect to do less well, set more stringent standards (especially for punishment), make depressive attributions about the causes of their behavior, evaluate their performance as poorer, use more self-punishment and recall their performance as poorer.

There were also very clear differences between clinic and normal children. These findings are encouraging to the strategy of considering self-management factors as a link between child and adult depression. However, many additional questions remain to be answered.

Developmental Trends

Our studies have found a fairly consistent pattern of depressive symptomatology across the age range studied. Minor developmental trends were found with regard to specific symptoms. For example, more depressed first graders were more likely to describe themselves as "bad," whereas, more depressed eighth graders were more likely to complain of poor relationships with parents. Assessments aimed more specifically at important developmental themes might provide evidence of situational factors which might be important considerations for intervention at different age levels.

Parental Influences

In our studies maternal depression has been clearly elevated much more than paternal depression and maternal depression correlates more with child's depression. However, depression in mothers does not strongly differentiate between depressed and non-depressed clinic children (see Table 3; Schultz, 1981). Many nondepressed clinical children also have depressed mothers. Our data hint that the relationship may be stronger if only biological mothers are considered. Correlations between parental and child self-management behaviors were positive though generally low.

INTERVENTION

Self-management (self-control) factors have been the targets of successful interventions for depression with adults in our research (Fuchs & Rehm, 1977; Rehm, Fuchs, Roth, Kornblith, & Romano, 1979; Rehm, Kornblith, O'Hara, Lamparski, & Romano, 1981; Kornblith, Rehm, O'Hara, & Lamparski, 1983). Follow-up of these studies suggests that future episodes of depression are reduced in frequency and intensity (Romano & Rehm, 1979). Our program has been administered in a group format of 10 weekly $1\frac{1}{2}$ hour sessions. As such, it is relatively low cost. The didactic format and emphasis on understandable behaviors and habits also makes the program relatively acceptable to depressed participants. Lewinsohn and his

Table 2 Social cognitive questionnaire data (Kaslow, 1981)

Item	Source	MSE	F	P
1. No. expected correct	Depression	62.839	9.91	.003*
	Grade	24.766	3.58	.03*
2. Amount of time expected	Depression	8.048	16.16	.001**
3. Expected level of performance	Depression	6.168	12.33	.001**
4. Std. setting for good score	Grade	694.112	3.4	.04
5. Std. setting for poor score	Depression	5373.826	6.99	.01*
6. Mother's Std. for good score	—	—	—	—
7. Mother's Std. for bad score	Depression	6656.508	10.18	.002*
8. Reward	—	—	—	—
9. Punishment	Sex X Dep.	32.585	4.45	.04*
10. Give/Take	Depression	1.587	11.28	.001**
	Sex	.772	5.5	.02*
11. Evaluation of performance	Depression	17.037	14.35	.001**
	Sex X Grade		3.45	.04*
12. Evaluation of amt. of time	Depression	9.801	20.31	.001**
13. Number correct	Depression	117.450	13.59	.001**
14. Assessment of performance compared	Depression	8.940	10.48	.002*

$p < .05*$
$p < .001**$

colleagues have similarly demonstrated the feasibility of a psychoeducational approach with groups of adults.

To date, only one study has been reported that employed a full self-control therapy program targeting depression in children. Stark, Kaslow and Reynolds (1985) reported on a carefully done evaluation of an adaptation of the self-control program for elementary school children. Twenty-nine moderately depressed children were seen in either self-control therapy, or a nonspecific therapy control condition or they were placed on a waiting list. The problem of reliable assessment was handled by having two separate pretherapy assessments and by the use of multiple assessment methods including two self-report scales, a clinical interview

Table 3 Relationship between mother SADS and child's DSM–III diagnosis (Schultz, 1981)

Child's DSM–III	SADS		
	Depressed	Nondepressed	Total
Depressed	14	14	28
Nondepressed	9	25	34
Total	23	39	62

rating and independent ratings by parent and teacher. Therapy consisted of 12 small group sessions over the course of a five week period. Therapists followed a structured manual and helped the children to acquire self-control skills with a variety of activities and cartoon examples. Results clearly indicated that the self-control program was helpful in ameliorating depression and that the effect was not due to simply participating in a group nor the passage of time. The effect was maintained at an eight week follow-up. While the intent of the study was clinical intervention not long-term prevention but the strength of these short-term effects suggests the possibility that the self-control skills acquired by these children might continue to serve them in later life in preventing depression.

Other than this study, the current literature on intervention with depressed children is rather sparse, consisting primarily of scattered case studies (Kaslow & Rehm, 1983). Self-control training is quite wide-spread in child therapy and the targets of training have frequently been aspects of depression e.g., social withdrawal, low self-esteem, self-depreciation.

In general, self-control behavior in children has become a rapidly expanding focus of work with children as exemplified by recent reviews (Craighead, Wilcoxin-Craighead, & Mayers, 1978; Karoly, 1977; Little & Kendall, 1977; Meichenbaum, 1977; Meichenbaum & Asarnow, 1977; Pressley, 1979). Although self-control therapy has not specifically been used with depressed children, there are a number of studies which demonstrate the effectiveness of various self-control strategies with children (Ballard & Glynn, 1975; Bolstad & Johnson, 1972; Broden, Hall & Mitts, 1971; Glynn & Thomas, 1974; Gottman, & McFall, 1972; Sagotsky, Patterson & Lepper, 1978; Thomas, 1976). In order to teach children to control their own behavior, it is first necessary to train them to monitor accurately their behavior and cognitions. There are a number of case reports and studies on self-monitoring with children (e.g., Broden, Hall & Mitts, 1971; Gottman & McFall, 1972; Sagotsky, Patterson & Lepper, 1978). These studies demonstrate that procedures designed to induce a child to self-monitor have also led to appreciable changes in the frequency of the target behavior. Self-evaluation involves a comparison between the individual's own performance and the performance criterion. Spates and Kanfer (1977) found that children trained in criterion setting improved significantly more than those trained in self-monitoring or control subjects who received no training. The addition of self-monitoring and self-reinforcement to criterion setting did not enhance treatment effects. In a complete self-management program, individuals need to set a target behavior, monitor the behavior, evaluate the progress made, and then reinforce this progress. Self-reinforcement has been found to be an effective procedure with children (e.g., Bolstad & Johnson, 1972).

Several other forms of therapy with children are related to self-management and have been used successfully with depressive target behaviors. For example, Dweck and her colleagues have conducted a research program relating deficits in problem-solving, helplessness and attributions (Diener & Dweck, 1978; 1979; Dweck, 1975; 1977; Dweck & Bush, 1976; Dweck, Davidson, Nelson & Enna, 1978; Dweck, Goetz & Strauss, 1978; Dweck & Repucci, 1973). Dweck & Repucci (1973) found that children who persisted in the face of failure attributed helplessness to a lack of effort, whereas children whose performance deteriorated after failure attributed this to a lack of ability. Diener and Dweck (1978) found that helpless children attributed their failure to lack of ability, their performance deteriorated after failure, and they demonstrated negative affect about the task. Diener and Dweck (1979) also found that in comparison to mastery-oriented children, helpless children were less likely to attribute success to ability, expected to do poorly in the future, and believed that other children would do better than they had done. Dweck (1975) gave children who had extreme reactions to failure one of two training procedures. One group was given success experiences only, and the second group was given attribution retraining which taught the children to take responsibility for their failure and to attribute it to lack of effort. Thus, they were taught to make an internal-unstable-specific attribution for failure. Results from this study revealed that after the training was complete, the performance of the children in the success only condition continued to deteriorate when they were confronted with failure. However, the children in the attribution retraining group maintained or improved their performance.

Social skill procedures have been used in a few cases of depression in children (Calpin & Cincirpini, 1978; Calpin & Kornblith, 1977; Matson, Esvelt-Dawson, Andrasik, Ollendick, Petti, & Hersen, 1980; Petti, Bornstein, Delamater, & Connors, 1980). Spivak, Platt and Shure (1976) have described a cognitive behavioral problem-solving program with children which has been used to increase social interaction among withdrawn children. These authors stress the importance of different skill programs for children at different levels of development.

Another strategy for improving overall self-control skills in children is self-instruction training (Meichenbaum, 1977). It is currently receiving a great deal of attention as a training method in the child cognitive-behavior therapy literature. Verbal self-regulation (self-instruction training) is one type of self-control strategy in that the verbalizations are intended to increase the probability of the corresponding overt behavior. Cole and Kazdin (1980) describe self-instructional training as a multifaceted intervention technique which is used to teach children to monitor their progress, to compare what they are doing to what they should be doing, and to self-reinforce contingently. Self-verbalizations are developed through modeling, overt and covert rehearsal, prompts, feedback and reinforcement. Self-instruction training has been used with children demonstrating a variety of behavior problems including impulsivity, hyperactivity, delinquency, social withdrawal (an aspect of depression) and learning disabilities.

All of these programs are consistent with a general self-management conception of problems in children. They all aim at modifying proximal skill targets on the assumption that these will help the child deal with a variety of life problems. Skill for dealing with classes of problems are taught. Many of these appear to be skills and problems closely related to depression. Programs teaching children these skills in a psychoeducational format in clinics or schools could be effective, preventative, cost efficient and popular.

CONCLUSION

This paper is premised on the idea that intervening with depressed children may be a feasible way to prevent depression in these same individuals as adults. This strategy is based on a number of assumptions and inductive leaps which may not be justified. A number of empirical questions need to be answered before this approach can be solidly justified.

First, the field needs better epidemiological data on the incidence, prevalence and course of depression in children. There continue to be controversies over the nature and significance of depression in children. Little progress can be made on settling these issues and developing a data base until reliable and valid assessment techniques can be developed. Assessment methodology is intimately tied to progress in this area.

Second, a major issue affecting any prevention intervention strategy is the specificity or lack of specificity of childhood depression. Does depression in childhood increase the individual's risk for depression in adulthood? Does childhood depression increase the individual's risk for a variety of forms of psychopathology in adulthood or does any childhood psychopathology increase the risk for depression in adulthood? Data on the natural course of depressive psychopathology are necessary before strategies for assessing the success of preventive intervention can be planned.

This paper has argued that intervening with depression in children can best be accomplished by targeting basic self-control behaviors which theoretically underly depressive behavior. Teaching self-control skills may represent an intervention strategy with applicability beyond depression. To the extent that improving self-control provides the individual with skills for coping with stress, a sense of competence or efficacy may develop which would aid in resistance to many forms of psychopathology.

Much of the research on self-control training with children has focused on applications to academic tasks. Children monitor their work, compare it to a self-evaluative standard and self-administer reward for work accomplished. Dweck's (e.g., 1975) self-attribution training with children was also done in the context of academic tasks. It would seem that the basic concepts of positive self-control skills could be taught to all school children with relative ease and economy. Extensions of the basic concepts specifically relevant to depression or other forms of psychopathology might be added for high risk groups. That is, interpersonal problem solving and self-control strategies for coping with loss or lack of reinforcement might require special training. Self-control or self-management training in elementary schools could well be a prevention strategy which would be credible and acceptable as well as being effective and inexpensive.

REFERENCES

Ballard, K. D., & Glynn, T. (1975). Behavioral self-management in story writing with elementary school children. *Journal of Applied Behavior Analysis, 8,* 387–398.

Bandura, A. (1977). Self-efficacy: Toward a unifying theory of behavior change. *Psychological Review, 84,* 191–215.

Bolstad, O. D., & Johnson, S. M. (1972). Self-regulation in the modification of disruptive classroom behavior. *Journal of Applied Behavior Analysis, 5,* 443–454.

Broden, M., Hall, R. V., & Mitts, B. (1971). The effect of self-recording on the classroom behavior of two eight-grade students. *Journal of Applied Behavior Analysis, 4,* 191–199.

Calpin, J. P., & Cincirpini, P. M. (1978, May). *A multiple baseline analysis of social skills training in children.* Paper presented at Midwestern Association for Behavior Analysis, Chicago.

Calpin, J. P., & Kornblith, S. J. (1977). *Training of aggressive children in conflict resolution skills.* Paper presented at the meeting of the Association for the Advancement of Behavior Therapy, Chicago.

Carver, C. S., & Scheier, M. F. (1982). An information processing perspective on self-management. In P. Karoly & F. H. Kanfer (Eds.), *Self management and behavior change: From theory to practice.* New York: Pergamon.

Cole, P. M., & Kazdin, A. E. (1980). Critical issues in self-instruction training with children. *Child Behavior Therapy, 2,* 1–21.

Craighead, W. E. (1980). Away from a unitary model of depression. *Behavior Therapy, 11,* 122–128.

Craighead, W. E., Wilcoxin-Craighead, L. W., & Meyers, A. W. (1978). New directions in behavior modification with children. In M. Hersen, R. M. Eisler, & P. M. Miller (Eds.), *Progress in behavior modification* (Vol. 6). New York: Academic Press.

Diener, C. I., & Dweck, C. S. (1978). An analysis of learned helplessness: Continuous changes in performance, strategy, and achievement cognitions allowing failure. *Journal of Personality and Social Psychology, 36,* 451–462.

Diener, C. I., & Dweck, C. S. (1979). *An analysis of learned helplessness: (II) The processing of success.* Unpublished manuscript, University of Illinois.

Dweck, C. S. (1976). The role of expectations and attributions in the alleviation of learned helplessness. *Journal of Personality and Social Psychology, 31,* 674–685.

Dweck, C. S. (1977). Learned helplessness and negative evaluation. In E. R. Keisler (Ed.), *The educator: Evaluation and motivation, 14,* (pp. 44–49).

Dweck, C. S., & Bush, E. S. (1976). Sex differences in learned helplessness: Differential debilitation with peer and adult evaluators. *Developmental Psychology, 12,* 147–156.

Dweck, C. S., Davidson, W., Nelson, S., & Enna, B. (1978). Sex differences in learned helplessness: II. The contingencies of evaluative feedback in the classroom and III. An experimental analysis. *Developmental Psychology, 14,* 268–276.

Dweck, C. S., Goetz, T. E., & Strauss, N. (1978). *Sex differences in learned helplessness: (IV) An experimental and naturalistic study of failure generalization and its mediators.* Unpublished manuscript, University of Illinois.

Dweck, C. S., & Repucci, N. D. (1973). Learned helplessness and reinforcement responsibility in children. *Journal of Personality and Social Psychology, 25,* 109–116.

Fuchs, C. S., & Rehm, L. P. (1977). A self-control behavior therapy program for depression. *Journal of Consulting and Clinical Psychology, 45,* 206–215.

Glynn, E. L., & Thomas, J. D. (1974). Effect of cueing on self-control of classroom behavior. *Journal of Applied Behavior Analysis, 7,* 199–306.

Gottman, J. M., & McFall, R. M. (1972). Self-monitoring effects in a program for potential high school dropouts: A time series analysis. *Journal of Consulting and Clinical Psychology, 39,* 273–281.

Kanfer, F. H. (1970). Self-monitoring: Methodological limitations and clinical applications. *Journal of Consulting and Clinical Psychology, 35,* 148–152.

Kanfer, F. H., & Hagerman, S. (1981). The role of self-regulation. In L. P. Rehm (Ed.), *Behavior therapy for depression: Present status and future directions.* New York: Academic Press.

Kanfer, F. H., & Karoly, P. (1972a). A behavioristic excursion into the lion's den. *Behavior Therapy, 2,* 398–416.

Kanfer, F. H., & Karoly, P. (1972b). Self-regulation and its clinical application: Some additional conceptualizations. In R. C. Johnson, P. R. Dokecki, & O. H. Mowrer, *Socialization: Development of character and conscience* (pp. 428–437). New York: Holt, Rinehart & Winston.

Karoly, P. (1977). Behavioral self-management in children: Concepts, methods, issues, and directions. In M. Hersen, R. Eisler, & P. Miller (Eds.), *Progress in behavior modification,* Vol. 5, New York: Academic Press.

Kaslow, N. J. (1981 August). Social and cognitive correlates of depression in children from a developmental perspective. In L. P. Rehm (Chair), *Empirical studies in childhood depression.* Symposium presented at the annual meeting of the American Psychological Association, Los Angeles.

Kaslow, N. J. (August, 1983). *Depression in children and their parents.* Unpublished doctoral dissertation, University of Houston.

Kaslow, N. J., & Rehm, L. P. (1983). Childhood depression. In R. J. Morris and T. R. Kratochwill, *The practice of child therapy: A textbook of methods.* (pp. 27–52). New York: Pergamon Press.

Klinger, E. (1982). On the self-management of mood, affect and attention. In P. Karoly, & F. H. Kanfer (Eds.), *Self-management and behavior change: From theory to practice.* New York: Pergamon.

Kornblith, S. J., Rehm, L. P., O'Hara, M. W., & Lamparski, D. M. (1983). The contribution of self-reinforcement training and behavioral assignments to the efficacy of self-control therapy for depression. *Cognitive Therapy and Research, 7,* 499–527.

Kovacs, M., & Beck, A. T. (1977). An empirical-clinical approach toward a definition of childhood depression. In J. G. Schulterbrandt & A. Raskin (Eds.), *Depression in childhood: Diagnosis, treatment and conceptual models.* New York: Raven Press.

Lazarus, R. S. (1981). The stress and coping paradigm. In C. Eisdorfer, D. Cohen, A. Kleinman, & P. Maxim (Eds.), *Models for clinical psychopathology.* New York: Spectrum.

Little, V.L., & Kendall, P. C. (1979). Cognitive-behavioral interventions with delinquents: Problem solving, role-taking, and self-control. In P. C. Kendall & S. D. Hollon (Eds.), *Cognitive-behavioral interventions: Theory, research, and procedures.* New York: Academic Press.

Matson, J. L., Esvelt-Dawson, K., Andrasik, F., Ollendick, T. H., Petti, T. A., & Hersen, M. (1980). Observation and generalization effects of social skills training with emotionally disturbed children. *Behavior Therapy, 11,* 522–531.

Meichenbaum, D. (1977). *Cognitive behavior modification.* New York, Plenum.

Meichenbaum, D., & Asarnow, J. (1977). *Cognitive-behavioral interventions: Theory, research and procedures.* New York: Academic Press.

Meichenbaum, D., & Cameron, R. (1974). The clinical potential of modifying what clients say to themselves. In M. J. Mahoney & C. E. Thoresen, *Self-control: Power to the person* (pp. 263–290). Monterey, California: Brooks/Cole.

Petti, T. A. (1978). Depression in hospitalized child psychiatry patients: Approaches to measuring depression. *Journal of the American Academy of Child Psychiatry, 17,* 49–59.

Petti, T. A., Bornstein, M., Delamater, A., & Conners, C. K. (1980). Evaluation and multimodal treatment of a depressed pre-pubertal girl. *Journal of the American Academy of Child Psychiatry, 19,* 690–702.

Pressley, M. (1979). Increasing children's self-control through cognitive interventions. *Review of Educational Research, 49,* 319–370.

Puig-Antich, J., & Chambers, W. (1978). *Schedule for affective disorders and schizophrenia for school-age children (6–16 years)—Kiddie–SADS.* New York: New York State Psychiatric Institute.

Rehm, L. P. (1977). A self-control model of depression. *Behavior Therapy, 8,* 787–804.

Rehm, L. P., Fuchs, C. Z., Roth, D. M., Kornblith, S. J., & Romano, J. M. (1979). A comparison of self-control and assertion skills treatment of depression. *Behavior Therapy, 10,* 429–442.

Rehm, L. P., Kornblith, S. J., O'Hara, M. W., Lamparski, D. M., Romano, J. M., & Volkin, J. (1981). An evaluation of major components in a self-control behavior therapy program for depression. *Behavior Modification 5,* 459–489.

Romano, J. M., & Rehm, L. P. (1979, April). Self-control treatment of depression: One-year follow-up. In A. T. Beck (Chair), *Factors affecting the outcome and maintenance of cognitive therapy.* Symposium presented at the meeting of the Eastern Psychological Association, Philadelphia.

Sagotsky, G., Patterson, C. J., & Lepper, M. R. (1978). Training children's self-control: A field experiment in self-monitoring and goal-setting in the classroom. *Journal of Experimental Child Psychology, 25,* 242–253.

Schultz, H. T. (1981, August). Correlates of depression in a clinical sample of children and their mothers. In L. P. Rehm (Chair), *Empirical studies of childhood depression.* Paper presented at the American Psychological Association, Los Angeles.

Schwartz, G. E. (1977). Psychosomatic disorders and biofeedback. In J. D. Maser & M. E. P. Seligman (Eds.), *Psychopathology: Experimental models* (pp. 270–307). San Francisco: Freeman and Company.

Skinner, B. F. (1957). *Verbal Behavior.* New York: Appleton-Century Crofts.

Spates, C. R., & Kanfer, F. H. (1977). Self-monitoring, self-evaluation, and self-reinforcement in children's learning: A test of multistage self-regulation model. *Behavior Therapy, 8,* 9–16.

Spivak, G., Platt, J. J., & Shure, M. B. (1976). *The problem solving approach to adjustment.* San Francisco: Jossey-Bass.

Stark, K. D., Kaslow, N. J., & Reynolds, W. M. (1985, March). *A comparison of the relative efficacy of self-control and nonspecific therapies for the treatment of childhood depression.* Paper presented at the National Conference on Clinical Applications of Cognitive Behavior Therapy, Honolulu.

Thomas, J. D. (1976). Accuracy of self-assessment of on-task behavior by elementary school children. *Journal of Applied Behavior Analysis, 9,* 209–210.

5

Prevention of Childhood Depression

Sheila D. Ginsburg
University of Rochester

Craig T. Twentyman
University of Hawaii

INTRODUCTION

If treatment of childhood depression is a research area that is considered to be in an early stage of development, then preventive programs might be characterized as being in a late gestational period. Thus, in the preparation of this paper, we had little experimental work to guide us. However, a considerable amount of experimental and theoretical work now exists on the assessment of childhood depression as well as prevention in mental health. We drew heavily on these areas in our conceptualizations.

This paper examines a number of questions relating to childhood depression. Discussion centers on theoretical questions concerning the existence and manifestation of this disorder. Methodological issues such as those relating to the assessment of children at various age levels are examined. Finally, prevention models are presented and their applicability to childhood depression is discussed.

DEFINITIONAL ISSUES

Chapters devoted to examining prevention of a childhood disorder rarely raise the question of the existence of that disorder. Ordinarily, questions may be formulated about the incidence rate for a particular *subtype* of the disorder or whether a given subtype exists. However, in the area of childhood depression, discussions of the existence of the syndrome itself dominate the literature. Prevention and treatment issues have been postponed by the necessity of the more pressing and complex task of identifying developmental and psychopathological phenomena. The efforts of researchers and theoreticians during the past twenty years have yielded considerable progress. In this review of the literature, Cantwell (1982) articulates four distinct positions on the existence and manifestation of the disorder.

Historically, the reason for questioning the existence of depression in children comes from the work of the early psychodynamically oriented theorists who argued that limitations posed by the child's psychosexual development make it impossible for children to experience depression. In a review of the early literature, Rie (1966) suggested that children do not have adequate superego development to experience the internalization of feelings that is theorized to be a prerequisite for depression. Within this conceptualization, authors hypothesized that children, restricted by their limited capacities for visualizing and anticipating events in the future, are unable to experience profound hopelessness, which is often assumed to be a major component of depression. In the normal course of development the requisite cognitive structures implied by these capacities unfold during adolescence, thus disqualifying children of all ages from receiving a diagnosis of depression.

The second major position is articulated by proponents of the concepts of "masked depression" or "depressive equivalents" (Glaser, 1948; Cytryn & McKnew, 1974). They suggested that depression exists in children but differs in appearance from the adult syndrome. While this position has been widely criticized on a number of fundamental issues, it appears that at least some supporters of this position have been particularly sensitive to the possible effects and limitations imposed by developmental phenomena on the expression of depressive symptomatology. The assumption, however, that the school age child's enuresis or conduct disorder is related to an underlying depression has been confusing to many. Moreover, this theoretical position does not seem to allow for the identification of symptoms that are unique to childhood depression. For example, it is not clear how children suffering from masked depression could be differentiated from those merely suffering from a similar set of dysfunctional behaviors. Also, no clear theoretical rationale is presented for how such a diverse set of symptomatic behaviors as have been associated with masked depression are related to the underlying depressive state.

The third and fourth positions summarized in Cantwell's (1982) review reflect the emphasis in the more recent literature on the similarities in the child and adult depressive syndromes. While the third position, first clearly articulated by Kovacs and Beck (1977) posits the existence of associated features of depression that are unique to children, the fourth position suggests that clinical depression appears as an identical disorder in adults and children (Puig-Antich, Blau, Marx, Greenhill, & Chambers, 1978; Puig-Antich & Gittelman, 1982).

Kovacs and Beck (1977) surveyed symptom lists reported in studies on childhood depression and found they corresponded fairly closely to those identified in Beck's (1967) categories for depressed adults: (1) affective changes; (2) cognitive changes; (3) motivational changes; and (4) vegetative and psychomotor disturbances. Thus, their position is that similarities in the manifestations of child and adult depression vastly outweigh differences. Careful assessment reveals that symptoms others described as "masking" an underlying depression may be analogous to those reported by adults who are depressed or may represent other existing disorders in children.

A pilot study conducted by Puig-Antich, Blau, Marx, Greenhill, and Chambers (1978) led to their hypothesis that the depressive disorder in children and adults represents an identical illness. These investigators applied the Research Diagnostic Criteria (Spitzer, Endicott, & Robins, 1978) for major depressive disorder in adults and found they were appropriate for prepubertal children. In addition to the clinical similarity to adult depressives found among these 13 children, findings from this study suggested that depressed children and adults responded similarly to the drug imipramine and that the family histories of these children yielded some history of psychiatric disorder. This study highlights the importance of diagnostic criteria in delineating pathology and suggests that similarly applied criteria yield similar clinical pictures and illness patterns for depression in children and adults.

Positions emphasizing the similarity of adult and child depressive symptoms continue to receive empirical and theoretical support. Of particular interest is the work by Kazdin, French, Unis, Esveldt-Dawson, and Sherick (1983) who developed the Hopelessness Scale for Children. By adapting the items on Beck's (1974) Hopelessness Scale for Adults, these authors created a 17-item scale validated on children between the ages of 8 and 13. As predicted, they found hopelessness correlated positively with severity of depression and negatively with self-esteem. Their results indicate that hopelessness, which is a central feature of adult depression, is also a meaningful construct for children, at least in this relatively restricted age range. Their findings address theoretical objections cited earlier concerning children's hypothesized difficulties experiencing hopelessness. This study directly evaluates a theoretical position, and as such is an example of the type of research needed to further clarify definitional issues in childhood depression.

The most far-reaching statement regarding the status and definition of childhood depression is reflected in the DSM III of the American Psychiatric Association (1980). Although the inclusion of such a category does not argue for or against the existence of depression, the widespread application of adult diagnostic criteria for affective disorders to children and adolescents suggests that the view that similarities in adult and childhood depression exist has found wide contemporary support on a practical basis.

DEVELOPMENTAL ASPECTS
OF CHILDHOOD DEPRESSION

In developing preventive and treatment programs for child psychiatric disorders, developmental phenomena must be considered. In the area of childhood depression, questions remain about the relationship between a child's depressed status and that child's cognitive and affectional structures. That is, if depression is viewed as a complex affective state, what are the necessary cognitive and affective preconditions for feeling this emotion? Also, what are the effects of developmental factors on the subjective experience of childhood depression? Answers to these questions could significantly influence a number of prevention and treatment issues including (1) selection of age groups to be treated; (2) identification of associated symptomatology in screening criteria; and, (3) choice of intervention.

Although there appears to be some consensus that developmental stage influences the manifestation of depression, there is currently little empirical evidence to support this view (Kazdin & Petti, 1982). In a theoretical paper, Bemporad and Wilson (1978) address developmental issues and their effect on depression-like states in children. They point out the particularly elusive nature of depression in infancy and early childhood.

One methodological issue of considerable importance is that younger children also tend to be poorer informants not only about feelings but also about temporal and causal relationships between mood states and observable events. Another methodological issue concerns the specificity of the relationship between behavioral symptoms in young children and the presumed causative factors of the depression. Thus, while depression-like states seem to appear in children as early as infancy, it is not clear that observed behavioral patterns actually result from the child's subjective experience of depression. An example could be illustrated by examining the concept of "anaclitic depression." Spitz (1946) utilized this term to describe the pattern of apathy and withdrawal evidenced by infants after prolonged separation from the mother. However, withdrawal could be multiply determined and result from understimulation, or in some cases, organic disease or nutritional deficiency.

The paucity of empirical studies makes it difficult to evaluate the positions stated by Bemporad and Wilson (1978). For example, they note that while the preschool or early school age child has the capacity to experience prolonged sadness, this child has not developed adequate internalization capacities to experience a negative self image that is maintained independently of external situations. They indicate that a true sense of self and others develops in the later childhood years as does the child's ability to mediate emotional states through personal interpretative thought processes:

> . . . the child has now crystallized a sense of self which can be dissociated from the effects of immediate experience and conceptualized as a separated entity. The child can form a stable opinion of his own worth, an ability which, given the child's developmental immaturities, might result in self-deprecatory conclusions. [Bemporad & Wilson, 1978, p. 342]

These suggestions underscore the necessity of considering developmental phenomena in developing assessment, treatment, and prevention programs. While one might reasonably assume that children's cognitive and affective complexities develop over time, it is not reasonable to assume that a linear relationship between age and the expression of clearly defined depressive symptoms exists or that older children are necessarily better candidates for programs because of their abilities to articulate feelings. Self-report measures exist for children as young as seven years (Kazdin & Petti, 1982) suggesting that even young children have the capacity for reporting on their internal states. Elementary school age children may also be receptive to an intervention that involves educational components and there may be a period during the school years when they are particularly receptive to learning to identify and articulate their feelings more clearly, for example. Finally, while the adolescent's capacities for hypothetical and abstract reasoning are closer to the adult's, adolescents manifest some depressive symptomatology that is unique to their age group. Inhelder and Piaget (1958) describe the adolescent's "cognitive egocentrism" marked by attribution of heightened or unlimited power to one's own thought processes. Bemporad and Wilson note the adolescent's sense of power "can easily become transformed into deep depression if he concludes that he is worthless or his problems are insurmountable" (Bemporad & Wilson, 1978, p. 345). The authors suggest that adolescents may arrive at their conclusions on the basis of limited evidence or as a result of their limited experiences. Additionally, the adolescent's symptoms may be influenced by increased societal pressures for achievement during this developmental phase.

Clearly, different age groups have varying levels of cognitive and affective complexity. Moreover, children and adolescents are subject to differential societal demands as a function of developmental phase. At this time, however, a clear theoretical account of childhood depression does not exist and further work is needed to clarify whether developmental factors result in *qualitative* differences in the subjective experience of depression or its associated symptomatology.

A STEP TOWARD THE PREVENTION
OF CHILDHOOD DEPRESSION

While work in the area of childhood depression has promoted general agreement on the existence and definition of the construct, research has also highlighted many more questions that must be addressed before we have a clear understanding of etiological and developmental issues. Thus, while the area of prevention of childhood depression is compelling, as are all efforts to prevent and eradicate childhood disorders, there are a number of factors that preclude the establishment of broadly-based effective prevention programs. However, the literature on primary prevention provides a framework for beginning considerations on how such endeavors might be conceived and developed in the future.

Cowen (1983), one of the major voices in the primary prevention movement, defines the goal of primary prevention in mental health as the promotion of psychological adjustment and the prevention of maladjustment. He delineates the structural requirements for a primary prevention program (1982):

1. It must be group or mass- rather than individually oriented (even though some of its activities may involve individual contacts).

2. It must have a before-the-fact quality, i.e., be targeted to groups not yet experiencing significant maladjustment (even though they may, because of their life situations or recent experiences, be at risk for such outcomes).

3. It must be intentional, i.e., rest on a solid knowledge base suggesting that the program holds potential either for improving psychological health or preventing maladjustment [Cowen, 1982, p. 132].

Additional considerations apply in developing preventive interventions for children. Of primary importance is a developmental perspective (Roberts & Peterson, 1983). Children have special needs and vulnerabilities at various life phases that must be considered in developing and applying prevention programs. Unlike adults, who may experience relatively stable levels of skills and environmental demands, children's abilities, repertoires, and demands from others change over time. Therefore, it is necessary to develop intervention and assessment strategies that take into account phase-related developmental issues for children. Downward extensions of strategies that have been successful with adults will not suffice.

Despite these additional requirements, there are a number of reasons why preventive interventions with children may prove particularly effective. First, a mass- or group-oriented intervention can be easily applied to children in an educational setting, who are already primed for learning. Thus, it may be easier in preventive work with children than with adults to actually implement an intervention. Also, as many disorders of adulthood have their roots in childhood and adolescence, targeting children may increase the likelihood that interventions are applied before the onset of disorder. Finally, interventions with children may have a widened sphere of influence, positively impacting the individual during the childhood years and thereby improving the quality of life in adulthood as well. Thus, while most prevention efforts have focused on the problems of adulthood, child-oriented strategies represent promising avenues for further study (Roberts & Peterson, 1983).

For guiding the process of developing prevention interventions, Cowen (1984) has outlined a series of steps:

1. Identification of the program's generative knowledge base that justifies a particular type of primary prevention intervention.

2. Translation of that base into guiding program concepts that suggest how the program's objectives can best be achieved.

3. Development of a concrete program methodology appropriate for the intended target group.

4. Implementation of the program including quality-control mechanisms to maximize its effectiveness.

5. Program evaluation with an emphasis on the assessment of the program's intended adjustive outcomes.

The survey of the literature on childhood depression reveals that we are currently at stage one in this developmental process. Much of the work of deriving a generative knowledge base regarding the etiology and appearance of the syndrome of childhood depression is currently in progress. Therefore, it may be impossible, or at least premature, to delineate linkages between independent variables such as circumstances, events, competencies, and deficits, and dependent variables such as psychological adjustment or disorder, defined in this instance as the absence or presence of depression.

It may be useful, however, to examine the existing data and speculate about how preventive interventions may be designed in the future. Cowen (in press) delineates two major subtypes of primary prevention programs that require different foci and approaches: (1) situation-focused approaches, and (2) competence enhancement approaches. The justifying knowledge bases for these approaches differ somewhat.

Situation-focused approaches seek to prevent otherwise likely maladjustment in groups at risk for later difficulties due to the life circumstances and events they have experienced. In the area of childhood depression, such programs would necessitate our ability to identify circumstances or life events that predispose a child to the development of depression.

The most promising area of focus for programs of this nature may rest with interventions targeted to children of parents who have been identified as having psychiatric disorders. In their review of existing family studies, Orvaschel, Weissman, and Kidd (1980) note that children of depressed parents, for example, are themselves a subgroup at risk for the development of depression and other types of psychopathology. The authors indicate, however, that methodological difficulties in studies prevent conclusions regarding etiology. They recommend longitudinal investigations on the offspring of depressed parents. These studies would help clarify linkages between psychiatric disorder among parents and their children and would necessarily precede the development of effective preventive interventions targeted to children-at-risk.

If such linkages are actually observed, however, primary prevention programs of this nature may be difficult to implement for other reasons. Cowen (1985) notes that recent concrete stressful events (such as divorce, death of a loved one, etc.) may have more potential than chronic situations for effective primary prevention programming. The chronic stresses that children with psychiatrically ill parents experience in their environments may produce actual symptomatology and disorder, therefore precluding the possibility of actual prevention of maladjustment as stipulated in the definition of primary prevention. Thus, there is a thin line in some situation-focused interventions between primary and secondary prevention.

A discussion relevant to situationally-focused prevention interventions appears in Petti's (1983) book on childhood depression. O'Brien (1983) targets the young children of depressed mothers as a group at risk for the development of behavioral disturbances such as difficulty in eating, difficulty in obtaining bladder control, and a high accident rate. He suggests the most important aspect of secondary prevention for the dyad is the detection and treatment of depression among the mothers. He stresses the importance of education among professionals providing the bulk of services to young children (e.g., pediatricians, visiting nurses, well-baby clinic staff) regarding the manifestations of depression among mothers of young children. When depression is identified and treated in these mothers, the quality of child care and the well-being of the child may improve.

This type of intervention is an example of what may be programmatically possible considering the stage of development of the literature on childhood depression. A program of this nature that includes careful data collection utilizing multimodal assessment procedures to identify and diagnose mothers and their children as well as the inclusion of matched controls and relevant outcome measures may help advance our understanding of the relationship between disorder among parents and their children. Education among allied professionals may open opportunities for interdisciplinary collaboration. Perhaps most importantly, such a program may serve to enhance adjustment among a subgroup of children that is clearly at risk.

The other category of primary prevention approaches outlined by Cowen (1985) is the competence-enhancement approach. These programs seek to impart age- and situationally-relevant skills and competencies to enhance adjustment. By identifying and providing competencies before-the-fact of mental disorder, individuals may be less likely to develop particular difficulties.

With a construct as complex as childhood depression, it may be impossible to identify particular skills and competencies that can be considered equivalent to the disorder. The assessment data in the area of childhood depression indicates that a combination of characteristics including low self-esteem, anxiety, social withdrawal, unassertiveness, poor academic achievement, and problems with attention and concentration are associated with the disorder (Strauss, Forehand, Frame & Smith, 1984). However, an investigator developing a program focusing on the building of any or even all of these skills would be hard-pressed to demonstrate its efficacy in preventing childhood depression. While such an intervention may enhance adjustment, childhood depression, according to more widely-held theories, is more than a collection of symptoms or "depressive equivalents."

Perhaps a competence-enhancement approach could focus on independent variables that are more integral to the child's personality than individual symptoms associated with childhood depression. For example, evidence indicates that childhood depression may be associated with the manner in which the child cognitively structures experiences (Kissel, 1970; Kovacs & Beck, 1977). More specifically, hopelessness has been highlighted as a central feature of childhood (as in adult) depression. The child who feels hopeless is likely to cognitively structure experiences in a negative manner. This child shows negative attitudes toward the self, the world, and the future, and is likely to assume that current suffering will continue indefinitely. On the positive side, then, the child's tendency to positively structure experiences may serve to promote adjustment and may be related to the prevention of childhood depression.

A primary consideration in implementing this type of intervention strategy concerns age and developmental issues for the target population. In the area of childhood depression investigators continue to explore features associated with depression at various developmental levels. There is general consensus that late elementary school age children have developed many of the cognitive structures that may account for the similarities in the manifestations of depression seen in children and adults. Hopelessness has been identified as a construct that is relevant for children as young as eight (Kazdin, French, Unis, Esveldt-Dawson, & Sherick, 1983). However, an approach based on cognitive-restructuring may not be as effective with younger children.

While the approach described above is more consistent with current views about the definition of childhood depression than is an approach targeting particular symptoms, it is highly questionable that this approach would represent an effective preventive strategy. Additional research must be completed including studies linking particular qualities of cognitive style with childhood depression. However, if it is clearly demonstrated that a particular cognitive style is a *necessary* component for childhood depression, it is unlikely that any one or two independent variables will be demonstrated as *sufficient* or defining variables for a construct as multifaceted as childhood depression.

SUMMARY AND FUTURE DIRECTIONS

After years of controversy and study, researchers and theoreticians have arrived at some agreement on the existence of childhood depression. The complexity of the disorder is highlighted by the continuing discussion regarding etiology and developmental manifestations. Much of the emphasis in the literature has been on assessment, which has yielded numerous tools for identifying children who are experiencing depression. These instruments include interviews with children and their parents (Carlson & Cantwell, 1979, 1980; Kuperman & Stewart, 1979; Puig-Antich, Blau, Marx, Greenhill, & Chambers, 1978); parent ratings (Achenbach & Edelbrock, 1979; Leon, Kendall, & Garber, 1980); peer nomination techniques (Lefkowitz & Tesiny, 1980), projective tests (Cytyrn & McKnew, 1972, 1974); and self-report measures (Birelson, 1981; Kovacs & Beck, 1977; Lang & Tisher, 1978). Due to the multifaceted nature of childhood depression, investigators have recommended multimodal assessment procedures. Petti (1983) emphasizes the importance of evaluating contributions from the home, neighborhood, and school that culminate in the child's experience of depression.

In the current account, a survey of the literature on childhood depression was presented followed by a presentation of prevention models and a consideration of their applicability to childhood depression.

Difficulties were noted in pursuing situationally-focused and competence-enhancement approaches that are related to the status of the literature in the area of childhood depression. However, a more crucial deterrent to the development of primary prevention programs for childhood depression may relate to the broad and ambitious nature of the task. The most successful programs in prevention research appear to be those that involve specific, targeted interventions rather than more global interventions, such as an intervention aimed at the prevention of schizophrenia (Roberts & Peterson, 1983). In the case of the former, there are more clearly delineated independent variables, dependent measures, and conceptualizations of etiology that are crucial for effective preventive interventions.

For researchers in the area of childhood depression, the path is clear. Additional attention must be focused on the etiology and nature of the disorder. Treatment and preventive interventions may be begun on a small, controlled scale and must be closely tied to theoretical formulations. Prevention interventions that are specific and targeted to a particular age group may fall short of our dreams of preventing childhood depression. However specific interventions targeted to children at risk and others designed to build skills and competencies may serve to both enhance adjustment and provide the essential building blocks for future, larger scale endeavors.

REFERENCES

Achenbach, T. M., & Edelbrock, C. S. (1979). The child behavior profile: II. Boys aged 12–16 and girls aged 6–11 and 12–16. *Journal of Consulting & Clinical Psychology, 47,* 223–233.

American Psychiatric Association (1980). *Diagnostic and Statistical Manual of the Mental Disorders* (3rd Ed.) Washington, DC: American Psychiatric Association.

Beck, A. T. (1967). *Depression: Clinical, Experimental, and Theoretical Aspects.* New York: Harper & Row.

Beck, A. T., Weissman, A., Lester, D., & Trexler, L. (1974). The measurement of pessimism: The hopelessness scale. *Journal of Consulting & Clinical Psychology, 42,* 861–865.

Bemporad, J. R., & Wilson, A. (1978). A developmental approach to depression in childhood and adolescence. *Journal of the American Academy of Psychoanalysis, 6,* 325–352.

Birelson, P. (1981). The validity of depressive disorder in childhood and the development of a self rating scale: A research report. *Journal of Child Psychology and Psychiatry, 22,* 73–88.

Cantwell, D. (1982). Childhood depression: A review of current research. In B. B. Lahey & A. E. Kazdin (Eds.), *Advances in Clinical Child Psychology, 5.* New York: Plenum Press.

Carlson, G. A., & Cantwell, D. P. (1979). A survey of depressive symptoms in a child and adolescent psychiatric population. *Journal of the American Academy of Child Psychiatry, 18,* 587–599.

Carlson, G. A., & Cantwell, D. P. (1980). A survey of depressive symptoms, syndrome, and disorder in a child psychiatric population. *Journal of Child Psychology and Psychiatry, 21,* 19–25.

Cowen, E. L. (1982). Primary prevention research: Barriers, needs, and opportunities. *Journal of Primary Prevention, 2,*(3), 131–137.

Cowen, E. L. (1983). Primary prevention in mental health: Past, present, and future. In R. D. Felner, L. Jason, J. Moritsugu, & S. S. Farber (Eds.) *Preventive Psychology: Theory Research and Practice.* (pp. 11–25). New York: Pergamon Press.

Cowen, E. L. (1984). A general structural model for primary prevention program development in mental health. *Personnel and Guidance Journal, 62,* 485–490.

Cowen, E. L. (1985). Person centered approaches to primary prevention in mental health: Situation focused and competence enhancement. *American Journal of Community Psychology, 13,* 87–98.

Cytryn, L., & McKnew, D. H. (1972). Proposed classification of childhood depression. *American Journal of Psychiatry, 129,* 149–155.

Cytryn, L., & McKnew, D. H. (1974). Factors influencing the changing clinical expressions of the depressive process in children. *American Journal of Psychiatry, 131,* 879–881.

Glaser, K. (1968). Masked depression in children and adolescents. *Annual Progress in Child Psychiatry and Child Development, 1,* 345–355.

Inhelder, B., & Piaget, J. (1958). *The Growth of Logical Thinking from Childhood to Adolescence.* New York: Basic Books.

Kazdin, A. E. (1981). Assessment techniques for childhood depression: A critical appraisal. *Journal of the American Academy of Child Psychiatry, 20,* 358–375.

Kazdin, A. E., French, N. H., Unis, A. S., Esveldt-Dawson, K., & Sherick, R. B. (1983). Hopelessness, depression, and suicidal intent among psychiatrically disturbed inpatient children. *Journal of Consulting & Clinical Psychology, 51*(4), 504–510.

Kazdin, A. E., & Petti, T. A. (1982). Self-report and interview measures of childhood and adolescent depression. *Journal of Child Psychology and Psychiatry, 23,* 437–457.

Kissel, S. (1970). Reflections on depression in children. *Interaction, 3*(2), 104–107.

Kovacs, M. (1980/1981). Rating scales to assess depression in school-aged children. *Acta Paedopsychiatria, 46,* 305–315.

Kovacs, M. (1983). *The Children's Depression Inventory: A self-rated depression scale for school-aged youngsters.* University of Pittsburgh School of Medicine, Unpublished Manuscript.

Kovacs, M. & Beck, A. T. (1977). An empirical-clinical approach toward a definition of childhood depression. In J. G. Schulterbrandt & A. Raskin (Eds.), *Depression in Childhood: Diagnosis, treatment, and conceptual models.* (pp. 1–25). New York: Raven Press.

Kuperman, S., & Stewart, M. A. (1979). The diagnosis of depression in children. *Journal of Affective Disorders, 1,* 213–217.

Lang, M., & Tisher, M. (1978). *Children's Depression Scale.* Victoria, Australia: The Australian Council for Educational Research.

Lefkowitz, M. M., & Tesiny, E. P. (1980). Assessment of childhood depression. *Journal of Consulting & Clinical Psychology, 48,* 43–50.

Leon, G. R., Kendall, P. C., & Garber, J. (1980). Depression in children: Parent, teacher, and child perspectives. *Journal of Abnormal Child Psychology, 8,* 221–235.

O'Brien, J. D. (1983). Intervention and prevention strategies for children with depressed mothers. In T. A. Petti (Ed.), *Childhood Depression.* (pp. 69–77). New York: Haworth Press.

Orvaschel, H., Weissman, M. M., & Kidd, K. K. (1980). Children and depression: the children of depressed parents; the childhood of depressed patients; depression in children. *Journal of Affective Disorders, 2,* 1–16.

Petti, T. A. (1978). Depression in hospitalized child psychiatry patients. *Journal of the American Academy of Child Psychiatry, 17,* 49–59.

Petti, T. A. (1983). The assessment of depression in young children. In T. A. Petti (Ed.), *Childhood Depression.* (pp. 19–28). New York: Haworth Press.

Puig-Antich, J., Blau, S., Marx, N., Greenhill, L. L., & Chambers, W. (1978). Prepubertal major depressive disorder. *Journal of the American Academy of Child Psychiatry, 17,* 695–707.

Puig-Antich, J. & Gittelman, R. (1982). Depression in childhood and adolescence. In E. S. Paykel (Ed.), *Handbook of Affective Disorders.* New York: The Guilford Press.

Rie, H. E. (1966). Depression in childhood. *Journal of the American Academy of Child Psychiatry, 5,* 653–686.

Roberts, M. C., & Peterson, L. (1984). *Prevention of Problems in Childhood: Psychological research and applications.* New York, Wiley and Sons.

Spitz, R. (1946). Anaclitic depression. *Psychoanalytic Study of the Child, 2,* 113–117.

Spitzer, R. L., Endicott, J., & Robins, E. (1978). Research diagnostic criteria: rationale and reliability. *Archives of General Psychiatry, 35,* 773–782.

Strauss, C.C., Forehand, R., Frame, C., & Smith, K. (1984). Characteristics of children with extreme scores on the Children's Depression Inventory. *Journal of Child Clinical Psychology, 13*(3), 227–231.

6

Autonomy and Self-Control: Key Concepts for the Prevention of Depression in Adolescents

Marjorie H. Klein, John H. Greist, Sandra M. Bass,
and Mary Jane Lohr
University of Wisconsin

INTRODUCTION

Our research and prevention programs for adolescents have been based on three familiar assumptions: (a) that an interpersonal perspective is essential in understanding the etiology and treatment of depression, regardless of whether genetic, biochemical, environmental, or cognitive factors are also involved; (b) that depression is a complex phenomenon, sometimes associated with attributions of external control, sometimes with internal control, and (c) that freedom from external demands that is won through tight and oppressive self-control is not equivalent to genuine autonomy and self-direction.

Most effective prevention and intervention strategies for depression are based on the laudable assumption that it is helpful to enhance self-esteem and autonomy, i.e., to help people effectively control external stressors and realize personal goals. A focus on the interpersonal context of such programs, however, reminds us that it is as essential to consider the interpersonal style or climate in which specific prevention or intervention strategies are implemented, as to be concerned with the content of the strategies themselves. Consider the paradoxical case where an intervention protocol calls for a depressed person to be vigorously persuaded to take steps for change (i.e., take "control" of his/her own behavior). Although the immediate impact of the change may be to lessen depressed affect or behavior, the simultaneous underlying message of the external control necessary to effect the change and the implied comparison with the effective "others" may remain unchanged and unchallenged.

Questions raised by this paradox are:

1. Will intervention strategies that stress self-control inadvertently perpetuate or reinforce depressogenic tendencies to internal causal attributions? Will stress on

This work was supported by the Prevention and Wellness Grant Program, Wisconsin Department of Health and Social Services and the Wisconsin Psychiatric Research Institute. We wish to thank Judith Wilcox, Pat Kane, and Roger Eischens for their tireless work at the schools; the teachers, administrators and boards of the schools (who must remain anonymous); and Jean Clatworthy and Martha Quimby for assistance in preparing this manuscript.

personal responsibility, self-monitoring and self-management feed into or reinforce feelings of guilt and obligation?

2. Will intervention strategies where direct and firm external pressure is used to change attitudes and behavior inadvertently reinforce depressogenic perceptions of external control—i.e., feelings of helplessness? If the depressed person views the intervention or the power of the intervener as having caused the change, is not another kind of dependence established? If so, how can the initial dependence be transformed (i.e., internalized) over time?

Just as effective intervention must ultimately focus on restoration of esteem and efficacy, it follows in the long run that the most effective intervention will be one that promotes these aims in the style and form as well as in its content. Even if strong pressure for compliance is necessary to initiate behavior change, the person must ultimately internalize or take personal responsibility for the change so that positive results and new behaviors can be personally owned and incorporated.

While the concepts of personal autonomy and self-control may appear and be used synonymously in theories of the etiology and treatment of depression, this analysis suggests that a more differentiated view may be necessary. We have already made a distinction between depression resulting from uncontrollable external factors and that resulting from a tendency to excessive internal control. The same distinction might be applied to a view of depression as developing in phases, i.e., depression that is set off initially by uncontrollable external events may be maintained and further reinforced by increasingly internalized blame for this inability to cope. The concept of self-control is also more complex than a superficial glance at the self-control literature would suggest. It potentially encompasses behaviors that range from friendly and positive (e.g., self-efficacy, self-management, planning) to rather unfriendly forms of coercive self-control (e.g., self-restraint and self-blame).

Given this complexity and the likelihood that depression is heterogenous, there is a real possibility that prevention or intervention strategies that stress self-control may misfire. Many of the self-control techniques in current use seem to have been developed for cases where depression has developed in the face of uncontrollable external circumstances. When applied to individuals whose depression stems from excessive internal control, the self-control emphasis may feed into or reinforce the tendency for internalization in the form, for example, of tight and oppressive self-management. Thus while we would all probably agree that the goal of prevention-intervention strategies is to enhance or maintain autonomy, we must be mindful of the quality and impact of the self-control strategies that are used to implement these aims.

CHARACTERISTICS
OF THE ADOLESCENT SAMPLE

The main focus of this paper is on our intervention trials with high school students carried out in the context of a "Wellness Program" in a Midwestern suburban high school. The data presented in this section describes students from two high schools in two communities: the target school where the Wellness Program was later carried out; the second, a control or comparison school where pre and posttesting only was done. Both communities are within 20 miles of a metropolitan area, with a blend of rural and urban residents.

Initial and final testing in both schools was done in physical education classes. Measures included the Symptom Checklist-90-Revised (SCL-90), the Social Adjustment Scale (SAS) with some questions adapted for adolescents, the Structural Analysis of Social Behavior (SASB) self-image scale, and a questionnaire for health risk assessment.

1. The SCL-90-R is a widely-used measure of symptomatology, with cluster scores for nine empirically derived factors (somatization, obsessive-compulsive, interpersonal sensitivity, depression, anxiety, hostility, phobic anxiety, paranoia and psychoticism) as well as scores for additional items and total scores (Derogatis, Lipman, & Covi, 1973). Analyses here will be focused on depression cluster and Global Severity Index (GSI) scores. Norms are available for psychiatric outpatients and community survey respondents (Derogatis, 1983).

2. The SAS was developed for research on depression and its treatment (Weissman & Paykel, 1974; Weissman & Rothwell, 1976). Questions cover functioning within five life areas (worker/student, social-leisure, family, dating, and economic). High scores indicate high impairment.

3. The SASB self-image scale was developed by Benjamin (1974; 1984), based on her work on the structural analysis of social behavior. The items and structure of the self-image (introject) scale are based on the assumption that feelings about the self are derived from one's history of relations with significant others (see Figure 1). The top surface of the figure (diamond) depicts interpersonal behaviors for which the focus is on the other person, and the middle surface displays interpersonal behaviors for which the focus is on the self. On each surface, the horizontal axis is affiliation and the vertical axis is interdependence. Opposite behaviors appear directly across from each other on the same surface (e.g., Chart Point 115, "friendly explore, listen," is the opposite of 135, "accuse, blame"). Complementary behaviors, those that tend to draw or prompt each other, are at corresponding positions on these two surfaces. The behavior complementary to "accuse, blame" is therefore "whine, defend, justify" (235). Antidotes are complements of opposites. Thus, the antidote to "whine, defend, justify" is the complement of "openly disclose, reveal" (215), namely, "friendly explore, listen" (115). The bottom surface portrays what happens when behaviors represented on the top surface are turned inward. Note that the Benjamin model depicts an entire spectrum of behaviors (mapped onto the top halves of the two interpersonal surfaces) involving the giving and taking of autonomy, either friendly or hostile, since dominance and submission are depicted as complementary forms of high interdependence. Scores, based on extensive factor analytic and construct validation studies, represent the major orthogonal dimensions of affiliation and autonomy (divisible into four quadrants and eight more specific cluster scores; see Figure 2) and a consistency coefficient which reflects cohesion vs. ambivalence of the self-image.

4. Assessment of health and health behavior was done using the Health Hazard Appraisal Method developed by Van Cura and others which covers family and personal medical history, tobacco, drugs, alcohol use, and lifestyle items needed to calculate health risk estimates (Van Cura, 1978; Van Cura, Jensen & Greist, 1976). For adolescents, health risk estimates are most heavily influenced by gender and motor vehicle use. To augment the standard global health risk scores in our

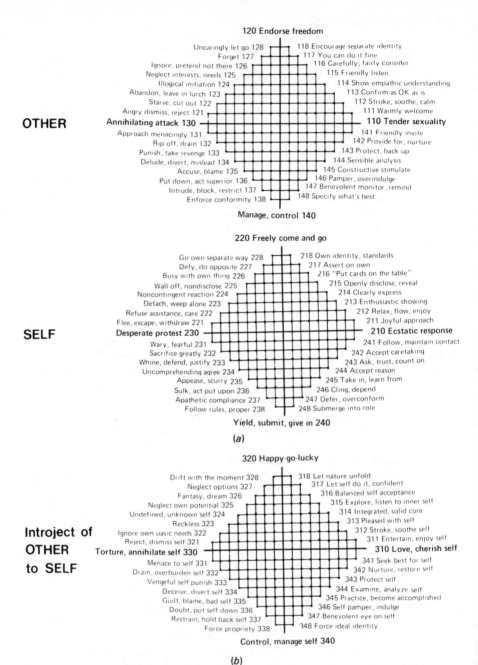

Figure 1 Most recent revision of Benjamin's "chart of social behavior." Note that the Benjamin model depicts an entire spectrum of behaviors (mapped onto the top halves of the two interpersonal surfaces) involving the giving and taking of autonomy, either friendly or hostile, since dominance and submission are depicted as complementary forms of high interdependence. (From "Structural Analysis of Differentiation Failure" by L. S. Benjamin, 1979, *Psychiatry, 42,* p. 6. Copyright 1979 by the William Alanson White Psychiatric Foundation. Reprinted by permission.)

(a) Interpersonal; (b) Intrapsychic

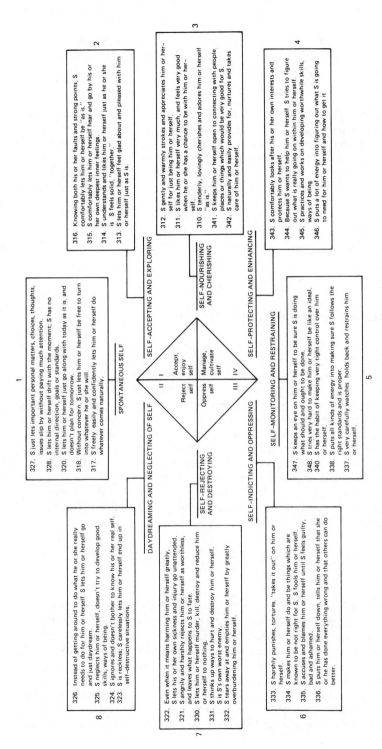

Figure 2 Three levels of complexity of the SASB model. The center presents the quadrant version. The middle contains the cluster names, and the boxes on the outer ring contain the questionnaire items for each cluster.

SPONTANEOUS SELF

1

327. S just lets important personal matters, choices, thoughts, issues slip by without paying much attention.
328. S lets him or herself drift with the moment; S has no internal direction, goals or standards.
320. S lets him or herself just go along with today as it is, and doesn't plan for tomorrow.
318. Without concern, S just lets him or herself be free to turn into whatever he or she will.
317. S freely, easily and confidently lets him or herself do whatever comes naturally.

SELF-ACCEPTING AND EXPLORING

2

316. Knowing both his or her faults and strong points, S comfortably lets him or herself be "as is."
315. S comfortably lets him or herself hear and go by his or her own deepest inner feelings.
314. S understands and likes him or herself just as he or she is. S feels solid, "together."
313. S lets him or herself feel glad about and pleased with him or herself just as S is.

SELF-NOURISHING AND CHERISHING

3

312. S gently and warmly strokes and appreciates him or herself for just being him or herself.
311. S likes him or herself very much, and feels very good when he or she has a chance to be with him or herself.
310. S tenderly, lovingly cherishes and adores him or herself "as is."
341. S keeps him or herself open to connecting with people, places or things which would be very good for S.
342. S naturally and easily provides for, nurtures and takes care of him or herself.

SELF-PROTECTING AND ENHANCING

4

343. S comfortably looks after his or her own interests and protects him or herself.
344. Because S wants to help him or herself S tries to figure out what is really going on within him or herself.
345. S practices and works on developing worthwhile skills, ways of being.
346. S puts a lot of energy into figuring out what S is going to need for him or herself and how to get it.

DAYDREAMING AND NEGLECTING OF SELF

8

326. Instead of getting around to do what he or she really needs to do for him or herself, S lets him or herself go and just daydream.
325. S neglects him or herself, doesn't try to develop good skills, ways of being.
324. S ignores and doesn't bother to know his or her real self.
323. S is reckless; S carelessly lets him or herself end up in self-destructive situations.

SELF-REJECTING AND DESTROYING

7

322. Even when it means harming him or herself greatly, S lets his or her own sickness and injury go unattended.
321. S angrily and harshly rejects him or herself as worthless, and leaves what happens to S to fate.
330. S lets him or herself murder, kill, destroy and reduce him or herself to nothing.
331. S thinks up ways to hurt and destroy him or herself. S is S's own worst enemy.
332. S tears away at and empties him or herself by greatly overburdening him or herself.

SELF-INDICTING AND OPPRESSING

6

333. S harshly punishes, tortures, "takes it out" on him or herself.
334. S makes him or herself do and be things which are known to be not right for S. S fools him or herself.
335. S accuses and blames him or herself until S feels guilty, bad and ashamed.
336. S puts him or herself down, tells him or herself that she or he has done everything wrong and that others can do better.

SELF-MONITORING AND RESTRAINING

5

347. S keeps an eye on him or herself to be sure S is doing what should and ought to be done.
348. S tries very hard to make him or herself be like an ideal.
340. S has the habit of keeping very tight control over him or herself.
338. S puts all kinds of energy into making sure S follows the right standards and is proper.
337. S very carefully watches holds back and restrains him or herself.

I Accept, enjoy self

II Reject self

III Oppress self

IV Manage, cultivate self

107

analyses we have turned to specific item scores for amount of exercise, tobacco use and alcohol consumption and to an estimate of overweight, based on the ratio of actual weight to ideal body weight, given height.

A total of 527 students (49% of the school's census) from the target school and 300 (45%) from the control school took part in the fall pretest. Because testing was done in physical education classes, grades 9–10 were better represented in the samples than grades 11–12 when many students were exempt. Spring posttesting was completed for 419 (39%) target and 272 (41%) control students. Because school policy had dictated that student participation be voluntary and anonymous, pre and post questionnaires for the repeated measures analyses were matched using date of birth, sex, and grade information. Using this method, 255 (48% of the pretest sample) target and 104 (35%) control questionnaires were matched (there was more missing grade information in the control school, especially among males).

Depression and Total Symptoms

The most complete information about the prevalence of depression and other problems in the two schools is based on SCL-90 and other data for all fall pretest participants. Table 1 shows the averages for depression and total symptom (GSI) scores and compares the percentile score distributions for the adolescents with community survey (n = 974; mean age = 46) and psychiatry outpatient (n = 1,002; mean age = 31) norms for adults (Derogatis, 1983). Generally, more than half of the adolescents scored above the 75th adult community percentiles for depression and overall symptomatology. Relative to psychiatry outpatients we found 3–14% of the respondents to be above the 50th percentile for depression. Even more extreme patterns were present when the overall symptom score was considered. Levels for the other SCL-90 scales were similar; the adolescents reported symptom levels that were considerably higher than community survey adults across all SCL-90 clusters.

Grade, Sex, and School

Analyses of variance of pretest SCL-90 data included school, sex and grade as factors. Consistent sex and school differences (p values significant at the .05 level or less) appeared for most SCL-90 scores, including depression and GSI. Females were consistently more symptomatic than males (except for hostility); the control school was more symptomatic (except for somatization) than the target school. (Because of these differences regressions were done separately for males and females.) Significant sex by grade interactions also emerged for depression, obsessive-compulsive, hostility, and GSI scores. While symptoms seemed to increase steadily with grade for females, males showed peaks at both 9th and 12th grades.

Table 1 Pretest depression and total SCL-90 scores for target and control schools

Scores	Target school		Control school	
	Male (*n* = 221)	Female (*n* = 306)	Male (*n* = 118)	Female (*n* = 182)
Depression				
Mean	.528	.865	.679	1.078
SD	.660	.553	.593	.741
Range	0–3.54	0–3.54	0–2.92	0–3.00
Community norms (%)				
0–25	19	11	12	5
26–50	14	9	10	13
51–75	24	28	23	13
76–100	43	52	55	69
Outpatient norms (%)				
0–25	73	73	82	64
26–50	20	18	15	22
51–75	5	7	3	10
76–100	2	2	0	4
Total symptoms (GSI)				
Mean	.574	.794	.699	.963
SD	.506	.530	.344	.555
Range	0–3.51	0–3.00	0–2.89	0–2.71
Community norms (%)				
0–25	6	4	9	4
26–50	12	8	9	5
51–75	25	11	9	13
76–100	57	67	73	78
Outpatient norms (%)				
0–25	70	63	67	46
26–50	19	21	14	28
51–75	7	10	14	16
76–100	4	6	5	10

Other Variables

Descriptive results for the other measures of health behavior, social adjustment and self-concept were also of interest as indicators of the overall functional level of adolescents. On the SAS, scores for most clusters fell within normal limits, but most distress was reported for the dating items. ANOVA results were generally similar to the SCL-90 pattern: poorer adjustment was reported by the control school and by females. The dating cluster provided the only exception: males' adjustment scores were significantly poorer. Dating adjustment scores also varied as a function of grade: interest in and frequency of dating increased over the 9–12 grade span, most steadily for females.

On the SASB self-concept measure the adolescent responses, in general, differed from norms reported for normal college students. This was especially the case with respect to self-esteem and consistency, which were considerably lower among the adolescents than among college students from Benjamin's (1984) normative sample. ANOVAs by sex, school, and grade revealed sex differences that were somewhat more complex than for other measures. Males were higher in self-esteem but *lower* in autonomy than females. Cluster detail indicated males were higher for the clusters associated with both friendly (2 and 3) and unfriendly power (4 and 5). School differences favored the target school. Unlike other measures the SASB showed quite consistent developmental change in that students became more self-accepting and self-consistent over grades 9-12.

Overall health risk scores varied significantly by sex, school and grade, with males, the control school, and the higher grades being at greater risk. As these differences were largely due to the greater frequency of males' driving, we thought it of greater interest to look at some specific "lifestyle" items that are crucial to teen-age health, namely exercise, cigarette use and alcohol consumption. Females reported less exercise than males (22% vs. 12% walked less than 5 blocks per day), were less likely to drink heavily (14% vs. 21% took seven or more drinks/day), but were more likely to be light smokers (28% vs. 17% reported smoking up to $\frac{1}{2}$ pack per day).

Predictors of Depression

Before discussion of the intervention program and its impact it is relevant to consider whether any aspects of the self-image, social adjustment and health measures predicted depression in these adolescents. First we present the results of regression analyses with *pretest* depression as the dependent variable, which depict factors associated with current depression. Next we turn to analyses where pretest variables are regressed on *posttest* depression levels, i.e., a more truly predictive model.

Predicting Pretest Depression

Table 2 presents the variables remaining in backwards stepwise regression equations, done separately for males and females with other pretest variables (4 self image scores, 6 social adjustment scores, 4 health behaviors, and grade) as independent variables. Depression in both males and females was associated with the SASB self-image quadrants that reflect self-management, self-oppression, and (negatively) self-acceptance (see Figures 1 and 2 for description of item content). Depression in both sexes was also associated with problems in school, social-leisure, and family adjustment. The importance of the additional social adjustment cluster (dating) for females suggests that opposite sex relationships may play a more important role for females. Finally, cigarette use was only associated with depression for females.

Predicting Posttest Depression

It was also possible to look at the predictors of depression over time by using pretest predictor variables (SAS, SASB, health) in regressions where posttest depression was the dependent variable. This approach is especially relevant to the prediction of depression and to prevention (as distinct from intervention or treatment). According to Table 3 the predictors of depression were quite similar to those that emerged for the pretest regressions. In females, posttest depression was again associated with pretest self-oppression and problems in school and social-leisure adjustment. In males, depression was again predicted by self-oppression vs. self-acceptance and problems with social-leisure and family adjustment. The

Table 2 Pretest variables remaining in regression equations (backwards stepwise) with pretest depression as dependent variable

Variables	B	r
Males (n = 229)		
Self-image		
Self-management	.174**	.344
Self-acceptance	−.142***	−.033
Self-oppression	.127*	.255
Social adjustment		
Student	.391**	.572
Social-leisure	.188***	.456
Family	.143*	.437
Multiple R	.665	
R Square	.443	
Females (n = 320)		
Self-image		
Self-oppression	.269***	.437
Self-management	.098†	.422
Self-acceptance	−.097*	−.173
Social adjustment		
Social-leisure	.270***	.488
Student	.197***	.507
Family	.142***	.416
Dating	−.086*	−.125
Health behavior		
Smoking	.118**	.267
Multiple R	.715	
R Square	.511	

†p < .10
*p < .05
**p < .01
***p < .001

relationship of depression to self-management dropped out for both sexes. Student role adjustment was replaced by alcohol consumption as a predictor for males. For females, depression was no longer associated with dating adjustment and cigarette consumption, but a relationship to financial difficulties emerged.

These findings have several implications for prevention-intervention programs. Most important, the generally high levels of depression, interpersonal concerns and problems and other symptoms suggest that adolescents were in need of prevention and intervention programs aimed at depression and other mental health issues. The fact that some students also reported behaviors associated with long range health risk (low exercise, smoking, heavy drinking) suggests that programmatic concern with wellness may also be appropriate. The consistent association of depression with a self-oppressing self-image also suggests that it will be important for prevention or intervention programs simultaneously to *raise* self-esteem and *lower* tendencies for tight, oppressive self-control. Intervention programs that stress self-monitoring and self-management may thus run the risk of further reinforcing characteristics of self-image that are precursors of depression. The consist-

Table 3 Pretest variables remaining in regression equations (backwards stepwise) with posttest depression as dependent variable

Variables	B	r
Males (n = 94)		
Self-image		
Self-oppression	.274***	.292
Self-acceptance	−.232**	−.193
Social adjustment		
Social-leisure	.346**	.485
Family	.164+	.393
Health behavior		
Alcohol consumption	.222**	.299
Multiple R	.650	
R Square	.423	
Females (n = 150)		
Self-image		
Self-oppression	.338***	.388
Social adjustment		
Student	.222**	.328
Social-leisure	.174*	.323
Financial	.127+	.243
Multiple R	.540	
R Square	.292	

+p < .10
*p < .05
**p < .01
***p < .001

ency with which some social adjustment factors were also associated with depression in our adolescent sample also points to the importance of addressing their salient interpersonal concerns, particularly with respect to school and social-leisure (primarily peer) activities.

THE INTERVENTION PROGRAM

The intervention program was designed to include elements of our earlier research on depression and computer applications in psychiatry (Greist & Klein, 1981). There were two foci: (a) an interest in extending our previous work with aerobic exercise (jogging) as a treatment for depressive symptoms in adults to adolescents in a prevention (as opposed to a treatment) setting (Greist et al., 1978; 1979) and (b) an interest in the impact of interactive computer techniques in facilitating dialogue and exchange of information about a range of health problems with adolescents (Greist, Klein, & Erdman, 1978).

Our previous experience developing and studying the effectiveness of interactive computer interviews as a means to gather and give information from adults in psychiatric outpatient settings had demonstrated that this is an excellent, often superior, medium for topics ranging from medical history (Slack, Hicks, Reed, & Van Cura, 1966) and medical complaints, venereal disease (Van Cura, Jensen,

Greist, Lewis, & Frey, 1975), psychological symptoms and target problems (Greist, Klein, & Van Cura, 1973), social adjustment, sexual functioning (Greist & Klein, 1980), drug-alcohol use (Greist, Klein, Van Cura, & Erdman, 1975), and other sensitive topics. In an earlier comparison of a computer interview and a questionnaire as a means of collecting information from high school students about alcohol and drug use-abuse, we found that adolescents preferred and were more responsive to the computer interview over the questionnaire, that they gave essentially equivalent information, and that the computer method (by virtue of branching and response-checking capabilities) guaranteed more complete and internally consistent data (Greist et al., 1975).

For these reasons we felt that interactive computer technology would provide an ideal entree into the adolescent setting, with the following advantages:

1. The novelty and liveliness of the technology would draw students into the Wellness Center initially.

2. The computer format of free choice, privacy and confidentiality would create a context in which adolescents would feel free and/or comfortable enough to engage in "dialogue" about personally sensitive topics (one consistent result of all of our research with computer interviews has been that people are *less embarrassed* about giving and receiving sensitive information with the computer).

3. The menu and branching capabilities of the computer would allow us to offer a wide range of materials in an individualized format.

4. The flexibility and openness of the system to modification and expansion would allow the adolescent users to build upon or modify existing programs to meet their own needs.

The basic philosophy that guided our approach and operating style was our desire to provide a system in which the adolescent users had maximum input, choice and control. This approach was not only consistent with our view of the basic psychological issues in depression but also with our preliminary findings that depressed adolescents were low in both self-esteem and "friendly" self-direction. As we first introduced the Wellness Program to the students we wanted to convey this philosophy. As part of the pretest we included a needs assessment in which students were asked to list any and all activities or health-related issues they would like to explore. The major categories of student interest were sexuality, peer and family relationships, planning for the future, communication with teachers and administrators, and health.

Shortly after the pretest and needs assessment, the Wellness Program opened its doors in rooms provided by the school in the nurses' area. The program was staffed by three women and a computer terminal. The staff had background in depression assessment and treatment research (Bass, Wilcox), use of exercise in depression treatment (Kane, Wilcox), community and youth organizing (Wilcox) and interactive computer interviews (Bass).

The computer terminal was connected by telephone with the UW Health Sciences Data General computer which operated a software system called CONVERSE (MIIS language) which is specially designed for the easy construction (textwriting and programming) and operation of computer-person dialogues or interviews. After signing on to the system, the user is offered a list or menu of available subjects. After taking the interview of choice, scoring, display and summary programs provide feedback. In addition all results can be permanently stored and retrieved for evaluation and summarization.

Within the broad scope of health, the Wellness Program focused on diverse issues and activities, in response to student interest. There were two operational formats:

1. Computer interviews. The Wellness office was open during school hours and students were free to drop in and take any of the available computer interviews. We especially encouraged interested students to form working groups to develop new interviews. Over the semester, 17 students were responsible for the creation and, to some extent, the programming of eight interviews.

2. Workshops and group activities. These ranged from school-wide surveys and information programs to small group workshops (e.g., running groups, relaxation and meditation classes, etc.).

Computer Interviews

Interviews on the following topics were available: health risk, venereal disease, diet, headache, alcohol use and suicide risk. These were supplemented by computer interviews designed by students which focused on sexuality, depression, drug and alcohol use, nutrition and skin care. As each interview is described we also summarize information that reflects the frequency of student concerns or problems in each area.

Contraception

This interview consisted of questions about attitudes toward contraceptive use and patterns of use with branching to additional information items as requested by users. Information was offered about effectiveness and long- and short-term side effects of various contraceptive methods. Judging from the responses of the 98 students who took the interview, 84% of the sexually active respondents *did not* use contraceptives.

Pregnancy

The focus of the pregnancy interview was on options to be considered and decisions to be made by pregnant women. The 40 questions covered contraceptive use, sexual activity, pregnancy detection, family history of hereditary disease, and issues involved in termination vs. continuation of pregnancy, including interpersonal issues (informing parents, relationship with father). A list of referral agencies was offered upon request. Of the 56 students who took the interview, 35% responded as if they were pregnant (we suspect that they were not all pregnant, but were curious about the interview). Their response patterns suggested that information about pregnancy would most likely be first shared with friends (71%) rather than with the sex partner (28%), a doctor (28%), or parents (9%) suggesting the importance of developing pregnancy counseling options and resources that teenage women can feel comfortable to approach.

Venereal Disease

This interview had been developed at the University of Wisconsin Hospital and its primary focus was on teaching. For any disease the student chose, the disease was defined symptomatically, followed by detail on diagnosis and treatment. The interview was taken by 23 students who most frequently requested information about gonorrhea, syphilis, crabs and scabies. In response to evaluation questions, most (67%) students found the interview interesting or fun and half of the respondents felt that comparable information would be difficult to obtain from other sources.

Depression

Because the pretest data suggested a fairly high level of depression among the students, we had gathered relevant self-help reading materials, including *Control Your Depression* (Lewinsohn, Muñoz, Youngren, & Zeiss, 1978). One of the students programmed the Beck Depression Inventory as a computer interview which was taken by 22 students. Scores averaged 20 (range 0–38) with significantly higher levels reported by females. Feedback was coupled with a discussion by staff of self-help and referral options.

Suicide Risk

Another interview we had provided was the suicide risk interview developed by Greist and colleagues for use in a psychiatric treatment setting (Greist et al., 1973; Gustafson, Greist, Stauss, Erdman, & Laughren, 1977). Questions about symptoms and behaviors relevant to suicide are followed by risk calculations which distinguish between serious and nonserious attempts and thoughts. Of the 52 students who took the interview, 37 gave enough information for risk estimates to be calculated. Six students had high (60% or more) probabilities for serious attempts, ten for nonserious attempts, three for suicide thoughts. When probabilities were high, referral sources were discussed with students by Wellness staff.

Alcohol

We also offered a computer version of the Alcohol Use Inventory (Wanberg, Horn, & Foster, 1977) and encouraged students to develop further programming in this area. While alcohol use was quite common and widespread there was little spontaneous student interest in preventive programming. Of the 28 students who took the interview, the majority reported frequent use of alcohol (61%), getting drunk (67%) and some reported other alcohol-related problems such as daily drinking (32%), recent increase in drinking (43%), loss of control (48%), hangovers (35%), etc.

Drug Use/Abuse

Two drug use interviews were designed by students with the help of a staff consultant and reference materials. One focused primarily on marijuana, which apparently was used frequently by 73% of the 44 students who took the interview, with "side effects" such as impaired school work (31%), blackouts (48%), truancy (52%) and suspension from school (36%). Interestingly, 69% of the students linked their own marijuana use to parental drinking. The second student-designed drug interview was more generally focused on chemical dependency based on material provided by the county drug abuse prevention center. The interview was not completed in time to be widely used.

Nutrition

The nutrition interview had been developed at UW Hospital for weight control counseling. Based on information about activity level and food intake patterns, an estimated caloric intake on a "typical day" is given. According to information given by 19 students, 32% of the daily caloric intake was provided by snacks, as compared with breakfast (15%), lunch (16%), and dinner (37%). Many respondents described themselves as overweight (56%) and as having struggled to lose weight (52%).

Skin Care

After skin care workshops and demonstrations attended by more than 200 students, one student put together a skin care computer interview which based specific care information on an evaluation of skin type.

Workshops and Group Activities

These varied from school-wide surveys, classes, classroom demonstrations and information tables to small group activities, sometimes done in cooperation with teachers and/or class projects. The focus was on activities and lifestyles that promote health, e.g., nutrition, exercise, sports, and environmental awareness.

Salad Bar

There had been considerable student interest in establishing a lunch-time salad bar as an alternative to the high carbohydrate, high calorie lunches provided by the school cafeteria. Student council members previously had met resistance from school administrators and were eager to enlist Wellness Program support. Students and Wellness staff developed a questionnaire about food preferences, collected, and tabulated (with help from the computer) responses from 600 students for presentation to the school administration. The extent of survey support for the salad bar concept was important in convincing the school to carry out a preliminary trial of an a-la-carte food bar which offered salad, soup and sandwich alternatives to the more traditional and fattening hot lunch.

Vegetarian Cooking

At student request, vegetarian cooking classes were offered two days a week for six weeks to 40 students and to interested home economics teachers. This was followed by workshops in all home economics classes, articles in the school newspaper, classes in some local women's groups, and a request from community members for student help in establishing a food co-op.

Exercise

In line with our previous research and treatment interests, we attempted to start before- and after-school jogging groups, targeted at students who were not otherwise active in physical education or sports. Due to a combination of harsh winter weather and student schedules these groups were short-lived.

There was more widespread and spontaneous student interest in indoor roller-skating (consistent with the national media interest in roller disco). Students requested program help in organizing a roller-skating club, which included a weekly Saturday bus trip to area rinks and a student contact with community business people to press for conversion of an unused building into a local rink. Similar Wellness Program support was also requested by students interested in promoting soccer (there were no school or local programs). Through information and liaison provided by the Wellness program, local physical education teachers were encouraged to run a series of spring soccer classes and workshops in which 250 10–12 year olds participated.

Canoeing and Nature Trips

Despite abundant local lakes, marshes, and woodlands few students had experience with canoeing. Wellness staff organized an overnight trip for 20 interested students that included vigorous canoeing, walking, and contact with nature. Several other events that combined outdoor activity and nature contact were: (a) a prairie burn (allowed by one science teacher as a final project) where students followed sessions with Arboretum staff where they learned about prairies and prairie management, with a "hands-on" attempt to use the ancient burn method on a local railroad track right-of-way; (b) a field trip to the International Crane Foundation was followed by a two-week student-conducted Crane count in local marshes (sponsored by several science classes); and (c) field trips and lectures at a nearby site that was being considered as an outdoor school nature laboratory were sponsored by the Wellness staff and taught by local naturalists.

Not all of the programs we planned or attempted succeeded. The more successful programs were those that flowed most directly from student need and interest and could be easily worked into the students' schedules, e.g., in ongoing classes or in distinct time periods outside of class when students were free. Participation and support of program staff was an essential ingredient in maintaining interest, particularly our ability to follow through and provide leaders, materials, resources, etc. needed to translate student ideas into concrete activities. The computer was a great asset not only in attracting the students to the program initially, but in providing a private and relaxed context in which students could confront sensitive issues. Programs that did not get off the ground or succeed involved sensitive subjects or fell victim to participant inertia. Student interest in classroom programs and computer interviews about sexuality ran afoul of resistance from parents. At the same time, our consultants from the University had unforeseen difficulty locating sex survey materials that they considered appropriate for the age group. Other areas of student concern proved difficult to translate into specific action. There was great interest for example, in exploring relationships, particularly with the opposite sex. Plans to develop a survey that would reflect what the students felt they were looking for in the opposite sex fell victim to the students' inability to formulate the characteristics in concrete terms.

PROGRAM EVALUATION

Participation Data

Student participation and evaluation data provides the most direct evaluation of the program. According to the records for all of the computer interviews, workshops, and other activities there were 2,542 contacts with the program, an average of 2.4 contacts per student registered in the school. Aside from the 811 of these contacts represented by participation in the salad bar and roller-skating surveys, we found that 17 students spent many hours planning and programming computer interviews and that 390 took one or more computer interviews. Another seven worked with Wellness staff to plan programs and demonstrations that were attended by more than 1,500 students.

Participation data was also reflected in the spring (posttest) survey which included detailed questions for the target school about student awareness and activity in the program. According to questionnaire responses 89% of the students had heard of the program, 34% said they had stopped by the Wellness office (69% of whom took a computer interview). Heaviest program participation was reported for 9th and 10th graders and females (which also corresponded to our records). The greater attraction of the younger students to the program was due, in our opinion, to their greater social insecurity coupled with the fact that they had less structured school (and after school) time than the upper-class persons. In addition it was our impression (confirmed by data analysis) that students who were attracted to the Wellness Program may have been somewhat more troubled than other students. The fact that the program was clearly defined as independent of school or parental authority and that staff members attempted to maintain an open, supportive nonjudgmental stance (and worked diligently to stay neutral in disputes between students, teachers and administrators) was also important. The fact that all of the permanent staff were female may well have contributed in part to the higher participation level for females. The greater ease we observed among male students with male visiting consultants was a clear indication of the importance of same-sex staff for programs that hope to involve adolescents in sensitive issues. This was probably further affected by the somewhat more "feminine" topics that the students chose (e.g., nutrition, cooking, skin care). For a young man to express interest in these activities might expose him to real or fantasied ridicule by male friends.

Impact on Depression and Other Symptoms at Posttest

Considering the variety of issues addressed by the Wellness Program and the wide range of student contact it may not have been entirely realistic to expect a strong school-wide effect on depression. Nevertheless data from the matched sample of students who took both pre and posttest surveys allowed us to consider whether there was any discernible program impact. This was examined by analyses of covariance of depression and GSI scores with pretest scores as covariates, and grade, sex, Wellness Program participation (none, low, high) and pretest depression status (low vs. high according to a cut-off at the 60th percentile for community adults) as independent variables. There was no main effect for program participation. Significant interaction of participation by grade reflected the tendency for program involvement to be associated with especially high posttest symptom levels among 10th graders. As there were no main effects associated with the classification by pretest depression levels or interactions of pretest depression with participation, there was no evidence of differential program impact by initial depression. Instead, as illustrated in the means in Table 4, it appeared more

Table 4 Means and standard deviations of pre- and posttest depression by level of program participation

Participation	Pretest			Posttest		
	n	*M*	*SD*	*n*	*M*	*SD*
None	146	.59	.56	143	.64	.60
Low	23	.78	.62	23	.97	.59
High	64	.84	.71	64	.87	.74

likely that differences in initial symptomatology led to differences in program attraction as opposed to program impact.

To explore this possibility we did an analysis of variance of *pretest* depression scores with sex, grade and participation as factors. Aside from sex and grade differences that have already been described, we found a monotonic relationship between *pretest* depression and program participation (i.e., a significant main effect for participation and a sex by participation interaction). When pretest means were compared with posttest we saw little program effect. Thus it was far more apparent that the program was attractive to the more depressed adolescents than it was clear that there was any substantial decrease in depression as a function of the program.

CONCLUSIONS

With Regard to Depression and Adolescents

Our data suggest that depression may be a significant problem among adolescents, particularly among younger students and females. Depression, however, was not the most important complaint in the adolescent's eyes. Interpersonal sensitivity and hostility were prominent concerns. Males were also higher in phobic avoidance. In addition to these symptoms, adolescents in our study seemed particularly high in problems with dating adjustment and had low self-esteem.

With Regard to Predictors of Depression

Depression was most clearly associated over time with an oppressive self-concept, i.e., in terms of Benjamin's (1974) model, a propensity for unfriendly control of self. In addition depression was sometimes associated with high self-management, a more benign facet of self-control, and with low self-acceptance. Depression was also related to social adjustment problems particularly in student, social leisure, and family domains. Finally smoking in females and alcohol consumption in males was related to depression. Notably absent was any relationship of depression to low exercise levels.

With Regard to Prevention Programs

In a "free choice" setting it was clearly the more depressed adolescents who were attracted to prevention program activities. In our setting, for example, it was our impression (confirmed by SCL-90 data) that the program appealed to and met needs in the less secure, more depressed, and less socially integrated students.

Computer technology proved to be a hopeful adjunct or "hook" for the students. Its novelty (probably more so at the time the program was begun than at present) helped lure the students into the program office. In addition, the interactive interview with its features of free choice, privacy, and branching options allowed the students to confront sensitive topics (e.g., sexuality, drug use, etc.) that they were typically loath to discuss with adults. Although time and resources did not allow us sufficient scope to develop the full range of programs the adolescents wanted or needed, the potential was great.

It was very important that the programming (both computer and human) was flexible and responsive to the students' interests and needs. That our exercise program fizzled while enthusiasm for roller disco thrived is but one example of how well-intentioned adults may fail to see possibilities for adolescent learning. The implication for prevention programming is that the medium and style of program delivery may be as or even more important than the content or message.

In short, the adolescents were responsive to the upbeat and different. They were put off by any implications that we, the experts, knew what was best. Our expertise and resources worked well when they could be used to help follow through in support of (rather than to direct and shape) their interests. While it was crucially important to "deliver" on promises, it was equally essential for us to let the students initiate the ideas, i.e., to hitch our expertise and organizational skill to their enthusiasm.

The style and personality of our program staff was extremely important in this regard. The warm, open, relaxed atmosphere in the office was invaluable. It was especially crucial that we were able to stay "neutral" in the school setting, i.e., not to become involved in school disputes. It was also important that we allowed some of the adolescents to become leaders and expert programmers in our settings.

In sum, our data suggest two important conclusions about the style and the content of prevention programs:

1. Adolescents are very likely to be turned off by and drop out of any program that is authoritarian or that smacks of adult do-gooding or threatens their already tenuous social comfort and esteem.

2. Depression was consistently associated with "unfriendly" self-oppressive feelings, reflecting endorsement of SASB items concerned with (see Figure 2) self-destruction (330, 331), self-punishment (322, 333), self-blame (334, 335), insecurity (336), restraint (337) and conformity (338). Pretest depression was also associated with "friendly" self-control as reflected in items of the self-management quadrant of Benjamin's (1974) model which includes items for self-control (340), self-improvement (348), self-monitoring (347), self-protection and enhancement (346–348). According to Benjamin's (1974) model behaviors from adjacent quadrants are especially likely to occur together or follow each other in time. The shift, for example, from self-monitoring (347) to restraint (337) involves only a shift in the amount of friendliness; the amount of control is identical. This suggests that some aspects of "self-control" programs could indeed reinforce depressogenic tendencies in the very people they are intended to help. It will be important in planning programs to find the line between friendly self-direction and self-protection on one hand, and hostile self-control with implications of guilt, blame and rigidity, on the other.

With Regard to the Results of Prevention Programs and Related Research Issues

It is very difficult to design and carry out research to demonstrate the benefits of prevention programs, especially programs that are offered on a free choice basis in naturalistic settings:

1. The effects of complex programs are bound to be themselves complex and difficult to capture in any one set of measures.
2. The effects of all the other events and influences on the participants are bound to be strong, particularly when dealing with milder levels of distress than are seen in treatment oriented settings.
3. Selection or attrition bias is a huge problem in prevention research. The fact that the more disturbed adolescents were the ones who were attracted to our program meant that we were probably not truly preventing but intervening, i.e., that we had established a quasi-therapeutic setting.

Thus, if the program is to be evaluated in a large and complex naturalistic setting, large effects will be unlikely, and significant changes within individuals may well be lost or obscured in a mass of data.

General Conclusions

We still do not know enough about how people naturally prevent, cope with, or intervene in their distress without the "help" of programs and interveners to adequately design prevention programs. Successful treatment strategies may not automatically translate to preventive settings and there is much more to be learned in the field.

To return to the theme of self-oppression and self-control: We must recognize that depression may be a complex or heterogenous phenomenon with different subtypes or phases of depression that are distinguishable with respect to the kind of disturbance in self-control. In some cases depression may be associated with too little self-control, in others with too much. When depression is the result of uncontrollable external factors, it will be beneficial to restore autonomy and internal direction through prevention or intervention strategies. When depression is associated with chronic internal attributions (i.e., self-oppression), the emphasis of self-control programs may simply reinforce depressogenic styles and make things worse. Thus, it may be especially important to consider where people start with respect to the variable of self-control, i.e., to know what their depressive process is like.

This distinction is particularly important in thinking about research and programming in treatment vs. non-treatment contexts where different phases of the depressive process may be involved: (a) Prevention or intervention efforts to strengthen internal direction and coping that take place early in situations where people face uncontrollable external circumstances may be helpful; (b) once depression has persisted, taken hold, and lowered self-esteem (e.g. Abramson, Seligman, & Teasdale, 1978) the phenomenology is different. At the point where blame and responsibility is internalized, self-control messages may make things worse; and (c) a later phase of depression is often seen in treatment settings. When people seek help for depression it may be because they have given up on self-control attempts and have accepted the fact that help from others is needed. For them, self-control strategies may indeed restore them to a relatively more autonomous level of functioning if the treatment is one that values and reinforces autonomy and self-esteem. In sum, the distinction between autonomy, which comes from inner direction and self-control which can lead to self-oppression, is one that must be kept in mind if genuinely helpful prevention programs are developed.

REFERENCES

Abramson, L. Y., Seligman, M. E. P., & Teasdale, J. D. (1978). Learned helplessness in humans: Critique and reformulation. *Journal of Abnormal Psychology, 87,* 49–74.

Benjamin, L. S. (1974). Structural analysis of social behavior. *Psychological Review, 81,* 392–425.

Benjamin, L. S. (1984). Principles of prediction using Structural Analysis of Social Behavior (SASB). In R. A. Zucker, J. Arnoff, & A. J. Robin (Eds.) *Personality and the prediction of behavior* (pp. 121–174). New York: Academic Press.

Derogatis, L. R. (1983). *The SCL-90-R administration, scoring and procedures manual-II* (2nd ed.) Baltimore: Clinical Psychometric Research.

Derogatis, L. R., Lipman, R. S., & Covi, L. (1973). SCL-90: An outpatient psychiatric rating scale: Preliminary report. *Psychopharmacology Bulletin, 9,* 13–27.

Greist, J. H., Gustafson, D. H., Stauss, F. F., Rowse, G. L., Laughren, T. P., & Chiles, J. A. (1973). A computer interview for suicide risk prediction. *American Journal of Psychiatry, 130,* 1327–1332.

Greist, J. H., & Klein, M. H. (1980). Computer programs for patients, clinicians, and researchers in psychiatry. In J. B. Sidowski, J. H. Johnson, & T. Williams (Eds.), *Technology in mental health care delivery systems* (pp. 161–182). Norwood: Ablex Publishing.

Greist, J. H., & Klein, M. H. (1981). Computers in psychiatry. In S. Arieti & H. K. H. Brody (Eds.), *American handbook of psychiatry (2nd ed.): Vol. 7. Advances and new directions* (pp. 750–777). New York: Basic Books.

Greist, J. H., Klein, M. H., Eischens, R. R., Faris, J. W., Gurman, A. S., & Morgan, W. P. (1978). Running through your mind. *Journal of Psychosomatic Research, 22,* 259–294.

Greist, J. H., Klein, M. H., Eischens, R. R., Faris, J. W., Gurman, A. S., & Morgan, W. P. (1979). Running as treatment for depression. *Comprehensive Psychiatry, 20,*41–54.

Greist, J. H., Klein, M. H., & Erdman, H. P. (1978). Computer interviewing: Beyond data collection. In F. H. Orthner (Ed.), *Proceedings of the Second Annual Symposium on Computer Application in Medical Care* (pp. 5–9). Washington, DC: Institute of Electrical and Electronics Engineers, Inc.

Greist, J. H., Klein, M. H., & Van Cura, L. J. (1973). A computer interview for psychiatric patient target symptoms. *Archives of General Psychiatry, 29,* 247–253.

Greist, J. H., Klein, M. H., Van Cura, L. J., & Erdman, H. P. (1975). The computer interview as a medium for collecting questionnaire data on drug use in predicting adolescent drug use: Predicting adolescent drug abuse. In D. J. Lettieri (Ed.), *Predicting adolescent drug use: A review of issues, methods and correlates* (pp. 147–164). Washington, DC: Government Printing Office.

Gustafson, D. H., Greist, J. H., Stauss, F. F., Erdman, H. P., & Laughren, T. P. (1977). A probabilistic system for identifying suicide attempters. *Computers in Biomedical Research, 10,* 83–89.

Lewinsohn, P. M., Muñoz, R. F., Youngren, M. A., & Zeiss, A. M. (1978). *Control your depression.* Englewood Cliffs, New Jersey: Prentice-Hall, Inc.

Slack, W. V., Hicks, G. P., Reed, C. E., & Van Cura, L. J. (1966). A computer-based medical history system. *New England Journal of Medicine, 274,* 194–198.

Van Cura, L. J. (1978). A self-administered health hazard appraisal. In F. H. Orthner (Ed.), *Proceedings of the Second Annual Symposium on Computer Applications in Medical Care* (p. 231). Washington, DC: Institute of Electrical and Electronics Engineers, Inc.

Van Cura, L. J., Jensen, N. M., & Greist, J. H. (1976). A self-administered health hazard appraisal. *Proceedings of the Mumps Users Group* (pp. 134–140). St. Louis, MO.

Van Cura, L. J., Jensen, N. M., Greist, J. H., Lewis, W. R., & Frey, S. R. (1975). Venereal disease interviewing and teaching by computer. *American Journal of Public Health, 65,* 1159–1164.

Wanberg, K. W., Horn, J. L., & Foster, F. M. (1977). A differential assessment model for alcoholism: The scales of the Alcohol Use Inventory. *Journal of Studies on Alcohol, 38,* 512–543.

Weissman, M. M., & Paykel, E. S. (1974). *The depressed woman: A study of social relationships.* Chicago: University of Chicago Press.

Weissman, M. M., & Rothwell, S. (1976). Assessment of social adjustment by patient self-report. *Archives of General Psychiatry, 33,* 1111–1115.

7

Running Therapy in the Treatment of Depression: Implications for Prevention

Wesley E. Sime and Mark Sanstead
University of Nebraska, Lincoln

INTRODUCTION

Recent studies suggest that exercise may be effective and somewhat more efficacious than verbal psychotherapy as an antidepressant treatment for some patients (Buffone, 1984; Sime, 1984). Running is by far the most prevalent form of exercise therapy, primarily because it requires no specific skills and it fosters the aerobic training and biochemical changes thought to be involved in the antidepressant effect. It is also a functional self-regulatory activity that enhances a physiological and biochemical homeostasis. The intensity, duration and frequency of training appear to be crucial variables influencing the extent of antidepressant effect. Exercise of moderate intensity for 3 times a week appears to be the minimum requirement though there are too few studies available to attempt to show a linear relationship between these variables and the extent of antidepressant effect.

Theories regarding the antidepressant mechanisms include: (1) the apparent increase in blood flow and oxygenation to the central nervous system, (2) increased norepinephrine levels and (3) increased endorphin levels. Most studies have been cross-sectional in nature looking at varied populations (sedentary, moderately active, and marathoners). The self-selection bias in these studies, as well as in the experimental studies that recruit interested subjects, is obvious. In spite of this problem there is sufficient evidence to suggest that exercise is the intervention of choice for some individuals, particularly those who have had some previous positive experience with exercise. Those individuals who experience the greatest antidepressant effect also develop a sense of "mastery" over their environment, which certainly has its own inherent therapeutic benefits relative to many psychogenic disorders including depression.

The role of exercise in the prevention and/or treatment of clinical depression is quite viable because of its active nature which provides, in addition to the feeling of "mastery," side benefits in the form of enhanced body image (weight loss, increased strength and fitness) with an apparent increase in self-worth. These additional outcomes of exercise would seem to facilitate the antidepressant response particularly among those individuals who value strength, fitness and weight control.

EFFECT OF EXERCISE ON DEPRESSION

Several recent review articles have summarized the research on the antidepressant effect of exercise (Mihevic, 1982; Folkins & Sime, 1981; Berger, 1984). The most comprehensive of these, by Folkins and Sime, (Folkins & Sime, 1981) compared seven studies dealing with exercise and depression. All of these (Kowal, Patton, & Vogel, 1978; Davidson & Schwartz, 1976; Folkins, 1976; Folkins, Lynch, & Gardner, 1972; Berger & Owen, 1983; Lynch, Folkins, & Wilmore, 1978; Tredway, 1978) showed significant improvements in mood state particularly where level of depression was higher than normal prior to training. However, only four of these showed documented evidence of simultaneous increase in fitness level attendant to the antidepressant effect (Kowal, Patton, & Vogel, 1978; Davidson & Schwartz, 1976; Folkins, 1976; Folkins, Lynch, & Gardner, 1972). Furthermore, as with the research on anxiety, the studies described above are quite encouraging, but are fraught with experimental design problems thus precluding any definitive statement.

EXERCISE AND DEPRESSION RESEARCH
DESIGN PROBLEMS

More recent research since those reviews has yielded a series of studies and somewhat better experimental control (Morgan, Roberts, Brand, & Feinerman, 1970; Joesting, 1981a; Joesting, 1981b; Wilson, Berger, & Bird, 1980; Wilson, Morely, & Bird, 1980; Buffone, 1980; Rueter & Harris, 1980). Two of these showed that exercise therapy was an effective treatment for depression (Morgan, Roberts, Brand, & Feinerman, 1970), particularly when used simultaneously with traditional psychotherapy (Rueter & Harris, 1980). Experimental control was still lacking; however, Joesting demonstrated in two cross-sectional studies that level of depression was lower in populations self-selected into vigorous activity, i.e., runners versus sailors (Joesting, 1981a) and distance runners (Joesting, 1981b). These results are inconclusive because of the self-selection bias. The counter-argument is that some depressed individuals seek out vigorous activity while others find it to be uncomfortable and ineffective treatment. Exercise may be considered one of a number of treatments which are differentially effective among various subgroups. As such, the results portray a need for a more sensitive diagnostic and a selective prescriptive process, thus developing criteria by which to assign patients to diverse treatments for greater likelihood of successful therapeutic outcome. Two other studies have provided data suggesting that the relative degree of distance/intensity and adherence is related to mood enhancement. Among three groups ranked according to intensity of exercise habits, there was a negative linear relationship between distance covered (versus no exercise control) and level of depression (Wilson, Berger, & Bird, 1981). Similarly, compliance was clearly associated (negatively) with level of depression in a long-term follow-up study over 4 years in cardiac patients (Kavanagh, Shepard, Tuck, & Qureshi, 1977). One of the most likely reasons why compliance still is a problem in exercise research is because one of the major symptoms of, or outcomes of, depression is a feeling of lassitude or even antipathy toward exercise of any sort. Thus exercise can be an aversive experience when used exclusively in the treatment of depression.

CLINICAL CONSIDERATIONS IN EXERCISE
AND DEPRESSION STUDIES

The most well-controlled clinical treatment research regarding exercise and depression has been done by Greist and colleagues (Greist, Klein, Eischens, Fairs, Gurman, & Morgan, 1978; Greist, Klein, Eischens, Faris, Gurman, & Morgan, 1979). They conducted a series of studies utilizing clinically depressed patients who, most importantly, were randomly assigned to treatment groups. They observed that exercise was equally as effective in reducing depression as time-limited psychotherapy (Greist, Klein, Eischens, Fairs, Gurman, & Morgan, 1978 & 1979). Their success with depressed patients is apparently due to the very slow, graduated exercise program. Apparently it fosters a sense of mastery, a new positive self-image and perhaps some cathartic release while minimizing strain and injury that would hamper compliance, particularly among a patient population.

While the clinical efficacy of antidepressant exercise awaits conclusive, definitive support, there is enough empirical evidence to pursue preventive strategies with much vigor. Brown embarked upon a very large study on a normal population regarding antidepressant exercise (Brown, Ramirez, & Taub, 1978). In a two phase project he worked with over 600 students who self-selected an activity varying according to aerobic work demands and according to frequency per week. Acknowledging the limitations associated with self-selection, it was still apparent that the reductions in depression were a function of intensity, duration and frequency of exercise.

It is apparent that design considerations are crucial in studying the effect of exercise for the prevention of depression. Unfortunately, the nature of exercise itself precludes any control for expectancy or any attempts at using a double-blind design. Thus wherein it is not feasible to use a matched control group, a single group design with multiple baseline and extensive follow-up is suggested.

Psychophysiological Correlates of the Antidepressant Effect
Cortical Blood Flow

From a physiological or biochemical standpoint there are several possible mechanisms to link exercise outcome with decreased depression. One practicing clinician in the field, Kostrubala, (1977) has suggested that increased blood flow and oxygenation might have a significant influence on the central nervous system causing mood changes. Laboratory research supporting this hypothesis showed a regional increase in cerebral blood flow in the area of the motor cortex of the hemisphere contralateral to the isolated hand that was exercised (Oleson, 1971).

Catecholamines (Epinephrine and Norepinephrine)

Another theory suggests that since exercise increases norepinephrine level (Howley, 1976) and since norepinephrine is known to be low in depressed persons (Schildkraut, 1965), perhaps it is the norepinephrine which accounts for the antidepressant effect of exercise. In contrast, however, those increased levels of catecholamines (norepinephrine and epinephrine) both at rest and during exercise are associated with higher level of trait anxiety (Peronnet, Blier, Brisson, Ladoux,

Volle, & deCarufel, 1982) particularly in persons with type A coronary-prone behavior pattern (Olewine, Thomas, Simpson, Ramsey, Clark, & Hames, 1981). Thus high levels of epinephrine and norepinephrine are associated with elevations in both positive and negative emotions and moods. This illustrates the influence perception and interpretation of stressors has upon arousal and catecholamine secretion.

Self-Concept and Depression

Others have suggested that it is the sense of mastery and self-control which leads many exercising patients out of their depression (Greist, Klein, Eischens, Faris, Gurman, & Morgan, 1978; Greist, Klein, Eischens, Faris, Gurman, & Morgan, 1979). Improved body image and increased feelings of self-concept and self-worth would also play a major role in the prevention of depression (Folkins & Sime, 1981). Distinctly different from typical anxiety and depression research, the studies on self-concept demonstrate much better experimental controls (presumably because they tend to focus upon normal populations). Subsequent to the review by Folkins and Sime (Folkins & Sime, 1981), two additional studies (both randomized and controlled) have come forth showing equally positive results. These are described below.

Collingwood showed significant increases in physical fitness, body attitude and self-acceptance in a clinical rehabilitation setting after 4 weeks of training (Collingwood, 1972). Further self-concept research by Jansonski and colleagues, demonstrated increased fitness and self-perception following a 10 week aerobic exercise class with randomized assignment to treatment versus wait-list control (Jasonski, Holmes, Solomon, & Agular, 1981). However, they failed to show a correlation between fitness changes and perceptual changes. They concluded that group participation and expectancies played a major role in the elevated self-concept. Fortunately exercise carries a strong expectancy factor inherent in its very nature (more so than most other behavioral or drug interventions), thus it should be considered a complementary aspect of the treatment. Self-concept has been treated as a factor somewhat related to depression, though it is generally considered to be a component of personality. Other dimensions of personality are reviewed in the next section.

EXERCISE PRESCRIPTION FOR CONTROL
OF DEPRESSION

The state of the art in exercise therapy has not advanced to the sophistication of prescribing specific exercises according to diagnostic criteria nor according to narrowly defined psychological problems. However, there are some basic guidelines that do apply to depression as indicated by the successes observed in some clinical programs. These guidelines are outlined in great detail by Eischens and Greist (1984) and Berger (1984).

Exercise Prescription Protocol and Contra-Indications

From the perspective of a very successful clinical practice and clinical research program, Eischens and Greist (1984) made the following recommendations. They suggest that the therapist provide a leadership program with a slow, progressively increasing exercise plan. The patient will have greater likelihood of symptom abatement when he or she has: 1) developed a regularly scheduled routine for daily exercise sessions, 2) considerable patience, thus allowing at least 4-6 weeks before expecting positive results, 3) a specific goal with the intent to accomplish something other than just symptom relief while appreciating the process as much as, or more than, the outcome, i.e., enjoyment and 4) developed a consciousness about physical and psychological responses, striving toward a feeling of self-mastery yet knowing when to use distractions and fantasies. He further suggests that the therapist will be more effective by: 1) ensuring that treatment never does more harm than good, acknowledging that exercise, like many therapies, is a double-edged sword, 2) ensuring that the treatment is, in fact, appropriate for this patient, acknowledging the contraindications for exercise based upon watchful concern for endogenous psychotic depressives, as well as patients with significant cardiovascular risk and 3) ensuring that the dosage is correct at the outset and throughout a preplanned program of graduated exercise instruction.

Berger has reviewed a larger volume of research that is relevant to an antidepressant exercise therapy (1984). She recommends a prescription specifying a minimum of 3 times/week (frequency), 20 minutes/session (duration), at 70-85% of maximal aerobic capacity (intensity) which is typical of a standard aerobic exercise program for development of cardiovascular fitness. However, Brown has shown that a frequency of 5 sessions/week is more effective than 3 sessions for reducing depression (Brown, Ramirez, & Taub, 1978). Furthermore, regarding duration of exercise, 40-60 minutes/session has been shown to be more effective in reducing depression than 20 minutes (Peronnet, Blier, Brisson, Ladoux, Volle, & deCarufel, 1976). At the other extreme, Dienstbier has shown that a moderate intensity (distance of 6 miles) is more effective in reducing depression than a full marathon, even in well-trained runners (Dienstbier, 1978). He also suggested that the exercise therapy should follow a scheduled routine which does not disrupt normal lifestyle, occupation or domestic patterns. Further practical considerations put forth by Berger (1984) include having the patient:

1. begin slow and run with a companion.
2. select good quality running shoes, use short comfortable leg stride and avoid hard uneven surfaces.
3. keep moving, even if fatigue precludes running and necessitates slow walking.
4. monitor intensity with the talk test (never exert beyond capacity to maintain conversation if it is desired) and decrease subsequent session intensity or duration if recovery from a single exercise bout exceeds one hour.
5. keep a log of activity for motivation, for immediate reinforcement and to chronicle progress.
6. make a behavioral contract with a substantial bonus for success and a meaningful penalty for failure.

Psychotherapy Combined with Exercise Therapy

Likelihood of success with antidepressant exercise therapy is greater if the therapist includes traditional counseling or psychotherapy during or in conjunction with exercise and if the therapist ensures that the patient always views his running experience in a positive sense (Rueter & Harris, 1980). Heaps (1978) showed that patients that ran with a faster confederate who made derogatory comments had lower self-acceptance and more negative feelings about their fitness and body functioning than those patients that ran with a confederate who was complementary regardless of the patients' actual fitness level (Schildkraut, 1965). These results seem obvious but they have great importance in the overall success of a program. Dienstbier (1978) had some additional insightful comments noting that novice runners need more extrinsic rewards at the outset of an exercise program. His observation was that novice runners do not experience the same immediate pleasures from running that habitual runners encounter. For example, they may not experience mood elevation, stress reduction, peak experiences and sense of accomplishment until after 2–3 months of exercise at progressively increasing duration and intensity. Thus the novice runner must be instructed to notice the short-term pleasures (tension relief, scenic outdoors, etc.) and to anticipate the long-term benefits to be derived in the near future.

Lastly the patient should be fully cognizant of the fact that exercise is a very aggressive, active therapy for depression and that it will lead him or her toward a feeling of self-responsibility. While much of the discussion above has dealt with clinical therapy, the principles are equally appropriate for prevention as for treatment. In an era where prevention, wellness and health promotion are emphasized, any treatment which shifts the burden of responsibility from the health-care treatment institution back to the patient is commendable and worth the additional efforts needed to foster it.

Adherence Problems in Exercise

It is evident that exercise is not the treatment of choice for some patients. The average attrition rate within six months after start of exercise is about 50% (Dishman, 1982). Some researchers (Beck, Rush, Shaw, & Emery, 1979; Wilson, Bergen, & Bird, 1981) have suggested that the problem of exercise adherence is quite analogous to that of medical compliance. Since the mechanism for the therapeutic benefit of exercise is not well understood, it has been extremely difficult to identify the most promising candidates for exercise interventions. Possible determinants in exercise therapy include motivation, exercise dosage, exercise format, age, and attitude toward exercise.

It is apparent that further research is needed to investigate the source and process of therapeutic benefits of exercise as well as the candidates who are most likely to benefit. Previous research suggests that studies on fitness training must be focused upon individual differences (Blumenthal, Williams, Needles, & Wallace, 1982) and must utilize innovative experimental designs such as time series analysis.

A SINGLE–CASE DESIGN
MULTIPLE–BASELINE STUDY

The purpose of this study was to examine and compare the process and nature of psychological change of individuals participating in a graduated exercise program for the treatment of depression. An intensive cross-sectional time series design was utilized to monitor depression on multiple levels throughout a two-week baseline and ten-week aerobic exercise program. Depression was assessed on a daily, weekly and pre- and post-questionnaire measures. In addition, subjects were interviewed weekly to investigate their reaction to the study procedures.

The focus of this study was on individual differences in response to exercise interventions. It was hypothesized that there are identifiable characteristics of individuals which can aid the practitioner in the prescription of exercise therapy. These positive indicators include: self-motivation level, ideal body weight, past pleasurable exercise participation, and a positive expectation for benefit from exercise. Secondly, it was assumed that a graduated exercise program would minimize attrition and encourage exercise maintenance. Finally, it was hypothesized that depression would be significantly reduced following the aerobic exercise intervention.

Population

The subjects were 14 women and one man ranging in age from twenty-six to fifty-three years, who sought help for symptoms of depression. All were employed, but eight worked only part-time. Five were divorced, seven were married and three were single. All subjects had completed high school. One subject had an M.S. degree, four had B.A. degrees and nine had some post high school training or college. Diagnostic information (DSM–III or RDC) were not available on these subjects.

Design

In this multiple-baseline across subjects design each subject acted as his or her own control. Multiple measures of depression were obtained over several weeks of screening and a two-week baseline which preceded the ten-week exercise portion of the study. The dependent variable, depressed mood, was assessed by interview and by daily self-report measures. Following the baseline period, the independent variable exercise was introduced in a graduated aerobic exercise program, which consisted of walking and/or jogging. Most of the subjects also participated in a two-week non-aerobic stretching program between the baseline and aerobic activity. This format was used to extend the baseline period and to control for a socialization effect and for expectancy.

Instruments

Beck Depression Inventory (BDI)

Is a 21-item self-report inventory (score range 0–63) developed to measure the intensity of depression. The higher the score, the more severe the depression. The validity and internal consistency of the instrument have been well established (Wilson, Morley, & Bird, 1980). The BDI was selected because it is a short and convenient screening tool in measuring the presence and level of depression.

Profile of Mood States (POMS)

Consists of 65, five-point adjective rating scales which are factored into six mood scores: tension-anxiety, depression-dejection, anger-hostility, vigor-activity, fatigue-inertia, and confusion-bewilderment. Each score is derived from the sum of ratings over 7 to 15 adjectives; there is no item overlap.

Reliability appears to be quite high and acceptable. The K-R 20 values range from .84 to .95. Test-retest correlations ranged from .65 to .74. The POMS scales have considerable face validity. Studies of predictive validity have shown that brief psychotherapy and minor tranquilizers produced a change in the expected direction of the POMS scores of experimental groups while there were no changes in the control groups.

The POMS was selected for use in this study because: 1) it is a valid measure of mood states, and 2) it provides a measure of depression couched among other variables so that the specific mood state of interest is not obvious to the patient.

Daily Mood Scale

Is a self-report measure constructed for this study. Mood was rated daily on a ten-point scale with each and grounded at "terrible" and "very good." Subjects were encouraged to jot down things that might have accounted for the mood of the day. Daily sleep and appetite were also recorded on a five-point scale grounded at "poor" and "good." There was also a space provided to record daily exercise activity.

Bicycle Ergometer Exercise Test

Is a means of estimating maximal oxygen uptake during an all-out physical effort. The measurement known as the maximum oxygen uptake (VO_2 max), or aerobic capacity is considered a prime indicator of physical fitness. As with fitness tests in general, the bicycle ergometer utilizes a large muscle group (legs). After the subject has warmed up on the bicycle, the work load is increased to a uniform standard and maintained for five minutes. The average heart rate of the fourth and the fifth minute is used to compute general level of fitness. The bicycle ergometer test was selected for this study to document physiological changes occurring as a result of treatment.

Self-Motivation Inventory (SMI)

Is a forty-item, true-false scale to assess self-motivation. Self-motivation was conceptualized as a behavioral tendency to persevere independent of situational reinforcements. Test-retest measures of reliability indicated a high degree of scale stability (r's ranged from 0.86 to 0.92). Measures of internal consistency have yielded an estimate = 0.91. Convergent evidence for construct validity was provided by the Self-Motivation Inventory relationship with the Thomas-Zander Ego-Strength Scale (r = 0.63) and more behaviorally specific attitudes (r's ranged

Table 1 Study Procedures

Activity	Initial meeting	Week 1	Week 2	Week 3-11	Final meeting
Screening interview	X				
Beck Depression Scale	X		X		X
Profile of mood states	X	X	X	X	X
Pre-fitness text		X			
Weekly interview		X	X	X	
Collect daily mood measure		X	X	X	X
Nonaerobic exercise				X	
Aerobic exercise				X	
Post-fitness test					X
Exit interview					X

from 0.47 to 0.58). Predictive validity was demonstrated in a variety of naturalistic settings in which perseverant behavior was easily quantified. These have included habitual exercise programs for exercise training, preventive medicine and acute exercise. Findings have provided considerable support for the valid and reliable assessment of self-motivation and the prediction of adherence to therapeutic exercise.

Procedure

The subjects were referred by psychologists from a local health maintenance organization, a university counseling center, a state vocational rehabilitation agency and a private fitness and diet center. Potential subjects were told of a university study investigating the process and effectiveness of exercise in the treatment of depression. The exercise program was described as appropriate for beginners and would consist of walking, running and stretching three to four times a week. Interested potential subjects were asked to contact the investigator.

The investigators conducted a screening interview with all patients who referred and utilized the Beck Depression Inventory as a screening instrument for depression. Two potential subjects were excluded because their Back score did not confirm mild to moderate depression. All 15 subjects were in this category.

The study procedures are outlined in Table 1. During the first meeting, the investigator met individually with each subject and explained that the study would last ten weeks and would require weekly contact with the investigator. Subjects were told they would be allowed to decide if they would exercise individually or in a group led by the investigator. The subjects completed the Profile of Mood States and Self-Motivation Inventory. In addition, they completed subject release forms which included a brief description of the study. Subjects were instructed about the procedure for filling out the Daily Mood Measure and were scheduled for a bicycle ergometer fitness test. The subjects were also interviewed regarding their expectations for the exercise. The investigator met with each subject one week later. The Daily Mood Measure was collected and another POMS was administered. Each subject was interviewed according to the Weekly Interview format.

During the second week of the baseline period, subjects were scheduled to take a submaximal fitness test with a bicycle ergometer at the Human Performance Laboratory at the University of Nebraska-Lincoln. Each subject was required to obtain the written consent of his or her physician prior to testing.

At the end of the second week and baseline period, each subject completed the BDI, POMS and handed in the Daily Mood Measure. Each subject was individually interviewed according to the Weekly Interview format. During this meeting, the investigator assisted each subject in planning an appropriate graduated exercise program. The first seven subjects who started the study were instructed to begin a non-aerobic two-week stretching program. The stretching program consisted of a ten-minute routine which utilized 25 exercises to stretch the major muscle groups. Subjects were encouraged to go through this routine four times a week on an individual basis.

All 15 subjects were assisted in their aerobic exercise program. Initial discussion covered proper footwear, advantages of walking or jogging, exercising, pacing and duration and frequency. Special emphasis was placed on the careful self-monitoring of a very graduated exercise program to avoid injury and reduce adverse experiences.

Subjects who were most comfortable starting a walking program were instructed to walk ten minutes a day four times a week. They were instructed to go slowly the first three to five minutes in order to gradually stretch their muscles and tendons.

Subjects who were in better physical condition and prepared to begin a jogging program were instructed using the model of Greist, Klein, Eischens, Faris, Gurman, and Morgan (1979). This model suggested a very gradual initiation for the novice runner. Subjects were taught to warm up by walking for a few minutes. This was followed by easy jogging to the point of dyspnea, followed by another bout of walking till dyspnea diminishes. This cycle is then repeated continuously, gradually lengthening the running time and decreasing the walking interval. Subjects were instructed to carefully self-monitor exercise to avoid muscular strain. Each week the total duration of jogging and walking was gradually increased.

All subjects were invited to join the investigator on Monday and Wednesday evenings and Saturday mornings at a local scenic park for aerobic exercise. During these periods, the investigator would jog a third-of-a-mile lap with the joggers and then walk a lap with the walkers. This alternating pattern allowed the investigator to monitor the exercise of subjects no matter what their pace.

Throughout the study, the investigator met all subjects each week on an individual basis to discuss exercise progress and collect mood data. These meetings occasionally included exercising with the subjects. These meetings took place at a variety of settings including the university, the subject's home and the subject's place of employment. These meetings were usually thirty minutes in duration.

At the end of the study, subjects were scheduled for post-training fitness at the Human Performance Laboratory at the University of Nebraska-Lincoln. In addition to laboratory testing, the investigator conducted an exit interview which probed the subjects' perceptions of progress in mood and exercise activity. Subjects were also tested on all the mood measures which had been utilized throughout the study. Data Analysis consisted of comparison of mood during the baseline period and the exercise period.

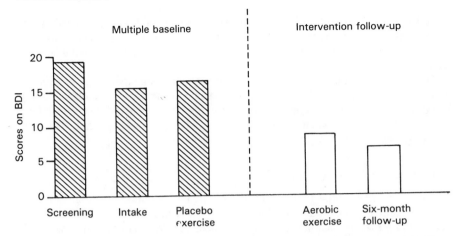

t-test of the differences between baseline and at six-month follow-up was significant
t = 3.47 (p < 0.02) (average of 2 or 3 scores); N = 13.

Figure 1 Mean scores on beck depression inventory (BDI) during multiple baseline placebo/exercise,
aerobic exercise and follow-up

Results

Of the 15 subjects who originally initiated treatment, three subjects dropped out
during the treatment phase. Reasons cited for discontinuing their participation
included moving to a new location, illness and accident to a spouse.

The subjects' scores on the Beck Depression Inventory at screening, baseline,
treatment and post-treatment are presented in Figure 1. These scores were computed by averaging the Beck scores for all subjects. The higher the score, the
greater the level of depression. In this study design, the multiple baseline measures
were not significantly different over three time periods of assessment which included screening, intake and a two-week placebo exercise treatment. Following
the exercise treatment there was a remarkable (though non-significant) decrease in
BDI scores but at six-month follow-up the scores were significantly lower. A t-test
showed that the differences were statistically significant (t = 3.47, p < 0.02). In
spite of small population sample, these data support the efficacy of exercise in the
treatment and secondary prevention of depression. Selected case study information
is provided below.

Selected Individual Reports of Antidepressant Effects

A 28-year-old, married Caucasian female who had been taking the prescription
medication (Ludiomil) for depression and had been seeing a psychologist and a
psychiatrist periodically for the past seven years.

When asked how she felt about exercise, after the study, she reported that she
had mixed feelings noting that exercising was hard and somewhat unpleasant but
so beneficial regarding her moods.

A 30-year-old, recently divorced Caucasian female said her depressive symptomatology included: insomnia, energy loss, lack of interest in usual activities, feelings of self-reproach, diminished ability to concentrate and occasional suicidal ideation.

One week after the termination of treatment, she summarized her experience with the study as follows: "I began to notice some of the causes and effects of my moods and in the end this helped me to control the depression with exercise. There was a time, however, when I noticed I could not force myself to run. This was when my depression was greatest."

Efficacy of Prevention Studies

Large scale, multilevel programs in the area of exercise are commonplace within Health Promotion and Wellness units. These are not specifically aimed at depression prevention but the spin-off benefits in that arena are evident. Two well-controlled studies evaluating such general health promotion exercise programs are of interest here. Both of these studies have dealt with normal, healthy subjects, one using a walk/jog model (Blumenthal, Williams, Needles, & Wallace, 1982) and the other swimming (Berger and Owens, 1984) to demonstrate the mood enhancement and antidepressant effect of exercise. Profile of mood state scores revealed dramatic changes in all six categories including depression.

CONCLUSION

The empirical evidence to support the use of exercise in mood enhancement and as an antidepressant is encouraging. Recent studies have demonstrated better experimental control conditions and more applicability in the role of prevention. Care must be taken in utilizing exercise given the contra-indications and the fact that it may not be appropriate for some individuals. More research is needed to characterize the appropriate candidates and the specific mechanism whereby the antidepressant effect occurs.

REFERENCES

Beck, A. T., Rush, A. J., Shaw, B. F., & Emery, G. (1979). *Cognitive therapy of depression.* New York: Guilford press.

Berger, B. (1984) Running away from anxiety and depression: A female as well as male race. In M. Sacks and G. Buffone (Eds.), *Running as therapy: An integrated approach.* University of Nebraska Press.

Berger, B., & Owen, D. K. (1983). Mood Alteration with swimming—Swimmers really do "feel better." *Psychomatic Medicine, 45,* (5), 425–433.

Blumenthal, J. A., Williams, S., Needles, T., & Wallace, K. (1982). Psychological changes accompany aerobic exercise in healthy middle-aged adults. *Psychosomatic Medicine, 44,* 529–536.

Brown, R. S., Ramirez, D. E., & Taub, J. M. (1978). The prescription of exercise for depression. *The Physician and Sports Medicine, 6,* 34–49.

Buffone, G. (1980). Exercise as therapy: A closer look. *Journal of Counseling and Psychotherapy, 3*(2), 101–115.

Buffone, G. (1984). Running and depression. In M. Sacks and G. Buffone (Eds.), *Running as therapy: An integrated approach.* University of Nebraska Press.

Carmack, M., & Martens, R. (1979). Measuring commitment to running: A survey of runners' attitudes and mental states. *Journal of Sport Psychology, 1,* 25–42.

Collingwood, T. (1972). The effects of physical training upon behavior and self-attitudes. *Journal of Clinical Psychology, 28,* 583–585.

Davidson, F. J., & Schwartz, G. E. (1976). The psychobiology of relaxation and related states: A multiprocess theory. In D. I. Mostofsky (Ed.), *Behavior control and modification of physiological activity.* Englewood Cliffs, N.J.: Prentice Hall.

Dienstbier, R. A. (1978). Running and personality change. *Today's Jogger, 2,* 30–33; 48–49.

Dishman, R. K. (1982). Compliance/adherence in health-related exercise. *Journal of Health Psychology, 1,* 237–267.

Eischens, R., & Greist, J. (1984). Beginning and continuing running: Steps to psychological well-being. In M. Sacks and G. Buffone (Eds.), *Running as therapy: An integrated approach.* University of Nebraska Press.

Folkins, C., & Sime, W. (1981). Physical fitness training and mental health. *American Psychologist, 36,* 373–389.

Folkins, C. H., Lynch, S., & Gardner, M. M. (1972). Psychological fitness as a function of physical fitness. *Archives of Physical Medicine and Rehabilitation, 53,* 503–508.

Folkins, G. H. (1976). Effects of physical training on mood. *Journal of Clinical Psychology, 32,* 385–388.

Greist, J. G., Klein, M. H., Eischens, R. R., Faris, J., Gurman, A. S., & Morgan, W. P. (1978). Running through your mind. *Journal of Psychosomatic Research, 22,* 259–294.

Greist, J. H., Klein, M. H., Eischens, R. R., Faris, J., Gurman, A. S., & Morgan, W. P. (1979). Running as treatment for depression. *Comprehensive Psychiatry, 20,* 41–54.

Heaps, R. (1978). Relating physical and psychological fitness: A psychological point of view. *Journal of Sports Medicine and Physical Fitness, 18,* 399–408.

Howley, E. (1976). The effect of different intensities of exercise on the excretion of epinephrine and norepinephrine. *Medicine and Science in Sports, 8,* 219–222.

Jasonki, M., Holmes, D., Solomon, S., & Agular, C. (1981) Exercise, changes in aerobic capacity and changes in self-perceptions: An experimental investigation. *Journal of Research in Personality, 15,* 460–466.

Joesting, J. (1981). Comparison of personalities of athletes who sail with those who run. *Perceptual and Motor Skills, 52,* 514.

Joesting, J. (1981). Running and depression. *Perceptual and Motor Skills, 52,* 442.

Kavanagh, T., Shephard, R. J., Tuck, J. A., & Qureshi, S. (1977). Depression following myocardial infarction: The effects of distance running. In P. Milvy (Ed.), *The marathon: physiological, medical, epidemiological, and psychological studies. Annals of the New York Academy of Science, 301,* New York: Academy of Sciences.

Kostrubala, T. (1977). Jogging and personality change. *Today's Jogger, 1,* 14–15.

Kowal, D., Patton, J., & Vogel, J. (1978). Psychological states and aerobic fitness of male and female recruits before and after basic training. *Aviation, Space and environmental Medicine, 49,* 603–606.

Lynch, S., Folkins, C. H., & Wilmore, J. H. (1978). Relationships between three mood variables and physical exercise. Unpublished manuscript.

Mihevic, P. (1982). "Anxiety, depression and exercise." *Quest, 32*(2), 140–153.

Morgan, W., Roberts, J., Brand, F., & Feinerman, A. (1970). Psychological effect of chronic physical activity. *Medicine and Science in Sports, 2.* 213–217.

Olsen, J. (1971). Contralateral focal increases of cerebral blood flow in man during arm work. *Brain, 94,* 635–646.

Olewine, D., Thomas, G., Simpson, M., Ramsey, F., Clark, F., & Hames, C. (1981). Exercise response of plasma and urinary catecholamines in young males with type A and B behavior patterns. *Medicine and Science in Sport and Exercise, 13,* 80.

Peronnet, F., Blier, P., Brisson, G., Ladoux, M., Volle, M., & deCarufel, D. (1982). Relationship between trait anxiety and plasma catecholamine at rest and during exercise. *Medicine and Science in Sport and Exercise, 14,* 172–173.

Reuter, M., & Harris, D. (September, 1980). *Effects of running on individuals who are clinically depressed.* Paper presented at the meeting of the American Psychological Association Convention, Montreal, Canada.

Schildkaraut, J. (1965). The catecholamine hypothesis of affective disorders: A review of supporting evidence. *American Journal of Psychiatry, 122,* 509–522.

Sime, W. (1984). Psychological benefits of exercise training in the healthy individual. In Mattazaro, Miller, Weiss, Herd, Weiss (Eds.) *Handbook of behavior health*. John Wiley and Sons.

Tredway, V. A. (August, 1978). *Mood effects of exercise programs for older adults*. Paper presented at the meeting of the American Psychological Association, Toronto.

Wilson, V. E., Berger, B. G., & Bird, E. I. (1981). Effects of running and of an exercise class on anxiety. *Perceptual and Motor Skills, 53,* 474.

Wilson, V. E., Morley, N. C. (1980). Mood profiles of marathon runners, joggers, and non-exercisers. *Perceptual and Motor Skills, 50,* 117–118.

8

Primary Prevention of Postpartum Depression and Its Sequelae among Low-Income Hispanic Women

Cynthia Telles
The Neuropsychiatric Institute, UCLA

INTRODUCTION

Pregnancy has been described as a period of developmental crisis which requires a significant emotional and physiological adjustment of the mother. The resulting psychological adaptation is a function of complex and multidetermined processes. Biological factors interact with the pregnant woman's personality functioning and interpersonal relations; furthermore, this equilibrium is continuously affected by the interplay of social, cultural and economic forces exerted by both the external environment and the family. Additionally, the pregnancy itself may impose certain stresses on each of the aforementioned areas of functioning and lead to a disequilibrium in the general system and its subsystems (Caplan, 1957).

Pregnancy is, thus, a period of increased susceptibility, during which any number of specific factors may trigger strong reactions, which can contribute to the occurrence of postpartum psychological disturbances. Estimates of the incidence of postpartum depression in mostly non-Hispanic white populations vary. On the average, it is reported that postpartum psychotic reactions occur at the rate of one or two per 1000 births (Kaij & Nilsson, 1972) and that less severe depressions can affect up to 65% of the childbearing population (Pitt, 1968). There are no published data on the incidence of postpartum depression among Hispanic women. Recent data suggest, however, that low-income Hispanic women are at greater risk than the general population for developing depressive symptomatology. Furthermore, fertility and birth rates are significantly higher for Hispanics; thus, they are exposed more frequently to the stressful experience of childbirth and to the risk of postpartum depression. Extrapolating from these vital statistics and epidemiologic data, one could expect Hispanics to be over-presented among women in the general population who recently have given birth and are experiencing depressive symptomatology.

Pregnancy is not only a time of increased stress and additional risk, but it is also an ideal time for preventive intervention. As in any crisis experience, the balance may be tipped in either direction, resulting in generally adaptive or maladaptive responses (Cohen, 1966). The manner in which the equilibrium of forces is resolved may have a long-lasting effect on any area of functioning of the mother. It is known that during periods of crisis, as opposed to periods of stability, preventive intervention has a greater impact in terms of influencing the problem-solving mechanisms of the participant and the ultimate outcome. An investment of minimal energy on the part of key caretaking agents can be used at maximum efficiency during this time (Caplan, 1957).

The importance of early recognition of potentially pathogenic factors and subsequent preventive intervention is underscored by research findings, which document the impact of maternal pregnancy and postpartum adaptation on the physical and psychological well-being of the fetus and the developing infant (Ferreira, 1965). It appears that the mother's ability to respond to the child can be adversely affected by psychosocial stress and subsequent depression which interfere with the tasks of developing an affiliative response to the fetus and a healthy social tie to the neonate (Cohen, 1966). Difficulties in postpartum psychological adjustment, specifically, have been related to a maternal attitude of rejection toward the infant and to the disruption of appropriate parenting (Cohen, 1966; Deutscher, 1970; Hemphill, 1952; Pollit, 1965). These abnormalities in early mothering due to postpartum disturbance have been found to have long-term consequences for the mother-child relationship and to contribute to severe personality and mental defects in the child (Bibring, et al., 1961; Stott, 1962; Talovic, Mednick, Schulsinger, & Falloon, 1980; Uddenberg, & Uddenberg & Englesson, 1978).

In order to develop effective and efficient primary prevention programs for postpartum depression and its sequelae, it is necessary 1) to develop a conceptual framework, which includes an understanding of the nature and etiologies of the postpartum depressive syndromes. Additionally, it is critical 2) to identify a population at risk, 3) to empirically define associated risk factors, 4) to develop a prenatal individual assessment procedure for the selection of women, who are most at risk though not yet significantly pathological and in need of clinical services, 5) to design comprehensive perinatal programs whose strategies are targeted specifically to reduce the negative impact of the modifiable risk factors and, finally 6) to implement an evaluation program.

POSTPARTUM DEPRESSION SYNDROMES: DEFINITIONS, INCIDENCE, AND ETIOLOGIES

Depression of the postpartum period may be broadly defined by the occurrence of dysphoric affect developing after or being exacerbated by the delivery. The affected individual should describe depressive symptomatology and experience it as a more or less unusual and disabling condition (Pitt, 1973). There is considerable variability, however, in terms of the severity and the specific symptomatology which can be manifested.

In its mildest form, postpartum depression is defined as "maternity blues," a transitory syndrome found to include anxiety and mild confusion, as well as depression and tearfulness. Hamilton (1962) lists the various common symptoms in the following order of frequency: fatigue, crying, anxiety, confusion, headaches, insomnia, hypochondriasis and hostility toward the husband. Compared to a group of controls, women with maternity blues tend to worry more about their babies and to be more distressed over difficulties with lactation or feeding (Pitt, 1973).

Postpartum "blues" are said to occur on one or two days during the early puerperium. It is considered a common condition reported to occur following 50% (Pitt, 1973) to almost 80% (Robin, 1962) of all deliveries. Though there is a general consensus regarding the high incidence of postpartum blues, there is some disagreement over the contributing factors. Sclare (1955) states that this depressive reaction is primarily experienced by primigravidae and can be understood as symptomatic of narcissistic loss suffered by the mother before she has rediscovered her child. Other investigators have attributed this condition to hormonal changes (Railton, 1961) and environmental stress (Telles, 1982).

Some authors make a distinction between "maternity blues" and the more neurotic form of puerperal depression. The latter is described as beginning mildly during hospitalization and becoming more evident after the return home. It may be characterized by tearfulness, despondency, some lability of affect, feelings of inadequacy and inability to cope with the baby. Guilt is often experienced with regard to not loving or caring for the infant. Anxiety usually accompanies the depression and is partly expressed in the form of excessive concern over the baby. Hypochondriasis and frequent somatic complaints are common. Anorexia reportedly occurs with consistent regularity, and sleep disturbance is found in about one-third of the neurotically depressed women. It is important to note that a considerable percentage of women with puerperal depression experience symptomatology for longer than a few weeks (Pitt, 1968). In an unselected sample of mothers, interviewed up to one year after childbirth, 25% had more than six symptoms which had developed postpartum. Most persistent symptoms included fatigue, irritability, tension, and some anxiety (Jacobson, Kaij, & Nilsson, 1965).

This more neurotic form of puerperal depression occurs after delivery in about 7–10% of the mothers (Pitt, 1968). It appears that there is an increase in the reported incidence of all types of postpartum neurotic reactions which possibly reflects a growing recognition of these conditions over the years (Madden, Luhan, Tuteur, & Bimmerle, 1958). While Strecher and Ebaugh (1926) only classified 2% of the postpartum reactions in hospitalized women as neurotic, Smalldon (1940) reported 12.7%, Boyd (1942) about 14.4%, and Madden, Luhan, Tuteur and Bimmerle (1958) about 20.7%. For the most part, these neurotic reactions were of a depressive nature.

Much of the literature on puerperal psychoses does not attempt to differentiate between the various clinical syndromes. They are described as having in common a particular time of occurrence, generally within a month or two after childbirth. Additionally, it has been suggested that the psychoses occur with such relative frequency during the postpartum period as to indicate that there is a significant relation between these conditions and circumstances particular to childbearing. The postpartum psychoses, however, do not constitute a uniform specific disorder. Instead, they can be conceptualized more accurately as a collection of disorders.

As reviewed by Thomas and Gordon (1959), the reported incidence of postpartum psychosis among women delivering in clinical hospitals varies from .8 per 1000 to 2.5 per 1000, with Hemphill's (1952) figure of 1.4 per 1000 probably being the most accurate. The average frequency of psychoses precipitated by childbirth is about 8 per 1000 female admissions to psychiatric hospitals. Most reports indicate there is a relatively greater frequency of postpartum psychoses related to the first pregnancy and delivery (Thomas & Gordon, 1959). Psychotic depression is the most common of the puerperal psychoses treated in psychiatric hospitals (Pitt, 1968).

Over the years, there has been some debate concerning the nature and definition of postpartum depression. Generally, the issue is whether this disorder is to be viewed as a separate clinical and nosological entity, or whether it constitutes a syndrome characterized by an association with childbirth. Hemphill (1952) stated that there is a psychological entity, puerperal depression, which differs from the manic-depressive disorder and is similar in many ways to involutional melancholia. Among women with puerperal depression, the personality tends to be rigid and restricted. In addition to depressive affect and motor activity, it is usually characterized by marked indecision, lack of concentration and guilt. This syndrome is considered by some authors to be more specifically a toxic-exhaustive state, subsequent to long, hard labor, which constitutes a distinct clinical entity.

Many authors have argued the other side of the controversy, stating that, although the postpartum depression might be connected with childbirth in some way, its clinical manifestations are quite diverse and not unlike those of depressive disorders and psychoses unrelated to childbirth in women and men. This position is supported by Zilboorg (1929) and Brew and Seidenberg (1950) who argue that postpartum psychoses are the result of ordinary stresses of pregnancy which operate in predisposed individuals and produce a non-specific mental disorder. The trend towards not considering postpartum depression a separate entity follows a more general trend in psychology to view any psychopathology as multidetermined; at the same time, though, it does not make much sense to consider depression following pregnancy as merely a coincidence in timing (Sherman, 1971).

HISPANIC POPULATION GROWTH: IMPLICATIONS FOR PREVENTION OF CHILDBIRTH RELATED DISORDERS

Hispanics constitute the second largest and fastest growing ethnic group in the United States. The rapid rate of expansion is reflected in the U.S. Bureau of the Census Reports which estimated a population of 9.6 million Hispanics in 1970, 11.2 million in 1975 and 14.6 million in 1980 (U.S. Bureau of the Census, 1973, 1976, 1982). There are other estimates, however, which suggest that the total Hispanic population is comprised of more than 23 million persons when census undercount, increase from birth, and legal as well as undocumented immigration are taken into consideration. Furthermore, it is projected that by the year 2000, Hispanics will number 55.3 million and, thus, will become the largest ethnic minority in the United States (Macias, 1977).

Birth and fertility rates computed from representative data of nine selected states indicate that those rates continue to be much higher for Hispanics than for non-Hispanics in the United States. In 1979, the Hispanic birth rate was 25.5 births per 1000 as compared to 14.7 for the non-Hispanic population. The Mexican birth rate was even higher (29.6 per 1000) and 31% greater than for the Puerto Rican population (22.6). The fertility rate for the Hispanic population was 100.5 births per 1000 women between the ages of 15 and 44, and it was 59% greater than the rate of 63.2 for non-Hispanic women. Again the fertility rate for Mexican women of 119.3 per 1000 surpassed that of other groups and was 48% greater than the rate for Puerto Rican women (80.7) and three times greater than the rate for Cuban women (National Center for Health Statistics, 1982).

These significant population changes have very important implications for social and governmental institutions, which have been mandated to provide adequate health care to all groups in our society. It is clear that the national health and mental health systems must make some adjustment to respond to the needs of a fast growing, linguistically and culturally diverse group. In setting priorities to meet these needs, not only should resources be shifted and allocated to the Hispanic population in proportion to its increasing size, but program policy should be designed to take into consideration the unique population characteristics of this group.

Among other things, these population characteristics require a focus on developing adequate prenatal and postpartum care interventions, which will prevent the potentially long-lasting pathogenic effects of psychological and physiological complications of childbirth. Considering that Hispanics constitute the youngest ethnic group with children and adolescents comprising 50% of the population, it makes sense to maximize prevention efforts by directing them toward mothers and youth during the earliest possible stage of intervention.

DEFINING A HIGH RISK POPULATION FOR PREVENTION INTERVENTION: LOW–INCOME HISPANIC WOMEN

In order to maximize primary prevention efforts, it is necessary to identify high risk populations as the target, given that the relatively vulnerable groups are more likely than others to contribute disproportionately to the incidence of psychopathology and to benefit the most from the intervention. As discussed by Heller, Price and Sher (1980), the concept of a population or a group "at risk" is an integral part of prevention theory and can be defined as "any group which based on epidemiological evidence shows a higher probability of developing psychological distress or disorder compared with the general population" (p. 293).

Given the paucity of psychiatric epidemiologic studies of Hispanic populations, early reports on the mental health status of this group relied on information inferred from sociodemographic indicators. A review of this early literature by Padilla and Ruiz (1973) suggested that, as a group, Hispanics are disproportionately subject to the deleterious effects of poverty and acculturation which have been identified as high stress indicators correlated with psychiatric disorder and the need for treatment. These stressful conditions include high unemployment and underemployment, lower income, undereducation, poor housing, prejudice, discrimination and cultural/linguistic barriers.

The Report to the President's Commission on Mental Health (1978) identifies Hispanic women as a subpopulation that is particularly at high risk for developing emotional problems. They are considered to be in double jeopardy in that they are both women and members of an ethnic minority. There is some evidence which suggests that acculturation stress creates greater anxiety among Hispanic women than men (Torres-Matrullo, 1976; Warren, Olmedo & Go, 1976). Consequently, the Report to the President's Commission on Mental Health recommends that "the particular socio-cultural stresses faced by Hispanic women be researched and the consequent findings be used to develop and implement counseling programs and other interventions designed to prevent emotional disorders in this subpopulation" (p. 40).

In recent years, a few epidemiologic or community survey studies have been reported which generally support the identification of lower-income Hispanic women in the United States as a group at high risk for psychological distress and depression. Roberts (1980, 1981) presented data from surveys conducted in Alameda County which suggest that Mexican-Americans have rates of psychological disturbance at least as high as those of Anglos and that the prevalence of depression may be higher than it is in other groups. Consistent with findings are the results of a more recent psychiatric epidemiologic survey on a multiethnic probability sample of 1003 adults in Los Angeles County. The data indicate that the prevalence of depression was greatest among Hispanics compared to Anglos and Blacks; furthermore, women were twice as likely to be depressed as men. The ethnic differences did not reach significance, however, when selected demographic and socioeconomic variables were controlled; therefore, the authors conclude that the reported psychological distress was mostly a function of socioeconomic strain (Frerichs, Aneshensel & Clark, 1981).

The increased risk of psychological distress associated with a lower socioeconomic status among Hispanics is further supported by data from a binational community survey conducted in El Paso, Texas and Juarez, Mexico. As compared to Anglos, persons of Mexican origin, whether they lived in Mexico or in the United States, reported more severe symptomatology associated with psychiatric disturbance. Similar to the results of the aforementioned study, the difference between the ethnic groups was eliminated after controlling for the effects of socioeconomic status (Burnam, Hough & Timbers, 1983).

Additionally, an epidemiologic field survey of 1345 adults was conducted in Santa Clara County among recent Mexican immigrants, as well as more acculturated Mexicans, second generation Mexican-Americans and Anglos. Overall, the data indicate that the Mexican origin groups had higher symptomatology and dysfunction levels than Anglos. Among the Mexican origin sample, the three high risk groups were comprised of the monolingual Spanish-speaking, especially women in their late teens and early twenties; Spanish-speaking females between the ages of 40–49; and Spanish-speaking immigrants (Vega, Warheit, Buhl-Auth & Meinhardt, 1982).

In summary, it appears that epidemiological data indicate that low-income Hispanic women are at risk for developing psychological disturbance and depression. The deleterious effects of poverty and recent immigration, as well as minority group status, all seem to contribute to the increased vulnerability of this group.

In addition to generally being at risk for depression, low-income Hispanic women may be at risk more specifically for developing psychological disturbance or depressive symptomatology, as a function of perinatal physiological complications. Boulette (1980) states that effective mental health promotion cannot ignore the physical health correlates of the postpartum psychological condition, given the Hispanic population's high rate of physical and neurological disorders associated with birth and infancy. According to the National Center for Health Statistics (1982), only 60% of all Hispanic mothers, as compared to 81.2% of non-Hispanic mothers, began receiving prenatal care in the first trimester of pregnancy. Mothers of Hispanic origin also received fewer prenatal care visits than all other groups.

Results of a survey on access to prenatal care at the University of California at

Irvine Medical Center indicate that 93.7% of women receiving inadequate care (no care or not until 3rd trimester) were Spanish-speaking. Of particular concern is that among this sample, inadequate care was significantly related to low birth rate, neonatal mortality rates, and death of a child during the first year (Colon, 1984). These observed relationships between lack of adequate prenatal care and birth-pregnancy outcome are consistent with the large body of literature of higher mortality rate and other childbirth related complications among low-income and minority women (Hirsch, 1969).

In addition to the physical trauma incurred as a result of pre- and peri-natal complications, an indirect psychological impact on the fetus and neonate has been postulated by some authors. Sugarman (1977) suggested that obstetric complications, which require medical intervention and/or create additional pain and postpartum discomfort, may negatively affect the mother's reaction to the infant by inhibiting the milk letdown during breast feeding and by causing her to feel less willing and able to care for her infant. In sum, as Pasamanick and Knobloch (1961) have suggested, the evidence of linking pre-, peri-, and post-natal complications with neurological and psychological impairment in the child is strong enough to warrant the institution of preventive programs in the prenatal period.

IDENTIFYING HIGH RISK HISPANIC INDIVIDUALS AS THE PREVENTION TARGET: MULTIFACTORIAL ASSESSMENT OF BIOPSYCHOSOCIAL RISK FACTORS

Much of the psychiatric epidemiologic literature has not yielded information which is very useful for the precise targeting of high-risk individuals based on relative risk factors associated with psychiatric disturbance or depression. In discussing the current gap between large scale psychiatric epidemiologic research and clinical practice, Hough (1981) underscores the need to develop multivariate models of the impacts of socio-cultural variables on impairment, such that the cumulative, interactive, reciprocal, and multilevel effects of those variables can be assessed. He convincingly argues that those models can be used effectively for more precise targeting of high risk groups, as well as specific problem areas and promising points of intervention, through the early identification of patterns of stress and strain, adaptive resources and coping skills associated with psychological adaptation.

This approach to the identification of risk factors is particularly appropriate for the study of pregnancy and childbirth adaptation which is clearly a multifactorial process. This method allows for the possibility of discovering combinations of variables and patterns of interaction which can assist in the identification of individuals and groups at risk for depression and in need of primary prevention.

A useful model for the investigation of risk factors, associated with post-partum depression among low-income Hispanic women involves the construct of environmental stress and related mediating variables. The methodological weakness of most investigations of the effects of environmental stress on psychological and physical dysfunction have been discussed by other authers (See reviews by Dohrenwend & Dohrenwend, 1978; Rabkin & Struening, 1976; and Rahe & Arthur, 1978). Taken together, however, the studies provide additive evidence, which suggests that environmental stress, as mediated by perceived social support, personality adaptation, affective state, premenstrual tension and level of acculturation, have a significant impact on psychological and physiological adaptation to pregnancy and childbirth.

A recent study was designed to investigate the independent and joint effects of selected sociocultural, psychosocial and physical factors related to psychological and physiological adaptation to pregnancy and childbirth among low-income Hispanic women. More specifically, the investigator attempted to empirically validate high risk factors found in studies of non-Hispanic populations (Telles, 1982). Psychological adaptation to pregnancy focused on the prediction of the severity of postpartum depression on the basis of biomedical and sociodemographic variables and greater prenatal difficulty in the areas of environmental (life) stress, perceived social support, personality adaptation, premenstrual tension and acculturation. The participants included 110 low-income Hispanic women who were interviewed twice prenatally and twice postpartum. Information regarding all predictive variables was collected prenatally. Medical records data were also obtained and scored in terms of the severity of physiological complications of pregnancy, labor, delivery and the puerperium. (For a more complete description of the design and measurement of constructs see Telles, 1982).

The purpose of the investigation was to compile preliminary data that later might be useful in developing a comprehensive screening device to identify women potentially at risk for developing psychological and/or physiological problems related to childbirth. Of particular interest was the possibility of discovering mediating variables, which could suggest areas of preventive intervention with the distal goal of reducing the incidence of problematic adaptation to pregnancy and childbirth.

Environmental Stress

The study of environmental stress as a contributing factor to pregnancy complications and postpartum depression is particularly important in examining a low-income Hispanic population. Based on consistent observations in epidemiological studies of high rates of psychopathology symptoms in the lowest social class, Dohrenwend & Dohrenwend (1969) have proposed that stress situations will be more frequent and more severe in a lower class environment. Furthermore, they propose that within a socioeconomic stratum, stress situations will be more frequent and more severe among members of disadvantaged than advantaged ethnic groups. They state that stressors such as the birth of a first child are experienced by most people as a developmental crisis and that the impact of this event is strongly influenced by mediating factors related to social status.

The results of the aforementioned study of Hispanic women confirmed the prediction that women with greater prenatal life stress would have higher depression scores 2–3 day postpartum and two months postpartum (Telles, 1982). Life stress was measured by the Yamamoto and Kinney scale (1976), a modified version of the Social Readjustment Rating Scale (Holmes & Rahe, 1967). The bivariate relationships of life stress with depression during both periods of time were greater in magnitude than those produced by any other predictor. These findings are consistent with a growing body of literature which demonstrates that the experience of recent stressful life events is related to psychiatric impairment (Andrews, Tennant,

Hewson, & Vaillant, 1978), psychiatric symptomatology (Lin, Simeone, Ensel & Kuo, 1979; Myers, Ludenthal & Pepper, 1975) and depression (Lloyd, 1980; Warheit, 1979).

The results also concur with those of studies specifically related to pregnancy adaptation. Grossman and her associates (1980) reported that women experiencing greater life stress before pregnancy had greater difficulty with postpartum adjustment; experienced (multiparous) mothers, in particular, appeared more vulnerable to external pressures. Earlier studies have also documented the significant effects of social factors on the severity and duration of postpartum emotional problems, and some have even suggested a relationship to the onset of psychoses following childbirth (Gordon & Gordon, 1967; Gordon, Kapostins, & Gordon, 1965; Karnosh & Hope, 1937; Paykel, Fletcher, & Rassaby, 1980; Shereshefsky & Yarrow, 1973). It appears that the cumulative impact of multiple stressors may be of little significance in themselves, yet of sufficient magnitude that a single added stressor, such as pregnancy, "tips the scale" (Thomas & Gordon, 1959). The resulting maladaptive psychological reactions in the puerperium are, thus, partly a function of specific stressors, which deplete the woman's energy and interfere with a developmental step necessary for a positive adjustment and a healthy tie to the baby (Cohen, 1966).

Perceived Social Support

Among the most important mediating variables of stress is the availability, utilization and perception of social support. It has been suggested that an individual's capacity to cope with life stress is dependent, to a substantial degree, upon the adequacy of his/her social support structures, which can be relied on to provide emotional sustenance, assistance, and resources (Caplan, 1974). Many authors have indicated that the social groups to which an individual belongs, not only serve to react effectively to crisis, but are important in supporting and sustaining everyday life. While an effective support system attenuates the impact of stress, deficiencies or impairments of such a system may create or exacerbate stress (Caplan, 1974; Rabkin & Streuning, 1976).

The results of the study on Hispanic women suggested that the perception of a lack of social support during the prenatal period is related to higher depression scores 2–3 days postpartum among Hispanic women. These results are in accord with the growing number of empirical studies which have documented the importance of social support from close relatives and/or friends in moderating the severity of psychiatric symptoms (Cobb, 1976; Caplan & Killilea, 1976; Lin et al., 1979; Silberfeld, 1978) and depression (Surtees, 1980).

The vital function of support from significant others specifically during pregnancy and childbirth has also been observed repeatedly. A focus of discussion has often been the role of the husband in alleviating the pregnant woman's anxiety and assisting her in adapting to a stressful experience (Benedek, 1970; Wenner & Cohen, 1968). A woman's ability to accept change, to deal with a natural anxiety and to accept her new dependency is closely related to her ability to ask for help and to her husband's ability to respond adequately (Grossman, et al., 1980). The occurrence of postpartum blues, in particular, has been related to an absence of support from the husband and, more specifically, the degree to which the woman could talk to her spouse about problems and the extent to which he listened (Paykel, Emms, Fletcher, & Rassaby 1980).

Premenstrual Tension

Consistent with the literature on non-minority groups, Hispanic women who reported greater premenstrual tension also were more depressed two months postpartum; however, premenstrual tension did not predict to depression immediately following childbirth (Telles, 1982). This former finding relating premenstrual tension to depression two months postpartum is consistent with some studies, which suggests that puerperal depression and premenstrual tension have a common underlying hormonal component possibly related to progesterone imbalance. Various authors have associated postpartum psychoses with endocrinological dysfunction and have reported success with hormonal treatment (Blumberg & Billing, 1942; Bower & Altschule, 1956). Furthermore, other investigators have attributed the premenstrual syndrome to a similar hormonal imbalance and have found an association between the two disorders (Dalton, 1971; Yalom, Lunde, Moos, & Hamburg, 1968). Warnes (1978) explained the association by stating that both premenstrual and postpartum disorders involve increased depression, anxiety and instability during periods of marked reductions in estrogen and progesterone production.

Additionally, given that the Premenstrual Tension score was also related to the Prenatal Depression score, it is possible that the women's perceptions and report of premenstrual difficulty were influenced by depressive character traits or mood. Higher levels of depression may have contributed to greater somatic problems or complaints in general.

Personality Adaptation

The prediction that low-income Hispanic women appearing to have more prenatal difficuly in the area of personality adaptation would experience greater depression was confirmed for the two months postpartum period but not for the few days following childbirth (Telles, 1982). This former finding is consistent with the literature which suggests that an individual's personality characteristics play a mediating role in the response to a life stress like childbirth. Understandably, persons with greater skills and resources, more versatile defenses and broader experience tend to adapt better (Rabkin & Struening, 1976). On the whole, the more competent an individual has been in the past, the more likely it is that he/she will deal effectively with later stressors.

Personality adjustment has been viewed by many authors as the primary factor contributing to a woman's adaptation to pregnancy and childbirth (Benedek, 1974; & Deutsch, 1973). Postpartum difficulties are attributed by some to chronic maladjustment; childbirth is considered one more event that a predisposed person has difficulty managing well (Brew & Seidenberg, 1950; Smalldon, 1940; & Zilboorg, 1929). More recent studies lend support to these formulations. Among a sample of mostly Anglo women, the best predictors of successful postpartum psychological adjustment were measures of ego strength and nurturance, rather than external factors (Shereshefsy & Yarrow, 1973). Various other studies also have found that psychological health predicted to a better postpartum adjustment in terms of lower levels of depression and anxiety (Grossman et al., 1980; Grimm & Venet, 1966; Meares et al., 1976; Seager, 1960; Zajicek & Wolkind, 1978).

The correlation between personality adaptation and depression in the immediate postpartum period approached but did not reach significance. Possibly, experiences directly related to childbirth may have temporarily overridden characterological factors. Two months following childbirth, the previous level of personality functioning, more closely related to pre-pregnancy and prenatal factors, may have been restored. Grossman et al., (1980) reported similar findings and suggest that the crises of childbearing is "sufficiently consuming" that factors associated directly with the pregnancy are most important during the early postpartum adjustment, but during the later postpartum phase more enduring character traits resume their prominent impact on a woman's adaptation.

Prenatal Anxiety

Results of the study on low-income Hispanic women suggest that higher levels of state anxiety prior to childbirth were associated with a greater degree of depression a few days and two months postpartum (Telles, 1982). Factors which contributed to disruptions of mood during one period most likely also affected the other. Possibly, the two measures of anxiety and depression were assessing fluctuations of similar affective states.

Various investigators have found that puerperal depression is heralded by anxiety in pregnancy (Dalton, 1971; Tod, 1964). In some studies, prenatal anxiety was the best predictor of the mother's postpartum psychological adaptation, in terms of depression and anxiety (Grossman et al., 1980). In another study of postpartum depression, the women formed a hierarchy of severity of mood change during the puerperim which appeared to correspond to a similar hierarchy of mean scores for anxiety during pregnancy. The authors conclude that there may be an underlying biological, presumably endocrinological, factor which contributes to this common pattern of mood change. Most other investigators, however, attribute these findings to psychosocial factors and concerns about pregnancy and childbirth.

SUMMARY OF MAJOR FINDINGS AND CONCLUSIONS

Adaptation of pregnancy and childbirth among low-income Hispanic women is indeed a multifactorial process involving complex interactions between psychosocial and physiological factors. On the whole, the psychosocial variables and premenstrual tension predicted the severity of postpartum depression and overall psychological adaptation to pregnancy. The high degree of interrelatedness between premenstrual tension, pregnancy symptoms, depression and anxiety suggests that these processes share a common underlying psychological component, as well as a possible endocrinological one. Multivariate analyses indicate that, the best predictor of more severe postpartum depression (two months) in the context of other variables was greater life stress. Life stress appeared to exacerbate difficulty in psychological adaptation, and social support acted as a mediator with a protective function.

The relation of prenatal depression and personality adaptation to postpartum adjustment suggests some contribution of characterological predisposition to psychological adaptation to pregnancy and childbirth; however, the effects of prenatal affective states are stronger predictors.

Additional analysis could focus on developing a screening instrument based on stressful life experience, perceived social support, prenatal depression and history of premenstrual tension for use in prenatal clinics. Women considered to be "at risk" for problematic psychological adaptation following childbirth and two months postpartum could then be identified and referred to a primary prevention program.

TOWARD THE CONCEPTUALIZATION OF A PRIMARY PREVENTION PROGRAM: SELECTION OF PRENATAL MODIFIABLE RISK FACTORS RELATED TO POSTPARTUM DEPRESSION

Given the multifactorial causation of most disorders, Heller and his associates (1980) recommend that preventive intervention programs aim at reducing as many modifiable risk factors as possible. Although research in prevention must yield information on the separate effects of individual risk factors, prevention programs will need to consider a group of contributing risk factors simultaneously, in order to maximize the probability of reducing the incidence rates of psychopathology.

A postpartum depression prevention program for low-income Hispanic women optimally would be offered as part of a comprehensive health services delivery model within the hospital/clinic setting, conveniently arranged for women attending regularly rescheduled prenatal visits. Undoubtedly, bilingual-bicultural staff should be utilized with an unacculturated Hispanic population.

Most importantly, the intervention strategies should be aimed at reducing the impact of empirically validated risk factors. Given the important contribution of environmental (stress, social support) factors to the psychological adaptation of these women, the intervention model should be multifaceted and responsive to their social environmental problems, as well as to their psychological needs. Some related areas of intervention could include: stress management, social support enhancement, health education, community outreach and consultation to hospital staff.

Stress Management and Depression Prevention

Given a target population of low-income Hispanic women, strategies should be developed which not only focus on the individual, but also take into consideration the social system with the goal of reducing the impact of environmentally induced stress, particularly as it relates to socio-economic status. As discussed by Caplan (1957), stress tends to impinge upon normal problem solving abilities; thus, it is important to strengthen the high-risk individual's coping abilities. Bloom (1985) suggests that "competence building," which increases a sense of mastery and control over one's life and enhances self-esteem is perhaps the single most effective prevention strategy.

Some specific objectives in relation to the prevention of postpartum depression and its sequelae might include:

1. The reduction of financial stress through advocacy and the dissemination of information related to a broad range of social services and community resources (i.e., employment referral, welfare assistance, child care facilities, church organizations, etc.) Printed materials could be distributed during the prenatal period and/or referrals and linkages could be made to appropriate agencies.

2. The reduction of pregnancy/childbirth related stress and fears through prenatal education programs which provide information regarding the physiological processes in pregnancy and birth. This is particularly important for primiparas and can be communicated in classes, which make use of literature and audio-visual aids.

3. An increased sense of competence and mastery through a skills training program for new parents regarding child caretaking and early childrearing techniques.

4. Direct prevention of depression through culturally-relevant skills training programs which impart knowledge with regard to stress management, in general, and methods of coping with depressive symptomatology. Useful interventions based on cognitive approaches have received theoretical and empirical support from the work of investigators such as Lewinsohn, Muñoz, Youngren and Zeiss (1978).

Social Support Enhancement

Though unexpected life events are not possible to control and endocrinological/physiological conditions are not always amenable to intervention, the literature suggests that efforts to mobilize the woman's social support system may succeed in positively altering her experience of physical discomfort and dysphoria during pregnancy and the postpartum periods. In this regard, special attention might be given to Hispanic women who have recently immigrated and are adapting to a different environment after having separated from their family of origin and, in particular, their mother. This is not to suggest that intervention in this sphere necessarily involves increasing the *size* of the active network. Larger social networks have been correlated with higher rates of psychopathology, although the directionality of this relationship is unclear.

Although it is necessary to investigate further the conditions which contribute to optimal social support during pregnancy, prevention efforts based on available information could be implemented and tested. Specific objectives could include:

1. The mobilization of existing natural support systems/resources, including the baby's father, parents, friends and others, as considered appropriate.

2. The creation of new support resources through prenatal mutual support groups. These groups could provide a forum for sharing concerns, information and coping strategies related to pregnancy, childbirth, childrearing, etc.

3. Provision of linkage to "natural caregivers" (community volunteers), especially women who have adapted well to childbirth and can act as role models and support resources. The use of this type of "linkperson natural support" among Hispanics has been described and recommended by Valle (1980).

4. The use of trained and supervised paraprofessionals or professional nurses,

who would visit the home to assure the mother's well-being and assess the mother-infant interaction during the postpartum period.

Reduction of Physiological Complications Associated with Postpartum Depression and Its Sequelae

As discussed earlier, physiological complications have been related to maternal psychological adaptation, the mother-infant interaction and a broad range of neuropsychiatric problems in the developing child. Consistent with the holistic viewpoint of the integrity of the emotions and the body, it is not conceivable that any one stress is limited to having an effect on physical well-being without having some effect on emotional well-being. The "psyche" and the "soma" are so inextricably interrelated and mutually resonant "that it would not make sense, even if it were possible, to divide stresses which affect one system to the exclusion of the other" (Thomas & Gordon, 1959, p. 363). A comprehensive postpartum depression prevention program would include techniques aimed at reducing the incidence of physiological complications of pregnancy, labor, delivery and the puerperium, such as:

1. Dissemination of information related to pregnancy, labor and delivery which focuses on reducing pain and facilitating childbirth. The prevention package could include relaxation training.
2. Health promotion through dissemination of information related to diet, exercise, weight, and other physical factors associated with a positive adaptation to childbirth.
3. An aggressive community outreach program, which includes public education through the mass media regarding the importance of early prenatal care. Spanish-speaking radio and television programs could be utilized.

Overcoming Structural/Environmental Barriers to Quality Care

The prevention program for low-income Hispanic women should also include interventions which reduce the barriers to quality care in the prenatal clinics and hospitals. A lack of communication between the primary caregivers and the clients, as well as misinformation and misunderstanding, contribute to increased stress and problematic adaptation to pregnancy and childbirth (Scrimshaw, Engle & Horsley, 1985). The intervention package, thus, should focus also on:

1. Consultation and education to clinic and hospital staff, including physicians and nurses, to reduce the socio-cultural distance which undermines effective health care.
2. Consultation to administrative hospital/clinic staff regarding personnel/ employment policies which include the hiring of bilingual-bicultural staff when unacculturated Hispanic women constitute a significant proportion of the patient population.
3. Reduction of financial and geographic barriers which limit the accessibility of adequate health care in the prenatal clinics.

EVALUATION OF A POSTPARTUM DEPRESSION PREVENTION PROGRAM: PROXIMAL PROGRAMMATIC OBJECTIVES AND DISTAL GOALS

The effectiveness of prevention efforts in reducing the incidence of postpartum depression and its sequelae could be assessed through the use of a prospective, longitudinal experimental design with repeated measures. Hispanic women who are identified as being "at risk" by means of a prenatal screening device, but who are not yet clinically depressed, would be assigned randomly to the experimental and control groups.

Following implementation of the primary prevention program, proximal programmatic objectives could be assessed to determine whether the interventions were successful in modifying some of the assumed risk factors. Pre-post outcome measures could be developed to ascertain acquisition of new coping strategies and skills; increased satisfaction with perceived social support; greater knowledge of pregnancy and childbirth processes; and increased knowledge of and sensitivity toward Hispanic patients on the part of primary caregivers.

The distal goals could include the evaluation of the program's effect on the incidence, severity and duration of postpartum depression as measured by an instrument, which yields information on symptomatology, as well as diagnosable disorders, such as the NIMH Diagnostic Interview Schedule (Robins, Helzer, Croughan, & Ratcliff, 1981). The assessment of the primary prevention efforts would involve analyses, not only of pre-post differences but also of the relationship between attainment of proximal objectives and depression.

Postpartum depression could be considered both an outcome and a predictor variable to be measured periodically (one week, two months, six months and one year postpartum). More specifically, a path analysis model could be developed which identifies conditions that precede (predict), as well as follow from, postpartum depression. Some distal outcomes to be assessed are the possible sequelae of postpartum depression which would include: 1. the mother-infant interaction, as a function of risk factors, depression and the intervention; 2. the neonate's emotional and cognitive development; 3. the maintenance of the effects of the prevention program over time (skills, resources); and 4. the effects of postpartum events and changes in social support on the maintenance of the prevention effects and depression.

As discussed by Gruenberg (1981), preventive trials can be initiated to examine the main and interaction effects of different strategies. Each of the experimental groups of Hispanic women could be exposed to one type of intervention or a combination of these. In this manner, the outcome study could yield direct information on relative and attributable risk factors for postpartum depression among low-income Hispanic women.

REFERENCES

Andrews, G., Tennant, C., Hewson, D. M., & Vaillant, G. E., (1978). Life event stress, social support, coping style, and risk of psychological impairment. *Journal of Nervous and Mental Disease, 166,* (5), 307-316.

Anzalone, M. (1977). *Postpartum depression and premenstrual tension, life stress, and marital adjustment*. Unpublished doctoral dissertation, Boston University, Boston.

Benedek, T. (1970). Sexual functions in women and their disturbances. In S. Arieti (Ed.), *American Handbook of Psychiatry*. New York: Basic Books, Inc.

Benedek, T. (1970). The psychobiology of pregnancy. In E. J. Anthony and T. Benedek (Eds.) *Parenthood: Its psychology and psychopathology*. Boston: Little-Brown.

Bibring, G. L., Dwyer, T. F., Huntington, D. S., & Valenstein, A. F. (1961). A study of the psychological processes in pregnancy and of the earliest mother-child relationship: I. Some propositions and comments. *The Psychoanalytic Study of the Child, 16,* 9–24.

Bloom, B. L. (1985). Focal issues and prevention of mental disorders. In H. H. Goldman & S. E. Goldston (Eds.), *Preventing stress—related psychiatric disorders*. Rockville, Md.: National Institute of Mental Health.

Blumberg, A., & Billing, O. (1942). Hormonal influence upon puerperal psychoses and neurotic conditions. *Psychiatric Quarterly, 16,* 454–467.

Boulette, T. R. (1980). Priority issues for mental health promotion among low-income Chicanos/Mexicanos. In R. Valle and W. Vega. (Eds.), *Hispanic natural support systems* (pp. 15–23). Sacramento, Ca.: State Department of Mental Health.

Bower, W. H., & Altschule, M. D. (1956). Use of progesterone in the treatment of postpartum psychosis. *The New England Journal of Medicine, 254,* 157–160.

Boyd, D. A. (1942). Mental disorders associated with childbearing. *American Journal of Obstetrics and Gynecology, 43,* 148–163, 335–349.

Brew, M. F., & Seidenberg, R. (1950). Psychotic reactions associated with pregnancy and childbirth. *Journal of Nervous and Mental Disorders, III,* 408–423.

Burnam, M. A., Hough, R. H., & Timbers, D. M. (1984). Psychological distress among Mexican-Americans, Mexicans and Anglos from two border cities. *Journal of Health and Social Behavior, 25,* 24–33.

Caplan, G. (1957). Psychological aspects of maternity care. *American Journal of Public Health, 47,* 25–31.

Caplan, G. (1974). *Support systems and community mental health*. New York: Behavioral Publications.

Caplan, G., & Killilea, M. (Eds.) (1976). *Support systems and mutual help: Multidisciplinary explorations*. New York: Grune & Stratton.

Cobb, S. (1976). Social support as a moderator of life stress. *Psychosomatic Medicine, 38* (5), 300–314.

Cohen, R. L. (1966). Some maladaptive syndromes of pregnancy and the puerperium. *Obstetrics and Gynecology, 27,* 562–570.

Colòn, Jose (1984). Issues of access to prenatal care for Hispanic women in Orange County. *Children, youth and families in the Southwest*. Hearing Before the Select Committee on Children, Youth and Families, U.S. House of Representatives. U.S. Government Printing Office, (Pub. No. 35-1580).

Dalton, K. (1971). Prospective study into puerperal depression. *British Journal of Psychiatry, 118,* 689–692.

Deutsch, H. (1973). *The psychology of women*. New York: Grune & Stratton, Inc.

Deutscher, M. (1970). Brief family therapy in the course of a first pregnancy: A clinical note. *Contemporary Psychoanalysis, 7* (1), 21–35.

Dohrenwend, B. S., & Dohrenwend, B. P. (1969). *Social status and psychological disorder*. New York: Wiley Interscience.

Dohrenwend, B. S., & Dohrenwend, B. P. (1978). Some issues in research on stressful life events. *Journal of Nervous and Mental Disease, 166* (1), 7–15.

Ferreira, A. J. (1965). Emotional factors in prenatal environment. *Journal of Nervous and Mental Disease, 141,* 108–118.

Finegan, J., & Quarrington, B. (1979). Pre- peri- and neonatal factors and infantile autism. *Journal of Child Psychology & Psychiatry & Allied Disciplines, 20* (2), 119–128.

Frerichs, R. R., Aneshensel, C. S., & Clark, V. A. (1981). Prevalence of depression in Los Angeles County. *American Journal of Epidemiology, 113,* 691–699.

Gordon, R. E., & Gordon, K. K. (1967). Factors in postpartum emotional adjustment. *American Journal of Orthopsychiatry, 37,* 359–360.

Gordon, R. E., Kapostins, E., & Gordon, K. (1965). Factors in postpartum emotional adjustment. *Obstetrics and Gynecology, 25,* 159–166.

Grossman, F. K., Eichler, C. S., & Winickoff, S. A. *Pregnancy, birth, and parenthood*. San Francisco: Jossey-Bass.

Gruenberg, E. (1981). Risk factor research methods. In D. A. Regier & G. Allen (Eds.), *Risk factor research in the major disorders*. OHHS Publication No. (ADM) 81-1068). Washington, DC: U.S. Government Printing Office.

Hamilton, J. A. (1962). *Postpartum psychiatric problems*. St. Louis: The C.V. Mosby Co.

Heller, K., Price, R. H., & Sher, K. J. (1980). Research and evaluation in primary prevention: Issues and guidelines. In R. H. Price and Associates (Eds.), *Prevention in Mental Health: Research, Policy and Practice*. Beverly Hills: Sage.

Hemphill, R. E. (1952). Incidence and nature of puerperal psychiatric illness. *British Medical Journal, 2*, 1232-1235.

Hirsch, C. (1969). Child guidance services to the poor. *Annual progress in child psychiatry and child development*. New York: Brunner/Mazel.

Holmes, T. H. and Rahe, R. H. (1967). The social readjustment rating scale. *Journal of Psychosomatic Research, II*, 213-218.

Hough, R. L. (1981). Sociocultural issues in research and clinical practice: Closing the gap. In E. A. Serafetinides (Ed.), *Psychiatric research in practice*. New York: Grune & Stratton.

Jacobson, L., Kaij, L., & Nilsson, A. (1960). Postpartum mental disorders in an unselected sample. *British Medical Journal, 1*, 1965.

Jones, A. (1974). *Psychological assessment as an adjunct to obstetrical screening of high-risk pregnancies*. Unpublished doctoral dissertation, University of Iowa.

Kaij, L., & Nilsson, A. (1972). Emotional and psychotic illness following childbirth. In J. Howell (Ed.) *Modern perspectives in psycho-obstetrics*. New York: Brunner/Mazil.

Kane, F. J., Jr., Harman, W. J., Keeler, M. H., & Ewing, J. A. (1968). Emotional and cognitive disturbance in the early puerperium. *British Journal of Psychiatry, 114*, 99-102.

Karnosh, L. J., & Hope, J. M. (1937). Puerperal psychosis and their sequelae. *American Journal of Psychiatry, 94*, 537-550.

Knobloch, H., & Pasamanick, B. (1966). Prospective studies on the epidemiology of reproductive casualty: Methods, findings and some implications. *Merrill-Palmer Quarterly, 12*, 28-43.

Lewinsohn, P. M., Muñoz, R. F., Youngren, M. A., & Zeiss, A. M. (1978). *Control your depression*. Englewood Cliffs, N.J. Prentice-Hall.

Lilienfeld, A. M., & Parkhurst, E. (1952). A study of the association of factors of pregnancy and parturition with the development of cerebral palsy. *American Journal of Hygiene, 53*, 262-282.

Lilienfeld, A. M., & Pasamanick, B. (1954). Association of maternal and fetal factors with the development of epilepsy. *Journal of the American Medical Association, 155* (8), 719-724.

Lin, N., Simeone, R. S., Ensel, W. M., & Kuo, W. (1979). Social support, stressful life events and illness: A model and an empirical test. *Journal of Health and Social Behavior, 20* (5), 108-119.

Lloyd, C. (1980). Life events and depressive disorder reviewed: Events as precipitating factors. *Archives of General Psychiatry, 37* (5), 541-548.

Macias, R. F. (1977). U.S. Hispanics in 2000 A.D.: Projecting the number. *Agenda, 7*, 16-20.

Madden, J. J., Luhan, J. A., Tuteur, W., & Bimmerle, J. F. (1958). Characteristics of post partum mental illness. *American Journal of Psychiatry, 115* (1), 18-24.

Meares, R., Grinwade, J., & Wood, C. (1976). A possible relationship between anxiety in pregnancy and puerperal depression. *Journal of Psychosomatic Research, 20*, 605-610.

Myers, J., Lundenthal, J. J., & Pepper, M. P. (1975). Life events, social integration and psychiatric symptomatology. *Journal of Health and Social Behavior, 16*, 421-427.

National Center for Health Statistics: Births of Hispanic parentage (May, 1982). *Monthly Vital Statistics Report*, Vol. 31, No. 2, Supp. DHHS Pub. No. (DAS) 82-1120. Public Helath Service, Hyattsville, Md.

Padilla, A. M., & Ruiz, R. (1973). *Latino mental health: A review of the literature*. DHEW Publication No. (HSM) 73-9143. Washington, DC: U.S. Government Printing Office.

Pasamanick, B., & Knobloch, H. (1961). Epidemiologic studies on the complications of pregnancy and the birth process. In G. Caplan (Ed.). *Prevention of mental disorders in children*. New York: Basic Books.

Pasamanick, B., & Lilienfeld, A. M. (1955). Association of maternal and fetal factors with development of mental deficiency. *Journal of the American Medical Association, 159* (3), 155-160.

Pasamanick, B., Rogers, M. E., & Lilienfeld, A. M. (1956). Pregnancy experience and the development of behavior disorder in children. *American Journal of Psychiatry, 112*, 613-618.

Paykel, E. S., Emms, E. M., Fletcher, J., & Rassaby, E. S. (1980). Life events and social support in puerperal depression. *British Journal of Psychiatry, 136*, 339-346.

Pitt, B. (1968). A typical depression following childbirth. *British Journal of Psychiatry, 114,* 1325–1335.

Pitt, B. (1973). Maternity blues. *British Journal of Psychiatry, 122,* 431–433.

Pollit, J. (1965). *Depression and its treatment.* London: Heinemann.

Rabkin, J. G., & Struening, E. L. (1976). Life events, stress, and illness. *Science, 194,* 1013–1020.

Rahe, R. H., & Arthur, R. J. (1978). Life change and illness studies: Past history and future directions. *Journal of Human Stress, 11,* 341–345.

Railton, I. E. (1961). The use of corticords in postpartum depression. *Journal of the American Women's Association, 16,* 450.

Report to the President's Commission on Mental Health from the Special Populations Sub-Task Panel on Mental Health of Hispanic Americans (1978). Los Angeles: Spanish-speaking Mental Health Research Center.

Roberts, R. E. (1980). Prevalence of psychological distress among Mexican-Americans. *Journal of Health and Social Behavior, 21,* 134–145.

Roberts, R. E. (1981). Prevalence of depressive symptoms among Mexican-Americans. *Journal of Nervous and Mental Disease, 169* (4), 213–219.

Robin, A. M. (1962). Psychological changes of normal parturition. *Psychiatric Quarterly, 36,* 129–150.

Robins, L. N., Helzer, J. C., Croughan, J., & Ratcliff, K. The National Institute of Mental Health. Diagnostic Interview Schedule: Its history, characteristics and validity. *Archives of General Psychiatry, 38,* 381–389.

Sclare, A. B. (1955). Psychiatric aspects of pregnancy and childbirth. *Practitioner, 175,* 146–154.

Scrimshaw, S., Engle, D. and Horsley, K. (1955). *Use of prenatal services by women of Mexican origin and descent in Los Angeles.* Unpublished manuscript, UCLA, School of Public Health, Los Angeles.

Seager, C. (1960). A controlled study of postpartum illness. *Journal of Mental Science, 106* (442), 214–230.

Shereshefsky, P. M., & Yarrow, L. T. (Eds.) (1973). *Psychological aspects of a first pregnancy and early postnatal adaptation.* New York: Raven Press.

Sherman, J. (1971). *On the psychology of women.* Springfield, Illinois: Charles C. Thomas Co.

Silberfeld, M. (1978). Psychological symptoms and social supports. *Social Psychiatry, 13,* 11–17.

Smalldon, J. L. (1940). A survey of mental illness associated with pregnancy and childbirth. *American Journal of Psychiatry, 97,* 80–97.

Stott, D. H. (1962). Abnormal mothering as a cause of mental subnormality: II. Case studies & conclusions. *Journal of Child Psychology & Psychiatry, 6* (3), 133–148.

Stratton, P. M. (1977). Criteria for assessing the influence of obstetric circumstances on later development. In T. Chard, & M. Richards (Eds.), *Benefits and hazards of the new obstetrics: Clinics in developmental medicine.* London: William Heinemann Medical Books.

Strecker, E. A., & Ebaugh, F. G. (1926). Psychoses occurring during the puerperium. *Archives of Neurology and Psychiatry, 15,* 239–252.

Sugarman, M. (1977). Paranatal influences on maternal-infant attachment. *American Journal of Orthopsychiatry, 47* (3), 407–421.

Surtees, P. G. (1980). Social support, residual adversity and depressive outcome. *Social Psychiatry, 15,* 71–80.

Talovic, S. A., Mednick, S. A., Schulsinger, F., & Falloon, I. R. H. (1980). Schizophrenia in high risk subjects. *Journal of Abnormal Psychology, 89*(2), 501–504.

Telles, C. A. (1982). Psychological and physiological adaptation to pregnancy and childbirth among low-income Hispanic women. (Doctoral dissertation, Boston University).

Telles, C. A. (in press). Towards the prevention of biopsychosocial complications of childbirth among Hispanics. In R. L. Hough, P. Gongla, V. Brown, and S. Goldston (Eds.), *Psychiatric epidemiology and primary prevention: The possibilities.*

Thomas, C. L., & Gordon, J. E. (1959). Psychosis after childbirth: Ecological aspects of a single impact stress. *The American Journal of the Medical Sciences, 238,* 363–385.

Timbers, D., & Hough, R. L. (1976). Life change and illness on the border: Implications for prevention. In R. L. Hough, P. Gongla, V. Brown, and S. Goldston (Eds.), *Psychiatric epidemiology and primary prevention: The possibilities,* (In review).

Tod, E. D. M. (1964). Puerperal depression: A prospective epidemiological study. *Lancet, 12,* 1264–1266.

Torres-Matrullo, C. (1976). Acculturation and psychopathology among Puerto-Rican women in mainland United States. *American Journal of Orthopsychiatry, 40* (4), 710–719.

Uddenberg, N., & Englesson, I. (1978). Prognosis of postpartum mental disturbance. A prospective study of primiparous women and their 4 ½ year old children. *Acta Psychiatrica Scandinavia, 58* (3), 201–212.

U.S. Bureau of the Census (1973). *Census of Population: 1970 Persons of Spanish Origin* (Final Report DC (2)—1c). Washington, DC: U.S. Government Printing Office.

U.S. Bureau of the Census. (1976). *Persons of Spanish Origin in the United States: March, 1976* (Current Population Report, Series P-20, No. 310). Washington, DC: U.S. Government Printing Office.

U.S. Bureau of the Census. (1982). *Persons of Spanish Origin, 1980.* (Census of Population, Supplementary Reports, Series PC80-S1-7). Washington, DC: U.S. Government Printing Office.

Valle, R. (1980). A natural resource system for health-mental health promotion to Latino/Hispanic populations. In R. Valle and W. Vega (Eds.), *Hispanic natural support systems.* Sacramento, Ca.: State Department of Mental Health.

Vega, W. A. (1980). Defining Hispanic high-risk groups: Targeting populations for health promotion. In R. Valle and W. Vega (Eds.), *Hispanic natural support systems.* Sacramento, Ca.: State Department of Mental Health.

Vega, W. A., Warheit, G., Buhl-Auth, J., & Meinhardt, K. (1984). The prevalence of depressive symptoms among Mexican-Americans and Anglos. *American Journal of Epidemiology, 120,* (4), 592–607.

Yamamoto, K. J., and Kinney, D. K. (1976). Pregnant women's ratings of different factors influencing psychological stress during pregnancy. *Psychological Reports, 18,* 16–27.

Warheit, G. J. (1979). Life events, coping, stress and depressive symptomatology. *American Journal of Psychiatry, 136* (4B), 502–507.

Warnes, H. (1978). Premenstrual disorders: Causative mechanisms and treatment. *Psychosomatics, 19* (1), 32–40.

Warren, L. W., Olmedo, E. L., & Go, (1976). *The relationship of Chicano acculturation to self-report anxiety and attitudes toward counseling and psychotherapy.* Paper presented at the Western Psychological Association Convention, Los Angeles, Ca.

Wenner, N., & Cohen, M. (Eds.) (1968). *Emotional aspects of pregnancy.* First report of the Washington School of Psychiatry Project: Clinical study of the emotional challenge of pregnancy.

Werner, E., Simonian, K., Bierman, J. M., & French, F. E. (1967). Cumulative effect of perinatal complications and deprived environment on physical, intellectual, and social development of preschool children. *Pediatrics, 39* (4), 490–505.

Yalom, I., Lunde, D., Moos, R., & Hamburg, D. (1968). Postpartum blues syndrome. *Archives of General Psychiatry, 18,* 16–27.

Zajicek, E., & Wolkind, S. (1978). Emotional difficulties in married women during and after the first pregnancy. *British Journal of Medical Psychology, 51* (4), 218–228.

Zilboorg, G. (1929). The dynamics of schizophrenic reactions related to pregnancy and childbirth. *American Journal of Psychiatry, 8,* 733–767.

9

The Coping-with-Depression Course

Peter M. Lewinsohn
University of Oregon

INTRODUCTION

The Coping with Depression Course (CWD) has been offered through the University of Oregon Depression Research Unit since 1979 to over 300 depressed individuals. The efficacy of the Course has been evaluated in a number of treatment outcome studies (Brown & Lewinsohn, 1984; Steinmetz, Lewinsohn, & Antonuccio, 1983; Teri & Lewinsohn, 1981) and additional research is still in progress (Hoberman, Lewinsohn, & Tilson, 1985). It is quite clear that as a group individuals who participate in this course show marked improvement, both in terms of their depression level and diagnosis, and that these changes are maintained to six months post-treatment. We (Gonzales, Lewinsohn, & Clarke, 1985) are currently in the process of studying the effects of the Course for up to three years after treatment. This paper has several objectives. First, a brief description of the CWD Course will be provided. Next, the theoretical foundation upon which the intervention is based will be discussed, followed by a summary of the results of several treatment outcome studies. Finally, potential applications to prevention and directions for future research will be indicated.

DESCRIPTION OF COPING–
WITH–DEPRESSION COURSE

The CWD Course is a multimodal, psychoeducational group treatment for unipolar depression. The major vehicle for treatment is a *course,* i.e., an explicit educational experience. The approach is called a *course* because it teaches people techniques and strategies to cope with the problems that are assumed to be related to their depression.

The CWD Course consists of 12 two-hour sessions conducted over eight weeks. Sessions are held twice a week during the first four weeks of treatment, and once a week for the final four weeks. Follow-up sessions called "class reunions" are held one month and six months after treatment to facilitate the maintenance of treatment gains.

The first two sessions of the Course are devoted to the definition of Course ground rules, the presentation of the social learning view of depression, and in-

The investigations reported in this paper were supported in part by a research grant from the National Institute of Mental Health (MH335721).

struction in basic self-change skills. The next eight sessions are devoted to the acquisition of skills in four specific areas: 1) The relation between tension and depression and the use of relaxation in everyday situations; 2) The relation between pleasant activities and developing a plan for increasing pleasant activities; 3) The role of thinking in depression and formulating a plan for constructive thinking; 4) Improving social skills and increasing positive social interaction. Two sessions are devoted to each skill. The final two sessions focus on maintenance and prevention issues. Activities during these final sessions include developing a personal maintenance plan for each participant based on their specific problems and the skills and techniques they found to be most useful. The class reunions provide a sense of continuity for the participants, and help them to stay motivated to periodically monitor their depression level and make use of their new coping skills.

The course is a highly structured, time-limited, skill training program that makes use of a text, *Control Your Depression* (Lewinsohn, Muñoz, Youngren, & Zeiss, 1978), from which reading assignments are made; a *Participant Workbook* (Brown & Lewinsohn, 1984) which was developed to supplement the text; and an *Instructor's Manual* (Steinmetz, Antonuccio, Bond, McKay, Brown, & Lewinsohn, 1979) to insure comparability of treatment across instructors. A more detailed description of the course is provided in Lewinsohn, Antonuccio, Steinmetz, and Teri (1984).

Since the course, by definition, is an educational experience, we have deemed it appropriate to make use of a variety of outreach approaches to make the course widely known in the community and to encourage people to participate. These have included advertisements in newspapers, public service announcements, and interactions with local radio and TV programs. Some of the announcements we have used to publicize the course. These are included in Lewinsohn, Antonuccio, Steinmetz, and Teri, (1984).

Consistent with the educational philosophy of the course, exclusion criteria have been minimal. Individuals are excluded if they show evidence of mental retardation, dyslexia, serious visual or auditory impairment, bipolar disorder, schizophrenia or schizoaffective disorder, or acute substance abuse. Concurrent psychotherapy, counseling, or pharmacotherapy for depression or other problems are not exclusion criteria. While being depressed is not required for inclusion, approximately 80% of the participants meet criteria for a diagnosis of depression as per the RDC (Spitzer, Endicott, & Robins, 1978) and DSM–III (APA, 1980) criteria. Typical enrollment is 5 to 8. Attrition has been less than 10%. Demographic characteristics of participants are shown in Table 1.

The typical chain of events is for people to call in inquiring about the Course. They are then scheduled for an intake interview. The purposes of this interview are two-fold: 1) For us to determine whether to recommend the Course to the particular individual, and 2) To provide the individual with the necessary information to decide whether they want to participate in the Course. Our general criteria for recommending course participation have been guided by three considerations: 1) Is the individual going to be able to function well within the treatment format? e.g., can they do the readings, carry out the assignments, and function appropriately as a member of a structured group? 2) Is the individual likely to benefit from this treatment given the data we have about the particular individual and about those who tend to benefit from this treatment? 3) Is the individual felt to be in need

Table 1 Demographic characteristics of coping-with-depression course participants in the four studies

Study	N	Female %	Diagnosed depressed* at start of treatment %	Age Mean	Age Range	Age SD	Graduate training %	Completed college %	Attended some college %	High school graduate %	Attended some high school %	Married %	Separated, divorced, widowed %	Single %
Brown & Lewinsohn 1984	75	73	81	37	19–74	11.5	30	15	38	13	4	45	35	20
Steinmetz, et al., 1983. Antonuccio et al., 1982.	112	69	67	36	22–59	10.6	13	19	46	17	5	53	31	16
Teri & Lewinsohn 1981	84	62	71	33	20–60	13.9	10	32	39	18	1	46	29	25
Hoberman, Lewinsohn, & Tilson, 1984	40	60	100	37	18–57	9.9	7	28	43	23	0	55	22	23

*Diagnosed according to the SADS/RDC Major, Minor, or Intermittent Depressive Disorder.

of some other treatment? Approximately 50% of those who call are interested in being interviewed and about half of these decide to participate. Very few are judged to be ineligible as per the exclusion criteria.

The leaders of the CWD Courses have all been advanced doctoral students in clinical and counseling psychology. In addition to having had supervised experience in individual psychotherapy as part of their graduate training, these students have been carefully selected and trained to conduct the course. Others (Thompson, Gallagher, Nies, & Epstein, 1983) have successfully trained paraprofessionals to conduct the Course, by providing them with highly specialized training and expert supervision. The training program we have found satisfactory has included having student instructors actually take the CWD Course from a trained instructor. Potential instructors are expected to do all the things participants do, such as in-class exercises, homework, monitoring, tracking, and reading. They then co-lead the Course with a more experienced instructor and in this way obtain supervised experience. Finally they lead the Course. It has been very useful to have two novice instructors co-lead their first Course. Throughout training and thereafter Course instructors are provided with opportunities for clinical supervision.

In one of our studies (Antonuccio, Lewinsohn, & Steinmetz, 1982) we were specifically interested in identifying therapist variables that were related to treatment outcome. The assumption was that there would be systematic differences between therapists in the amount of improvement shown by their clients and that these differences would be related to therapist variables hypothesized to be important on the basis of a literature review. A repeated measurements design was used. Each of 8 Course leaders conducted two consecutive treatment groups consisting of 5 to 8 subjects per group. The leaders were evaluated on a large number of variables (pre-treatment therapist characteristics, therapist behavior and style during treatment, group behavior, and group process) which were hypothesized to be related to outcome. A major finding of this study was that even though the leaders differed significantly on many of the therapist variables (e.g., group cohesiveness, group participation, therapist warmth, therapist enthusiasm, therapist expectations, on task activities, etc.) the main effect in the ANOVA due to leader differences did not attain statistical significance. Since all the groups had shown substantial improvement pre to post, we interpret these results to indicate that our criteria for the selection of therapists and our therapist training procedures are quite adequate, i.e., by insuring a predictable and high level of therapeutic success and by minimizing any systematic effects that leader characteristics might have on outcome.

THEORETICAL BACKGROUND AND RATIONALE

Briefly, the CWD Course is anchored on several foundations.

1. It is based on the social-learning theory analysis of depression according to which depression is associated with a decrease in pleasant and an increase in unpleasant person-environment interactions (Lewinsohn, Youngren, & Grosscup, 1979).

2. The Course addresses areas which have been shown to be problematic for depressed individuals. To wit: (1) The occurrence of stressful life events and feelings of tension (Lewinsohn & Hoberman, 1983), (2) a reduced rate of engagement in pleasant activities, (3) problematic cognitions, and (4) social interactional problems.

3. The Course incorporates interventions which have been shown to be therapeutically effective singly or in combination, such as cognitive therapy (Muñoz, 1977), social skills training (Zeiss, 1977), increasing pleasant activities, and relaxation (Lewinsohn, Sullivan & Grosscup, 1980).

4. In addition, the Course incorporates elements which in a previous publication (Zeiss, Lewinsohn & Muñoz, 1979) were hypothesized to constitute critical components for successful short term cognitive-behavioral therapy for depression; to wit:

1. Therapy should begin with an elaborated, well-planned rationale. This rationale should provide initial structure that guides the patient to the belief that he or she can control his or her own behavior, and thereby his or her depression.

2. Therapy should provide training in skills which the patient can utilize to feel more effective in handling his or her daily life. These skills must be of some significance to the patient and must fit with the rationale that has been presented.

3. Therapy should emphasize the independent use of these skills by the patient outside of the therapy context and must provide enough structure so that the attainment of independent skill is possible for the patient.

4. Therapy should encourage the patient's attribution that improvement in mood is caused by the patient's increased skillfulness, not by the therapist's skillfulness (Zeiss, Lewinsohn, & Muñoz, 1979, p. 437–438).

The CWD Course was specifically designed to incorporate the above mentioned hypotheses.

EVALUATION

We have completed three treatment outcome studies (Brown & Lewinsohn, 1984; Steinmetz, Lewinsohn, & Antonuccio, 1983; Teri & Lewinsohn, 1981) and one is currently in progress (Hoberman, Lewinsohn, & Tilson, 1984). In each of these studies participants were carefully assessed on a wide range of variables at four points in time: pre-treatment, post-treatment, one month and six month post-treatment. Each of these studies assessed somewhat different variables depending upon the specific hypotheses under investigation. A core assessment battery, however, was constant across studies. Depression was assessed both through self-report and interviewer report. Self-report measures of depression included the Beck Depression Inventory (Beck, Ward, Mendelsohn, Mock, & Erbaugh, 1961) and the Center for Epidemiological Studies—Depression scale (CES–D; Radloff, 1977). Additional information was gathered from participants in a two-hour semi-structured, pre-treatment interview, the Schedule of Affective Disorders and Schizophrenia (SADS; Endicott & Spitzer, 1978). Diagnoses of depression and other psychopathological syndromes were obtained utilizing decision rules classified by the Research Diagnostic Criteria (RDC; Spitzer, Endicott, & Robins, 1978). For each episode of disturbance the interviewer recorded the diagnosis, age at onset, and duration of the episode. In addition, a second and much shorter version of the interview, the Schedule for Affective Disorders and Schizophrenia—Change version (SADS–C; Spitzer et al., 1978) was used to measure change from pre-treatment to post-treatment and follow-up. The first question, of course, is whether the Course is therapeutically effective. This is not an

easy question to answer unequivocally. Ideally one should have a randomly selected no-treatment control group; but ethically it is very difficult to not offer
treatment to people who are depressed and potentially suicidal. Our solution to this
problem was to randomly assign a proportion of the patients in the first study
(Brown & Lewinsohn, 1984) to a delayed treatment condition. Their treatment
was begun after an eight week waiting period during which time they were encouraged to call the course leader if they needed help. During these eight weeks, then,
these subjects received very little treatment. The results of this and other studies
are shown in Table 2.

As can be seen, results of this first study indicated more clinical improvement
by all of the active treatment conditions compared to the delayed treatment condition. The results also indicated that the improvement shown by depressed individuals participating in the CWD Course are substantial not only at post-treatment,
but are maintained at both one month and six month follow-up. Improvement has
been comparable in magnitude to those shown by patients in individual therapy in
our own as well as in other studies of cognitive-behavioral therapy for depression
(e.g., Bellack, Hersen, & Himmelhoch, 1981; Rush & Beck, 1978; McLean &
Hakstian, 1979; Schmidt & Miller, 1982) Further, these gains were replicated in
three subsequent studies (See Table 2). Recognizing the usual limitations about
generalizing and the need for cross validation by other centers, it appears that the
CWD Course format as currently constituted is a viable and cost effective treatment approach for depressed outpatients.

While our results show that a majority of depressed individuals are improved at
the end of treatment, it is also true that a significant proportion (approximately
20%) are still depressed at the end of treatment. This figure is fairly constant
across studies. It would obviously be valuable if one could predict which individuals do not respond to this treatment. In all of our studies we have included
overlapping participant variables with the goal of identifying and cross validating
positive and negative findings.

Prior to summarizing our findings in regard to patient characteristics predictive
of improvement, it needs to be emphasized that our dependent variable so far has
been post-course depression level. Post-course depression level has been made
independent of pre-course depression level by using analysis of covariance, computing residual gains scores, or by entering pre-course depression level as the first
variable into the multiple regression. We have used these particular analyses because our initial interest was in identifying distinguishing characteristics of participants who show the greatest amount of change (improvement) from pre to post.
What is being summarized, then, are the predictors of improvement as they have
emerged in our studies.

The results from our first two studies (Brown & Lewinsohn, 1984; Steinmetz,
Lewinsohn, & Antonuccio, 1983) are very tentatively summarized in Table 2. As
one might expect the single strongest predictor of post-course depression level (as
measured by the BDI) is pre-treatment depression level. Those who are the most
depressed at the beginning are still, relatively, the most depressed at the end of
treatment. This result supports Garfield's (1978) statement that pre-treatment severity should always be taken into account in the prediction of treatment outcome
because the correlation between pre and post-treatment scores is typically positive
and substantial.

Table 2 Beck depression inventory scores from four treatment outcome studies involving the coping-with-depression course

Study/Treatment	Pre-treatment		Post-treatment		1 month follow-up		6 month follow-up		Percent still meeting RDC criteria for depression at one month post-treatment
	X	S.D.	X	S.D.	X	S.D.	X	S.D.	
Brown & Lewinsohn, 1984									
Class (N = 31)	19.8	7.7	7.6	7.0	6.6	6.2	6.4	6.9	21%
Individual (N = 15)	24.4	8.6	9.5	7.7	11.1	9.4	7.4	7.5	
Phone (N = 12)	20.1	7.5	10.8	7.2	10.0	9.2	9.5	6.2	
Delayed (N = 13)	21.5	9.6	13.9	8.7					
Steinmetz, Antonuccio, Lewinsohn, 1983									
Class (N = 93)	21.1	9.4	6.8	6.1	6.5	6.1	7.9	8.5	22%
Teri & Lewinsohn, 1981									
Class (N = 56)	25.7	14.8	5.9	5.0	5.8	5.3	5.7	4.9	24%
Individual (N = 26)	18.7	10.7	6.2	7.1	5.8	5.5	6.5	4.8	
Hoberman, Lewinsohn, Tilson, 1984									
Class (N = 40)	24.4	9.0	6.0	8.7	7.3	6.1	8.3	8.4	15%

Note. Table includes subjects who did not meet criteria for unipolar depression at pre-treatment.

Table 3 Pre-treatment variables which predict improvement in CWD course

Variables	Approximate correlations
1. Pretreatment depression level (BDI)	−.45
2. Expected improvement (EBDI)	.34
3. Satisfaction with major life roles	.30
4. Concurrent treatment	−.25
5. Perceived social support from family	.20
6. Physical handicap, disabling disease, recent surgery	−.25
7. Suicidal behavior	−.40
8. Perceived control	.20

Correlations 2 through 8 are partial correlations with post-BDI after controlling for pre-BDI.

As shown in Table 3, seven variables accounted for outcome variance beyond that explained by pre-treatment BDI scores:

1. Expected improvement. This was measured by asking participants to complete, at intake, the BDI according to how they predict they will feel at the end of the course. Participants who expected to be the most symptom free at the end of treatment actually were the most improved.

2. Satisfaction with major life roles. Participants who had expressed more satisfaction (using a seven-point scale) with 18 life areas generally considered to be important were also the most improved.

3. Concurrent treatment. Participants who were *not* concurrently receiving additional treatment for depression (Psychotherapy and/or antidepressant medications) were more improved.

4. Perceived social support from family members. Better treatment outcome was obtained by individuals with more perceived social support.

5. Physical problems. Patients who did not have a physical handicap, a disabling disease, or recent surgery were more improved.

6. Suicidal attempts. Those who had a history of a suicidal attempt were less improved.

7. Perceived mastery. This was assessed via participants' ratings of three items designed to reflect perceptions of control over one's life (e.g., "I have little control over things that happen to me"). Participants who felt that they had greater mastery were more improved.

These eight predictors (including pre-treatment BDI level) have a multiple correlation with post-BDI of approximately .75 accounting for 56% of the variance in post-treatment BDI scores.

POTENTIAL APPLICATIONS OF THE CWD COURSE TO PREVENTION

Most of our work to date has been in what has been called tertiary prevention, i.e., the Course has been aimed at people who are already depressed and in whom depression is the major presenting problem. As mentioned earlier, the CWD Course seems to attract a certain percentage (approximately 20%) of people who are not currently depressed but who are taking the Course because they would like to avoid becoming depressed again in the future. As of yet we have no data as to whether or not taking the Course actually helps these nondepressed participants to accomplish this goal. However, it may be hypothesized that taking the Course serves as a preventive function in that by teaching coping skills, it reduces the probability for the occurrence of episodes of depression.

Before pointing to some of the potential applications of the CWD Course to *prevention,* I would like to digress briefly to consider the more general issue of what the specific objectives are when we talk about preventive interventions for depression. There is now a firmly established tradition to define (unipolar) depression as an episodic, all-or-none type of disorder analogous to suffering a heart attack, or a stroke, or having cancer. If one defines depression in this way then the objective of prevention is to reduce incidence, i.e., the number of people who are going to develop an episode of depression during a given period of time. However, in evaluating the potential usefulness and the effectiveness of any particular intervention for preventing depression, it may be important not to lose sight of the fact that unipolar depression can just as easily be conceptualized as being on a continuum (i.e., individuals differ in how depressed they are at any given point in time) and where one draws the line between those who are and those who are not depressed may be rather arbitrary. The continuum definition of depression involves at least two dimensions: 1) Severity level (how many symptoms are present and the frequency and degree of severity with which they are experienced), and 2) Duration (length of period during which depression symptoms are experienced). As can be seen in Figure 1 the values for the length of episodes are highly skewed with *most* people having relatively short, and a few people having relatively long episodes.

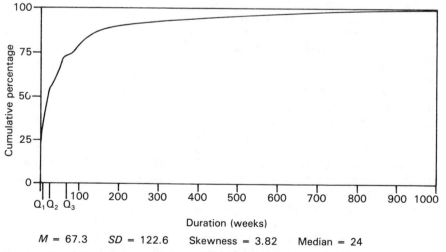

$M = 67.3$ $SD = 122.6$ Skewness = 3.82   Median = 24

Figure 1 Cumulative frequency distribution for all episodes combined. From Lewinsohn, P. M., Fenn, D. S., Stanton, A. K., & Franklin, J. (1986). Relation of age at onset to duration of episode in unipolar depression. *Journal of Psychology and Aging, 1,* 63–68.

Conceptualizing depression in terms of these types of continua allows one to define somewhat more modest but perhaps more consequential goals for prevention; namely, reducing the severity and the duration of episodes of depression. In other words, instead of evaluating a given intervention simply vis a vis the degree to which it prevents "an episode per se" of depression (it may be very difficult to avoid becoming at least somewhat depressed under many difficult and common life circumstances) an intervention might also have an important preventive role to the extent that it allows people to limit the degree of severity and the length of time for which they are depressed. In other words, preventive intervention might be useful if it results in people having relatively mild and short-lived episodes of depression instead of more severe and potentially chronic episodes. An intervention that is capable of doing this would be useful because it is well known that mild episodes have a much better prognosis (Steinmetz, Lewinsohn, Antonuccio, 1983; Keller, Shapiro, Lavori, & Wolfe, 1983). People who are mildly depressed are also much less incapacitated (e.g., they continue to be able to function in important life roles.)

The CWD Course might well serve as a means of preventing *episodes* of depression in the more traditional sense of prevention. However, we hypothesize the CWD Course's most effective and far reaching potential for prevention as being at the level of teaching people how to terminate episodes of depression quickly and before they become severe. Although the CWD Course might act to eliminate depression altogether in some persons, a more realistic goal might be to conceptualize it as a vehicle to provide people with skills they can use to terminate episodes of depression before they become very severe.

With these considerations in mind, research aimed at evaluating the preventive function of the CWD Course with groups of people known to be at elevated risk for depression appears warranted. On the basis of epidemiological studies such as our own (Lewinsohn & Hoberman, 1982) and of others (Hirschfeld & Cross, 1982) information is rapidly becoming available with which to select populations at risk. To wit, those who are a) female, b) have had previous episodes of depression, c) are mildly depressed, d) have weak social support systems, e) are unemployed and seeking employment; f) are experiencing marital conflict, g) have experienced recent life events, especially those involving social exits (e.g., divorce and separation) are at elevated risk for episodes of depression. Another population which is at risk for depression and for whom the CWD Course may serve a preventive role are individuals who are afflicted with medical illnesses (e.g., arthritis) which require major changes in their life styles (i.e., victims of illnesses which disrupt important components of these individuals' skill and behavioral repertoires that are important for their being able to maintain positive reinforcement and to avoid punishment in terms of their interactions with the environment). Such individuals might be well-served by being taught coping skills. Other groups of patients for whom the CWD Course might serve a preventive function are those who have other disorders (e.g., alcoholism) or who are on medications which are known to be accompanied by depression symptoms. Of relevance here is a study by Turner, Wehl, Cannon, and Craig (1980) in which techniques similar to those employed in the CWD Course were successfully employed to treat depression in alcoholics. A strength of the CWD Course is the fact that it can easily be adapted to fit the special needs of different groups as in the Turner et al. study, in treating the elderly (Thompson, Gallagher, Nies, & Epstein, 1982), and even with adolescents (Clarke, Lewinsohn, & Alexander, 1984).

In summary, given the increasing knowledge of the variety of populations at risk for depression and the apparent robust flexibility of the CWD Course, research aimed at examining the preventive functions of the CWD Course for these groups should be fruitful.

Finally, in regard to primary prevention, one could give one's imagination free rein and suggest offering the Coping Course as part of "Life Skills" or "Mental Hygiene" courses in high schools and in adult education. The CWD Course is designed to teach people skills they can use to deal with feelings of dysphoria. There are good reasons to hypothesize that possessing these skills to control, if not to eliminate these feelings, may be useful to many people.

REFERENCES

American Psychiatric Association. (1980). *Diagnostic and Statistical Manual of Mental Disorders, 3rd Edition.* Washington: Author.

Antonuccio, D., Lewinsohn, P. M., & Steinmetz, J. (1982). Identification of therapist differences in a group treatment for depression. *Journal of Consulting and Clinical Psychology, 50,* 433-435.

Beck, A. T., Ward, G. H., Mendelson, M., Mock, J., & Erbaugh, J. (1961). An inventory for measuring depression. *Archives of General Psychiatry, 4,* 561-571.

Bellack, A. S., Hersen, M., & Himmelhoch, J. (1981). Social skills training, pharmacotherapy, and psychotherapy for unipolar depression. *American Journal of Psychiatry, 138,* 1562-1567.

Brown, R., & Lewinsohn, P. M. (1984). A psychoeducational approach to the treatment of depression: Comparison of group, individual, and minimal contact procedures. *Journal of Consulting and Clinical Psychology, 52,* 774-783.

Brown, R., & Lewinsohn, P. M. (1984). *Participant workbook.* Eugene, OR: Castalia Publishing Co.

Clarke, G., Lewinsohn, P. M., & Alexander, C. (1985). *A psychoeducational approach to the treatment of adolescent depression.* Paper presented at the meetings of the Western Psychological Association, April 19, 1985 at San Jose, CA.

Endicott, J., & Spitzer, R. L. (1978). A diagnostic interview: The schedule for affective disorders and schizophrenia. *Archives of General Psychiatry, 35,* 837-844.

Garfield, S. L. (1978). Research on client variables in psychotherapy. In S. L. Garfield, & A. E. Bergin (Eds.), *Handbook of psychotherapy and behavior change. 2nd edition.* New York: Wiley.

Gonzales, L., Lewinsohn, P. M., Clarke, G. (1985). Longitudinal follow-up of unipolar depressives: An investigation of predictors of relapse. *Journal of Consulting and Clinical Psychology, 53,* 461-469.

Hirschfeld, R. M. & Cross, C. K. (1982). Epidemiology of affective disorders: Psychological risk factors. *Archives of General Psychiatry, 39,* 35-45.

Hoberman, H., Lewinsohn, P. M., & Tilson, M. (1985). *Group treatment of depression: Therapeutic process, client characteristics, and outcome.* Paper presented at the meetings of the Western Psychological Association, April 19, 1985, San Jose, CA.

Keller, M. B., Shapiro, R. W., Lavori, P. W., & Wolfe, N. (1982). Recovery in major depressive disorder. *Archives of General Psychiatry, 39,* 905-910.

Lewinsohn, P. M., Antonuccio, D., Steinmetz, J., & Teri, L. (1984). *The coping with depression course: A psychoeducational intervention for unipolar depression.* Eugene, OR: Castalia Publ. Co.

Lewinsohn, P. M., & Hoberman, H. (1982). *Stress moderator variables and depression: A prospective perspective.* Paper presented at Western Psychological Association meeting, Sacramento, April 1982.

Lewinsohn, P. M., Muñoz R., Youngren, M. & Zeiss, A. (1978). *Control your depression.* NJ: Prentice-Hall.

Lewinsohn, P. M., Sullivan, J. M., & Grosscup, S. (1980). Changing reinforcing events: An approach to the treatment of depression. *Psychotherapy: Theory, Research & Practice, 17,* 322-334.

Lewinsohn, P. M., Youngren, M. & Grosscup, S. (1979). Reinforcement and depression. In R. A. Depue (Ed.), *The psychobiology of the depressive disorders: Implications for the effects of stress.* New York: Academic Press.

McLean, P. D., & Hakstian, A. R. (1979). Clinical depression: Comparative efficacy of outpatient treatments. *Journal of Consulting and Clinical Psychology, 47*, 818-836.

Muñoz, R. F. (1977). A cognitive approach to the assessment and treatment of depression. *Dissertation Abstracts International, 38*, 2873B. (University Microfilms No. 77-26, 505, 154.)

Radloff, L. (1977). The CES-D scale: A self-report depression scale for research in the general population. *Applied Psychological Measurement, 1*, 385-401.

Rush, A. J. & Beck, A. T. (1978). Behavior therapy in adults with affective disorders. In M. Hersen & A. S. Bellack (Eds.), *Behavior therapy in the psychiatric setting*. Baltimore: Williams & Wilkins.

Schmidt, M. & Miller, W. (1982). *Amount of therapist contact and outcome for a multimodal depression treatment program*. Paper presented at Western Psychological Association, Sacramento, April 1982.

Spitzer, R. L., Endicott, J., & Robins, E. (1978). Research diagnostic criteria. *Archives of General Psychiatry, 35*, 773-782.

Steinmetz, J., Antonuccio, D., Bond, M., McKay, G., Brown, R., & Lewinsohn, P. M. (1979). *Instructor's manual*. Unpublished mimeo, University of Oregon.

Steinmetz, J., Lewinsohn, P. M., & Antonuccio, D. (1983). Prediction of individual outcome in a group intervention for depression. *Journal of Consulting and Clinical Psychology, 51*, 331-337.

Teri, L. & Lewinsohn, P. M. (1981). *Comparative efficacy of group vs. individual treatment of unipolar depression*. Presented at the Association for Advancement of Behavior Therapy, Toronto, 1981.

Thompson, L., Gallagher, D., Nies, G., & Epstein, D. (1983). Evaluation of the effectiveness of professionals and nonprofessionals as instructors of Coping with Depression classes for elders. *Gerontologist, 23*, 390-396.

Turner, R. W., Wehl, C. K., Cannon, D. S., & Craig, K. A. (1980). *Individual treatment for depression in alcoholics: A comparison of behavioral, cognitive, and nonspecific therapy*. Unpublished mimeo, VA Medical Center, Salt Lake City.

Zeiss, A. (1977). *Interpersonal behavioral problems of the depressed: A study of outpatient treatment*. Unpublished dissertation, University of Oregon.

Zeiss, A., Lewinsohn, P. M., & Muñoz, R. (1979). Nonspecific improvement effects in depression using interpersonal skills training, pleasant activity schedules, or cognitive training. *Journal of Consulting and Clinical Psychology, 47*, 427-439.

10

Stress Management Training: An Approach to the Prevention of Depression in Low-Income Populations

Betty Tableman
Michigan Department of Mental Health

INTRODUCTION

Although stress management training has become widely available in adult education and health promotion offerings, such opportunities for learning to modify behavior have been directed primarily at executive men concerned with health risks, and at professionals seeking to avoid burnout. Mental health agencies have been slow to adopt stress management training as a prevention strategy directed at populations at high risk for unipolar depression and depressive symptomatology. Yet stress management training directed at high risk adults, primarily women, has a more immediate linkage to mental health agency caseloads than more traditional prevention strategies directed at younger populations. The emerging conceptual and research base on treatment of depression would appear appropriate for prevention strategies designed to reduce the need for and utilization of mental health treatment services.

This article describes a cognitive-behavioral intervention, Stress Management Training (SMT), designed to enhance the management of stress by women on public assistance. This population characteristically experiences significant ongoing stressors and stressful life events and uses coping responses which tend to exacerbate rather than reduce stress (Pearlin & Schooler, 1978; Ilfeld, 1977).

SMT was developed as a prevention project of the Michigan Department of Mental Health. Since 1977, a small annual legislative appropriation for pilot demonstration projects permits the development and evaluation of service models for community mental health agencies. If there is evidence suggesting effectiveness, the project is transferred to continuation funding and the service model becomes available for replication in other community mental health centers (Tableman, 1980).

SMT resulted from an interest in stress management strategies shared by the prevention coordinator of the Ionia County Community Mental Health Services Board and a home economist from the Cooperative Extension service.* This inter-

Acknowledgement is made of the contributions of Carolyn L. Feis, William Redmon, Arnold Greenfield, and Dennis Howard in the evaluation analyses.

*STM was developed by Diane Johnson, now affiliated with the West Chester (Ohio) Counseling Center, and Roberta Rodgers, Michigan Cooperative Extension Service. Since 1980, it has been directed by Deborah Marciniak who has refined, stabilized and documented the content and process.

est was directed at women on public assistance in view of a needs assessment which indicated that the largest identifiable group of mental health center clients were economically deprived, depressed young women.

THE INTERVENTION

In developing SMT, the initial authors and their successor drew on existing conceptualizations and strategies; their contribution has been to translate available material from a varied literature (including such areas as stress management, values clarifications, child abuse and women's issues) into an intervention relevant for women on public assistance. The authors' experience with low income women in therapy and in educational outreach suggested that women on public assistance are characterized by low self-esteem and "learned helplessness" behavior (Seligman, 1975). They tend to be isolated by the circumstances of their lives, to be trapped in destructive interpersonal relationships, to assume that their problems are unique and unmanageable. They interpret their past histories (often fraught with traumatic events) and their present circumstances to mean that they are worthless. These behaviors associated with low self-esteem and hopelessness/helplessness, as well as the lack of a confiding relationship, were found by Brown and Harris (1978) to predispose women for depression in the face of a provoking event.

SMT was developed as a multi-dimensional intervention using both cognitive restructuring and behavioral training. Both approaches were felt to be necessary as a prevention strategy with low income women. Before behavior change was possible, the women must overcome their perception of themselves as worthless and incapable of affecting their own lives. This approach is consistent with theoretical work which suggests that prevention or treatment of depression requires modification of attributions of worthlessness and/or expectations of failure (Hollon & Garber, 1980).

Secondly, it was felt that specific skill training was needed to enable these women to take control of their lives and to modify maladaptive responses. SMT incorporated a wide range of techniques and strategies, consistent with research suggesting that use of a variety of coping responses is more important in reducing stress than any single identified response (Pearlin & Schooler, 1978).

Other formulations related to learning contributed to the design of the project. SMT was defined as a time-limited educational experience and used educational techniques. Significant support and reinforcement is provided to the participants by the group experience. Leaders present themselves as role models, participating as group members and sharing their personal experiences. Learning is reinforced by giving the women "self-discovery" exercises to do at home and a notebook to maintain handouts and exercises for future reference.

Participants attend 10 weekly $2\frac{1}{2}$ to 3-hour sessions. Each group consists of 6 to 12 women. Transportation and child care is provided, facilitating attendance. Churches and other community centers are used as informal and comfortable settings, avoiding any suggestion that participants were mental health center clients. A snack break during the sessions encourages socialization and provides opportunities for leaders to discuss nutrition.

SMT provides a broad introduction to life-coping skills. The ten session training is designed to help women to feel better about themselves, accept responsibility for their own behavior, take control of their lives, and handle stress more effectively.

The first three sessions are directed at enhancing self-esteem and identifying stress-producing aspects of personal relationships. The women explore the effect of perceptions on self-esteem, begin a process of self-discovery, and identify problems and goals on which to work. They learn to label feelings and to recognize the difference between feelings and action. They explore the impact of negative communication, and practice accepting and providing positive feedback. The sessions also review steps toward developing a positive mental attitude, strategies for self-acceptance, attitudes toward women and women's roles, dynamics of destructive behavior, and positive approaches with children. Women learn about communication and empathy in interpersonal relationships. They learn how to respond to negative statements and actions. Stress and relaxation through deep breathing are discussed in the third session.

The next five sessions on life planning emphasize acceptance of responsibility for one's behavior and techniques for taking control. Women clarify their values, needs, capabilities, and goals. Developing past and future "Life Lines" (Kirn & Kirn, 1978) are significant activities. The women explore decision making approaches. They practice problem solving and how to make changes one step at a time. Participants also assess key relationships in their lives, identify characteristics of "true" friends, and make lists of personal and community supports.

In the last two sessions, participants explore understanding stress and stress management strategies. They learn the signs of stress and how people tend to respond to stressful situations. The women identify sources of personal stress. They practice such stress resolution techniques as anticipatory role-playing, redefining the situation, and positive self-talk (Meichenbaum, 1975). They develop a list of positive coping strategies. Although relaxation techniques are presented throughout the manual, they are not always used during sessions because of time constraints.

The curriculum as currently packaged requires basic reading and writing skills to respond to visuals, handouts and home exercises. While leaders occasionally pair non-readers with a literate member, adaptation of the materials would be required for groups with substantial reading deficits.

The project uses available and specially developed written and visual materials. Sessions are structured and experiential. Leaders must be mature and nonjudgmental as participants react to the concepts presented and relate them to their own lives.

THE IONIA COUNTY PROJECT

SMT was evaluated in 1977–79 in Ionia County, Michigan,* an area with 50,000 population in scattered small communities between two metropolitan counties. Participants were white women on public assistance (Aid to Families of Dependent Children or General Assistance).

The Ionia project was staffed with a part-time prevention service coordinator with a professional background in counselling who handled overall arrangements

*Material on the Ionia county project was previously published in the *American Journal of Community Psychology,* Vol. *10*(3), 355–365.

and co-led the sessions; a co-leader with a professional background in adult education whose only responsibility was the sessions; and a full-time administrative assistant who carried out enrollment, data collection, and clerical functions. This staffing pattern made it possible to conduct three groups simultaneously. Total program costs per participant were about $300.

Experimental Design and Measures

From a population of 900 women, 209 were recruited by family service workers who thought the training would be beneficial. During a home visit, 65 women were enrolled as experimental subjects and 51 women as controls. Random assignment prior to the home visit was imperfectly implemented. Data was obtained from 39 of 45 women who attended 7 to 10 training sessions, 14 women who dropped out after attending an average of 2.7 sessions and 35 women who received no training.

Although women who were receiving mental health center services were excluded, a high proportion of participants had sought help with personal problems (63%) or used medication (50%) in the previous year. Average age was 28 years.

A pretest/posttest, nonequivalent control group design was used. Pretest data were collected within 30 days before the first workshop session. Posttest data were collected $2\frac{1}{2}$ months after the last workshop session, or about 6 months after the pretest data. Participants were paid $3 for returning test data.

SMT's impact on the mental health of participants was assessed through three standardized measures: *The Cornell Index* (Weider, Wolff, Brodman, Mittelmann, & Wechsler, 1948) is a 101-item checklist designed to assess neuropsychiatric and psychosomatic symptoms. The total score and subscores for Depression, Anxiety, and Fear/Inadequacy were used. *State-Trait Anxiety Inventory* (STAI) (Spielberger, 1968) has 20 test items rated on a 4-point Likert scale to indicate how often a subject experiences various anxiety related emotional states. Form X2 measuring trait-anxiety was used. *The 16 Personality Factor Test, Form C* (The Institute for Personality and Ability Testing, 1969) consists of 103 forced-choice items that measure 16 functionally independent, psychologically meaningful personality dimensions. Two dimensions were relevant to the training: Ego strength and Self-confidence.

Results

No significant group differences in demographic/experiential characteristics were found (all $ps > .05$) in a statistical comparison of the groups using an analysis of variance for mean scores and chi-square analyses for differences in proportions. Significant pretest differences, however, were present on the evaluation measures when separate analyses of variance were performed on each instrument and subscales for the three groups. Table 1 presents a comparison of pretest data for experimental, control, and dropout groups on each measure in the evaluation test battery. Post hoc analyses of these effects were done using the Least Significant Difference test for simultaneous mean comparison. The dropout group differed significantly from the experimental group on only one factor (16 PF-Ego Strength). The experimental and control groups differed significantly on six of nine factors, indicating nonequivalence prior to intervention.

Table 1 Pretest means and standard deviations for experimental and control groups and dropouts, Ionia County Project

Measure subscale	Experimental[a] (n = 39)		Control (n = 35)		Dropouts (n = 14)		Probability	
	Mean	SD	Mean	SD	Mean	SD	Experimental vs. control	Experimental vs. dropouts
Cornell index[b]								
Full score	28.6	14.02	18.9	15.17	29.5	14.61	<.01	NS
Depression	2.9	1.96	1.5	1.72	2.9	1.83	<.01	NS
Anxiety	3.1	1.75	1.9	1.64	3.1	1.69	<.01	NS
Fear, inadequacy	5.9	3.44	3.9	3.95	6.3	3.75	<.05	NS
STAI—								
Trait-anxiety[b]	52.1	7.22	41.9	11.96	53.5	10.09	NS	NS
16 PF								
C-Ego strength[c]	4.2	2.35	6.2	2.67	5.9	1.75	<.01	<.05
O-Self-confidence[b]	8.4	2.44	6.4	2.95	8.0	2.75	<.01	NS

[a]Completed 7–10 sessions.
[b]Lower scores denote better status.
[c]Higher scores denote better status.

Table 2 Mean change score and standard deviations for pretest to 6 month follow-up outcome
measures for experimental and control groups, Ionia County Project

Measure subscale	Experimental[a] (n = 39)			Control (n = 35)		
	Mean change[b]	SD		Mean change[b]	SD	p
Cornell index[c]						
Total	−8.74	12.80		0.06	7.53	< .001
Depression	−1.30	2.77		0.06	1.62	< .005
Fear, inadequacy	−1.74	3.93		0.00	1.92	< .005
Anxiety	−0.97	1.53		0.03	1.04	< .001
STAI—						
Trait-anxiety[c]	−9.15	10.84		0.83	7.66	< .001
16 PF						
C-Ego strength[d]	1.79	2.44		0.09	2.37	< .001
O-Self confidence[d]	−1.69	3.02		0.43	2.29	< .001

[a]Completed 7–10 sessions.
[b]From pretest to follow-up at 6 months, $3\frac{1}{2}$ months after termination of intervention.
[c]Negative change denotes better status.
[d]Positive change denotes better status.

Cook and Campbell (1979) suggest three types of analysis for nonequivalence
between groups: matching, analysis of covariance, and analysis of change scores.

Analysis of change scores was selected because alternative approaches recommended were not appropriate to this data. Matching would have required prior
knowledge of pretest differences. Valid use of covariance assumes comparable
regression lines for experimental and control groups when pretest scores are regressed on posttest scores (Cohen & Cohen, 1975). Neither situation was applicable.

On the analysis of change scores, pretest scores were subtracted from posttest
scores for each subject, and mean group change scores were compared for experimental and control groups using an independent-sample *t*-test. Dropouts, attending
an average of 2.7 sessions, were considered to be non-users of services and were
excluded in comparing service users with controls.

The effects of the training intervention are presented in Table 2, which shows
group means, standard deviations, and probability levels for pretest-posttest
change scores. Experimental subjects improved significantly more than controls on
total Cornell scores and on all three subscales, i.e., Depression, Anxiety, and
Inadequacy, as well as on the STAI trait-anxiety scale and the 16 PF scales for Ego
strength and Self-confidence. This data has been translated into effect sizes in
Table 7, permitting comparison between studies.

Anecdotal Data

In addition to the evaluation measures, after completion of the training, comments of professionals in contact with the women were noted. Department of
Social Services staff described SMT participants as more future-oriented, which is
uncharacteristic behavior in welfare recipients: they talked about what they intended to do with their lives, and when and how they would go about it. SMT

participants were seen as less dependent, making fewer requests for assistance. They were less devastated in times of crisis and were able to participate immediately with the services worker in problem solving.

It was also reported that women who had been uninvolved at Headstart meetings were now actively participating and communicating their concerns. In other individuals, attitude and behavior had changed from hostility and defensiveness to more productive involvement.

Information about the perceived impact of training was also collected from the women themselves. At the time posttest data was collected, the women were asked to put down in their own words what changes they had made in their lives as a result of participating in SMT. Table 3 gives this information.

For these women, SMT facilitated decision-making and change: 47 percent returned to school, obtained a job or a new place to live, resolved longstanding health problems, made a decision to divorce or to accept this life change.

One-third improved their relationships with children, husbands, boyfriends and mothers. For one-fourth, SMT resulted in better friendships, ability to use friends for support and willingness to take time for themselves.

Changes in cognition around problems and acquisition of problem-solving strategies were mentioned by 36 percent. Eight percent were more assertive in expressing their opinions and feelings. Twenty-two percent indicated they were more in control of their lives, recognized that change was up to them, and were setting attainable goals. Thirty percent indicated that their outlook on life had improved; they felt more self-confident.

According to the women, the training sessions provided a rare opportunity for

Table 3 Ratings of workshop and comments by participants on changes in their lives as a result of SMT, Ionia County Project

A. Formal rating of workshop	(%)
Very helpful—made a big difference in my life	39
Somewhat helpful—I did learn some things and made a few positive changes	53
An okay way to spend time but I didn't get much out of it	8
B. Comments on changes made as a result of SMT	
Facilitated life changes	47
School (21%), jobs (10%), place to live (4%), took care of health problems (6%), facilitated decision about, acceptance of divorce (6%)	
Improved relationships	34
With children (10%), husband, boyfriend, ex-husband (6%), mother (4%), in general (14%)	
Increased use of friends (20%), more activity (4%)	24
Changes in cognition, attitude and behavior	
Improved outlook, more self-confident, more assertive	30
Improved problem solving	36
Changed attitude about problems (12%), learned problem-solving strategies (24%)	
In control of life; more goal-oriented	22
More assertive	8
SMT did not make a difference	8
Not long enough to solve difficult problems (4%), made no changes (4%)	

Note. Percent will not add up to 100 because some women gave multiple comments.

social contact, sharing, and acceptance and for recognizing that other people were also struggling. The workshops apparently helped the women to step back and look at their lives from a new perspective, to talk over problems, and to find solutions in a way that they had never experienced before. Participants reported that they learned new concepts about letting go of the past, planning for the future. Training changed their expectations about their ability to be in control of their lives and their understanding of their own and other's needs. Training seemed to improve their ability to communicate and their problem-solving skills. It enhanced assertiveness and decision-making.

APPLICABILITY FOR OTHER POPULATIONS

With the availability of a replication manual (Marciniak and Tableman, 1981*), SMT has been utilized with other populations. The majority of these efforts have not been formally evaluated. A survey of agencies who purchased the manual indicated that SMT has been used with reported success with women in jail, pregnant adolescents in alternative schools, abusing parents, and women variously characterized as mothers, single, working, returning to work, or adapting to divorce. SMT has been installed in Ionia county's community education offerings as the first part of a parent training sequence.

In Ionia County, SMT has also been used with men on general assistance enrolled in work training; it was perceived by the training staff and participants as an effective motivational component. Little or no modification of material was required for use with men. However, the coordinator found it more difficult to work with men who, having failed in both work and interpersonal roles, had even more limited assets than the women and provided little or no responsive feedback during sessions. In 1985, SMT was adopted in several Michigan counties as a component of the Department of Social Services employment and training program.

Two additional valuations of SMT have been completed. In Ionia county, SMT was evaluated in 1982 as an alternative treatment for women seeking services from, or already on, the caseload of the mental health center. Excluded were women who were actively psychotic, severely depressed or of borderline intelligence. While this was not a preventive intervention, the results illuminate the impact of SMT. A comparison of women assigned randomly to traditional one-on-one therapy or to SMT found SMT equally effective in producing change in all aspects measured and more effective than individual therapy in improving feelings and moods and enhancing mastery (Feis, Tableman, Howard, & Marciniak, 1984).

THE DETROIT PROJECT

SMT was also evaluated in 1984 with predominantly black women on public assistance in inner city Detroit. With an average age of 36, this was an older group than the Ionia sample. Women were referred through the Department of Social Services employment and training program and assigned by alternate months to

---

*The SMT replication manual (Marciniak, D., and Tableman, B.) is available for $10 from the Ionia County Community Mental Health Center, 437 West Lincoln, Ionia, Michigan, 48846.

experimental and control groups. Illustrations were modified to reflect the race of the participants, and one homework exercise was deleted; there were no changes in content. Group sessions were held at the mental health center. Data was obtained during the first session (pretest), last session (posttest), and six months after the pretest (follow-up).

The Detroit project used five different evaluation instruments to expand information about the impact of the intervention. *Pearlin Mastery Scale* (Pearlin & Schooler, 1978), 7 items, scored 0 to 3, assesses the extent to which life changes are seen as being under one's own control versus fatalistically ruled. *Beck Depression Inventory* (Beck, Ward, Mendelson, Mock, & Erbaugh, 1961) is a 21-item instrument designed to measure symptoms of depression. Each item represents distinct symptom-attitude categories, with responses having values from 0 to 3. *Rosenberg Self-Esteem Inventory* (Rosenberg, 1965), a 10 item measure, is designed to assess the positiveness of one's attitude toward oneself. Although parenting skills are not specifically included in SMT, the *Parental Coping Scale* (Pearlin & Schooler, 1978), a 21-item measure, was included to explore the impact of SMT on parenting. The five subscales are: Selective Ignoring, Nonpunitiveness vs. Reliance on Discipline, Self-reliance vs. Advice Seeking, Positive Comparisons, and Exercise of Potency vs. Helpless Resignation. *Progress Evaluation Scales* (Ihilevich & Gleser, 1981) are seven scales each with five levels (maximum score of 5) which assess the most pathological to healthiest levels of functioning in regard to Family Interaction, Occupation, Getting Along with Others, Feelings and Mood, Use of Free Time, Problems, and Attitudes Toward Self.

Results

Pretest data was collected for 139 SMT participants in eight groups, and 67 controls in six groups. Follow-up data was obtained for 48 of 79 women who attended 7 to 10 training sessions, and for 32 controls. Because of a change in the group leader between groups 2 and 3, and recruitment difficulties, the first six groups were considered trial runs. Results are therefore presented for the last two experimental groups (pretest n = 61).

The two experimental groups resulted in complete data through follow up for 23 women. Three of the 32 control participants did not have complete data on various subscales of the Pearlin Parental Coping Scale and were therefore excluded from those subscale comparisons. Again, experimental and control groups scores were not comparable on evaluation measures at pretest (Table 4) and change scores were therefore used.

The experimental group showed significant pretest to posttest improvement on the following measures: Beck Depression; the Pearlin Mastery; Pearlin Parental Coping Positive Comparisons subscale; Progress Evaluation scales (PES) subscales Use of Free Time, Problems, and Attitudes Toward Self, and Rosenberg Self-Esteem Scale. Comparisons were made with controls on these measures. While the experimental group showed positive improvement from pretest to posttest, the control group barely improved on two measures and actually declined on the Pearlin Mastery Scale (Table 5). Differences were significant on all measures except the Rosenberg Self-Esteem.

Table 6 shows that by follow-up, the women in SMT had maintained significant improvement over controls on the Beck Depression, Pearlin Mastery and Pearlin

Table 4 Pretest means and standard deviations for experimental[a] and control groups, Detroit Project

Measure subscale	Experimental[a]			Control			Probability	
	N	Mean	SD	N	Mean	SD	t	p[b]
Beck Depression[c]	23	15.22	8.07	32	9.63	7.29	-2.69	<.05
Rosenberg self-esteem[c]	23	1.13	1.10	32	1.03	1.33	-0.29	NS
Pearlin Mastery[c]	23	8.48	4.27	32	6.41	3.48	-1.93	NS
Pearlin parental coping scale[d]								
Positive comparisons	23	4.70	0.82	31	6.71	1.79	5.03	<.001
Selective ignoring	23	6.57	1.44	31	5.81	1.28	-2.05	<.05
Nonpunitiveness vs. reliance on discipline	23	4.87	1.69	30	5.77	1.64	1.96	NS
Self-reliance vs. advice seeking	23	5.96	2.48	31	6.39	2.38	0.64	NS
Exercise of potency vs. helpless resignation	23	5.30	1.58	31	6.84	1.99	3.08	<.01
Progress evaluation scales[d]								
Use of free time	23	2.83	1.50	32	3.72	1.37	2.28	<.05
Problems	23	3.57	1.38	32	3.94	1.13	1.09	NS
Attitude toward self	23	3.96	0.88	32	3.97	1.17	0.03	NS
Family	23	4.52	0.79	32	4.72	0.57	1.11	NS
Occupation	23	3.78	1.51	32	4.25	1.50	1.15	NS
Getting along with others	23	4.61	0.50	32	4.46	0.58	-0.33	NS
Feelings and mood	23	4.35	1.15	32	4.44	0.95	0.32	NS

Note: Includes only participants with complete data through follow-up
[a]Completed 7–10 sessions.
[b]Two-tailed probability.
[c]Lower scores represent better status.
[d]Higher scores represent better status.

Table 5 Mean change scores, standard deviations, and t-tests for pretest to 10 week posttest outcome measures for experimental and control groups, Detroit Project

Measure subscale	Experimental		Control		Probability	
	Mean change	SD	Mean change	SD	t	p[a]
Beck depression[b]	4.26	5.43	0.13	7.67	2.21	< .01
Rosenberg self-esteem[b]	0.43	0.90	−0.09	1.33	1.63	NS
Pearlin mastery[b]	2.35	3.65	0.00	3.75	2.33	< .01
Pearlin parental coping						
Positive comparisons[c]	1.74	1.81	−0.45	1.81	4.38	< .005
Progress evaluation scales						
Use of free time[b]	0.65	1.75	−0.44	1.85	2.22	< .01
Problems[b]	0.65	1.30	−0.03	0.93	2.27	< .01
Attitudes toward self[b]	0.48	0.89	−0.13	1.31	1.91	< .05

Note: Positive change scores denote better status.
[a] One-tailed probability.
[b] n = 23 experimentals, 32 controls.
[c] n = 23 experimentals, 31 controls.

Table 6 Mean change scores, standard deviations, and t-tests for pretest to 6 month follow-up outcome measures for experimental and control groups, Detroit Project

Measure subscale	Experimental		Control			Probability	
	Mean change	SD	Mean change	SD	t	p^a	
Beck Depression[b]	7.78	9.19	2.06	5.27	2.92	<.005	
Rosenberg self-esteem[b]	0.43	1.14	0.16	1.14	0.843	NS	
Pearlin mastery[b]	2.78	3.48	0.22	3.44	2.72	<.01	
Pearlin parental coping							
Positive comparisons[c]	2.26	2.77	−0.13	1.57	3.98	<.005	
Progress evaluation scales							
Use of free time[b]	1.35	1.72	0.03	1.17	2.81	<.01	
Problems[b]	0.74	1.54	0.25	1.16	1.32	NS	
Attitudes toward self[c]	0.48	0.99	0.13	1.43	1.00	NS	

Note: Positive change scores denote better status.
[a] One-tailed probability.
[b] n = 23 experimentals, 32 controls.
[c] n = 23 experimentals, 31 controls.

Table 7 Effect sizes

Effect	Ionia County pretest- follow-up	Detroit	
		Pretest- posttest	Pretest- follow-up
Total (Cornell Index)	1.17		
Anxiety	.96		
Depression	.84	.54	1.09
Fear, inadequacy	.91		
Self-confidence	.92		
Ego strength	.72		
Mastery		.63	.74
Self-esteem		.39	.24

Note. Sizes are the experimental change score minus control change score divided by standard deviation of the control group.

Parental Coping Positive Comparisons subscale. The Use of Free Time subscale of the PES was the only subscale of the PES which continued to show significant improvement of experimentals over controls. Effect sizes are presented in Table 7.

DISCUSSION

The studies reported from two different populations suggest the strength of SMT for the prevention of depression with women on public assistance. In the context of a group caring experience, SMT provides participants with (1) cognitive restructuring toward a belief in one's power and potential; (2) a system for life planning, i.e., setting and accomplishing goals and reducing life changes to manageable levels; (3) a framework for problem solving and decisionmaking to change negative aspects of one's life; and (4) specific stress management skills and a repertoire of alternative approaches for reducing stress generated by unplanned or uncontrollable events.

While these can be powerful tools for the prevention of depression—and the data shows that gains continue to be made $3\frac{1}{2}$ months after the termination of training—their long run effectiveness may be flawed in a political environment which has increased stressors and made moving off dependency more difficult. Changes in expectations and life planning skills may be less than adequate when there are no training opportunities; when if training can be accomplished, there are no jobs; when if there are jobs in other communities, the welfare system provides disincentives to moving away from dependency.

SMT's greatest contribution to women on public assistance may well be its emphasis on control over one's response to events. By modifying self-attributions, improving modes of interaction with significant others, and increasing the coping repertoire, SMT positions a highly stressed population to use social support, to take advantage of formal assistance and thus to restabilize more rapidly.

While one can suggest from other research the relevance of various aspects of the training (Tableman, Marciniak, Johnson, & Rodgers, 1982), more definitive information on the contributions of the various components of the training and the behavior of participants over time requires a more complex research study. It would be useful to assess changes in attributions, in expectations, in interpersonal cognitive problem-solving ability, and in social support so as to have a better understanding of the relative contributions to change. Documentation of coping behavior pre and post training would be useful. Women should be followed over a longer period of time to determine the staying power for the intervention. It would also be interesting to assess the secondary impact of the intervention on the children of participants in view of research showing the deleterious impact of stress on parenting capability (Belle, 1979; Egelund, Phipps-Yonas, Brunnquell, & Deinard, 1979). The logistics and cost of more extensive data collection and tracking a public assistance population over time, however, are beyond the capacity of field research through a state department of mental health.

REFERENCES

Beck, A. T., Ward, C. H., Mendelson, M., Mock, J., & Erbaugh, J. (1961). An inventory for measuring depression. *Archives of General Psychiatry, 4,* 561–571.

Belle, D. (Ed.) (1979). *Lives in stress: A context for depression.* Cambridge, MA: Stress and Families Project, Graduate School of Education, Harvard University.

Brown, G., & Harris, T. (1978). *Social origins of depression: A study of psychiatric disorder in women.* New York: Free Press.

Cohen, J., & Cohen, P. (1975). *Applied multiple regression/correlation analysis for the behavioral sciences.* New York: Wiley.

Cook, T. D., & Campbell, D. T. (1979). *Quasi-experimentation: Design and analysis issues for field settings.* Boston: Houghton Mifflin Company.

Egelund, B., Phipps-Yonas, S., Brunnquell, D., & Deinard, A. (1979). A prospective study of the antecedents of child abuse. *Caring, 5,* (4), 1–4.

Feis, C. L., Tableman, B., Howard, D., & Marciniak, D. (1984). *Stress management training as an alternative treatment.* Lansing, MI: Michigan Department of Mental Health.

Hollon, S. D., & Garber, J. (1980). A cognitive-expectancy theory of therapy for helplessness and depression. In J. Garber & M. Seligman (Eds.), *Human helplessness: Theory and applications* (pp. 173–195). New York: Academic Press.

Ihilevich, D., & Gleser, G. (1981). *Measuring program outcome: The Progress Evaluation Scales.* Owosso, MI: Shiawassee County Community Mental Health Services Board.

Ilfeld, F. W. (1977). Current social stressors and symptoms of depression. *American Journal of Psychiatry, 134,* 161–166.

Institute for Personality and Ability Testing (1969). *16 Personality Factor Test, Form C.* Champaign, IL: Author.

Kirn, A., & Kirn, M. O. (1978). *Life work planning.* New York: McGraw-Hill.

Marciniak, D., & Tableman, B. (1981). *Stress management training for women on public assistance: A replication manual.* Lansing, MI: Michigan Department of Mental Health.

Meichenbaum, D. (1975). A self-instructional approach to stress management: A proposal for stress inoculation training. In C. D. Spielberger & I. G. Sarason (Eds.), *Stress and anxiety* (Vol 1). New York: Wiley.

Pearlin, L. A., & Schooler, C. (1978). The structure of coping. *Journal of Health and Social Behavior, 19,* 2–21.

Rosenberg, M. (1965). *Society and the adolescent self-image.* Princeton: Princeton University Press.

Seligman, M. (1975). *Helplessness: On depression, development and death.* San Francisco: W. H. Freeman.

Spielberger, C. D. (1968). *Self-evaluation Questionnaire: STAI X2.* Palo Alto, CA: Consulting Psychologists Press.

Tableman, B. (1980). Prevention activities at the state level. In R. H. Price, R. F. Ketterer, B. C. Bader, & J. Monahan (Eds.), *Prevention in mental health* (pp. 237–252). Beverly Hills: Sage.

Tableman, B., Marciniak, D., Johnson, D., & Rogers R. (1982). Stress management training for women on public assistance. *American Journal of Community Psychology, 10.* 357–367.

Weider, A., Wolff, H. G., Brodman, K., Mittelmann, B., & Wechsler, D. (1948). *Cornell Index.* New York: The Psychological Corporation.

11

The Life Satisfaction Course: An Intervention for the Elderly

Julia Steinmetz Breckenridge, Antonette M. Zeiss,
and Larry W. Thompson .
Center for the Study of Psychotherapy and Aging
Palo Alto Veterans Administration Medical Center

INTRODUCTION

The Life Satisfaction Course is a psychoeducational intervention modeled after the Coping with Depression Course developed by Peter Lewinsohn and his colleagues at the University of Oregon (Lewinsohn, Antonuccio, Steinmetz, & Teri, 1984), with modifications designed to address the unique needs and problems of the elderly. It is designed to serve either a primary preventive function with elderly who are currently asymptomatic and functioning adequately, or more commonly, a secondary preventive function. For the latter purpose, the target population is adults aged 55 and older who are dissatisfied or dysphoric but do not meet criteria for a major depressive episode. The course is currently being evaluated as a pilot project. This chapter will describe the rationale, procedures, and preventive implications of the work in progress.

The prevalence of clinical depression in the elderly has been variously estimated as 2 to 10% (Blazer & Williams, 1980; Gurland, 1976). Blazer and Williams (1980), in a recent epidemiological study, found substantial depressive symptomatology in 14.7% of a sample of 997 elderly community residents, and other community studies (e.g., Gaitz, 1977; Lowenthal & Berkman, 1967) have found the *majority* of elderly respondents to report symptoms of depression. George and Bearon (1980) and Larson (1978) have reported that the elderly have a low level of life satisfaction. This pervasive dysphoria and dissatisfaction in the elderly is not surprising, when one considers the number of stressors that increase late in life: Decreased financial resources, declining physical health, loss of friends and close relations through death, and many changes in habitual activity patterns due to retirement are only a sampling. Dysphoria and dissatisfaction, and the increasing potential for life stresses and physical and social-emotional difficulties, are factors which could easily set the stage for the emergence of clinical depression.

The research of Peter Lewinsohn has demonstrated a clear relationship between

James N. Breckenridge and Dolores Gallagher are co-investigators along with the authors. Lesley Parke and Julie Hill contributed to the development of the Life Satisfaction Course materials.

pleasant and unpleasant events and mood (Lewinsohn, Youngren, & Grosscup, 1979). Lewinsohn has hypothesized that interactions which result in a low rate of positive or a high rate of negative outcomes can be precursors of depression (Lewinsohn, Muñoz, Youngren, & Zeiss, 1978). A "vicious circle" sequence of events has often been associated with the development of depression: Few interactions with positive outcomes lead to low mood, and low mood reduces the likelihood of engagement in the types of activities which have positive outcomes. Decreased frequency of positive outcomes leads to a further drop in mood, leading to further inactivity and passivity, and so the downward trend continues. Early intervention in this sequence could reasonably be expected to interrupt and correct such a chain of events.

There is, however, evidence in the literature that the elderly are unlikely to seek psychological help (Blazer & Williams, 1980). A perceived stigma attached to "mental illness," and a lack of conviction that mental health professionals can be of assistance, are two explanations advanced for this situation (Feigenbaum, 1973). Thus, it seems likely that elderly individuals at risk for depression or in the early stages of its development will be unlikely to seek professional clinical assistance. In developing the intervention to be described here, we have assumed, on the basis of our experience with subject recruitment for a major therapy outcome study with the elderly, that elders who are reluctant to seek help from mental health professionals *may* be willing to seek or accept information about how to cope with problems in the future. This should be true particularly if that information is presented without the stigmatizing associations of mental health difficulties (i.e., as an educational class for increasing satisfaction and well-being).

The apparent utility of Lewinsohn's model of depression for the elderly prompted us to expect that interventions following that model would be effective for this population. The psychoeducational course developed by Lewinsohn and his colleagues could address both the special needs of the elderly and also their reluctance to seek and accept psychological treatment. Two of the three outcome studies evaluating Lewinsohn's Coping with Depression course, however, found elderly depressed participants to derive less benefit from the treatment than their younger counterparts (Steinmetz, Lewinsohn, & Antonuccio, 1983; Teri & Lewinsohn, 1981). Hypothesizing that the treatment covered too much material, too quickly, for elderly depressed, Thompson, Gallagher, Nies and Epstein (1983) modified the course to make it particularly suited to older adults. Their "Coping with Depression" course for the elderly focused primarily on basic self-monitoring of mood and activity, and self-change skills. This simplified treatment was found to be quite effective for treating elderly depressives. This course, however, was still designed for intervention with currently clinically depressed elders, and it required a willingness to label oneself with a potentially stigmatizing diagnosis.

The Life Satisfaction Course was developed to teach skills similar to those covered by the Coping with Depression course of Thompson et al. (1983), with a preventive twist. Similar to the earlier coping classes, this intervention teaches skills for monitoring mood, for identifying potential sources of increased pleasure, and for developing a systematic "self-change plan" to increase the frequency and enjoyment of salient activities. Basic behavioral strategies for self-change are covered in greater detail in this course, to provide participants with specific skills to be used in the future for effecting needed changes and coping with stressful life events and situations. This additional step-by-step emphasis on self-change proceeds at a much slower pace than in the Lewinsohn and Thompson interventions. We felt that a more detailed and leisurely treatment of this topic would maximize the elderly participants' capacity to absorb the material and implement the techniques within their daily routines. We expect subsequent use (and thus preventive effect) of these strategies to be more likely when the material is fully understood and applied to begin with.

Because Lawton (1982) has found life satisfaction in the elderly to be directly related to quality in the use of time, the course has a parallel theme of managing the use of time effectively so as to maximize positive outcomes and experiences. Time management is not advocated in the interest of being *efficient,* but rather in reference to arranging one's schedule to ensure that there is enough time for rewarding activity, to balance the inevitable neutral and unpleasant tasks and events. Self-change plans are introduced in terms of developing habits to assess one's daily routine and its effect on mood, and to rearrange those habits to enhance positive mood and satisfaction.

To summarize, the Life Satisfaction course was designed to provide elderly who are dysphoric or dissatisfied, and thus potentially at risk for depression, with specific skills of self-observation and self-change to be used to prevent a downward spiral of depressive affect and behaviors. An additional feature of the course is the socially acceptable procedures and nomenclature so as to make the intervention as accessible as possible to the elderly.

DESCRIPTION OF THE POPULATION

The intervention is designed for use with male and female community residents aged 55 and older. Participants are usually self-referred and learn of the course through senior centers, notices in senior newsletters, articles in general circulation newspapers, and by word of mouth. The course is held at senior centers and senior residences throughout the San Francisco Bay Area, and is offered as a regular class within each center's activity program. Prospective participants telephone our center, or they may register for the class at their senior center and receive a follow-up call from our staff. Applicants are given an individual "screening" appointment with one of the course instructors. The screening interview has three purposes: First, to inform prospective participants about the nature of the class, making sure they understand its psychoeducational nature and that their expectations are appropriate; second, to gather sufficient information to determine whether an applicant might better be referred to an alternative treatment (i.e., to assure absence of prohibitive organic or psychological impairment); and third, to gather pretreatment data to provide a basis for evaluating the impact of the course.

Applicants diagnosable as having major clinical depressions or evidencing other serious psychopathology are referred for more intensive treatment. Those meeting criteria for minor or intermittent depressive disorders are invited to participate in the class along with those not claiming any psychopathology other than low life satisfaction. Those not claiming any current adjustment problems are welcome in the class as well, but are less common.

PHILOSOPHY OF THE COURSE

The Life Satisfaction Course is based on a psychoeducational model. That is, there is an emphasis on learning specific material and applying it; there is no attempt to provide a "healing experience." Leaders are clearly designated as teachers rather than therapists, and the participants are seen as students rather than clients or patients. The students are told that the course will present specific skills that they can use at present and in the future to enhance their well-being and satisfaction with life.

The goals of the course, as delineated in the first session, are to provide students with the tools necessary to progress through a series of steps. The first step is to be aware of daily fluctuations in mood and life satisfaction. Next, students attend to their use of time on rewarding and unrewarding activity. After attending to current use of time, students assess potentially pleasant activities that are being neglected. This results in a recognition of the relationship between mood, life satisfaction, and daily activities and the consequent implications for self-change. Next, students identify problems that contribute to lowering mood and identifying strategies to work on them. Through this process, they become aware of steps to gain more control so that more pleasure and satisfaction can be experienced on a daily basis. Finally, students incorporate the skills learned in the class into personal approaches for coping with specific difficulties faced at present or in the future.

It should be noted that this intervention, although behavioral in nature, is quite different from what is customarily thought of as behavior modification. Thus, participants learn skills, are encouraged to view issues of life satisfaction in a certain way, and are supported by the group and instructors in implementing these skills and viewpoints. The instructors make little effort to rearrange the environmental contingencies related to students' mood, but rather attempt to teach the students the skills to assess the need for and bring about appropriate changes themselves.

STRUCTURE

The course consists of 9 two-hour sessions in 9 weeks, plus "reunions" at 1 month and 6 months posttreatment. Each class has two instructors, usually an experienced leader and a trainee. Class size is limited to 6 to 10 participants. A seminar format is arranged, with students and leaders seated around a table in a small room with a blackboard.

Leaders follow a detailed outline for each session, and students are provided with a "participant workbook" for each meeting, including an agenda listing material to be covered, a synopsis of the main ideas communicated during that session, and a homework assignment for the following week. The workbook contains all of the forms that will be needed during the class session and during the subsequent week to complete the homework assignment. A sample "agenda" page is outlined below. Students are also provided with a textbook (*Control Your Depression*, Lewinsohn et al., 1978) to supplement these materials. Textbooks may be either borrowed or bought by the participants.

Sample Agenda Page from Participant Workbook
Session #1

Agenda

1. Review of orientation: ground rules, materials, getting acquainted.
2. Goals of class
3. Lecture: Your Mood and Your Environment
4. Workshop: How to monitor your mood and life satisfaction
5. Preview of Session #2
6. Homework assignment
7. Quiz packet

Main Ideas to Remember

1. One of the goals of this class is to learn the relationship between our mood, events, and life satisfaction.
2. Events that occur each day can cause mood to go up or go down.
3. It is possible to learn skills so you can keep mood fluctuations within the "comfort zone."
4. *Awareness* and *application of skills* are the keys to increasing mood and life satisfaction.

Homework

1. Monitor mood and life satisfaction daily
   A. Mood is how you're feeling (your emotions) on any given day.
   B. Life satisfaction is how satisfied you are with your life that day.
2. Complete Pleasant Events (PE) exercise
3. Read chapters 1 to 3 in textbook (*Control Your Depression*)

The first meeting of the class is an "orientation" session. Pretreatment assessment packets are collected and checked for completeness, informed consent is obtained, and students are provided with a folder for organizing the course materials. An important item on the agenda for the orientation session is a "getting acquainted exercise" to allow participants and leaders to introduce themselves and to foster a spirit of congeniality and collaboration in the class. A final task of the orientation session is to review the "ground rules" for the course: (1) Be supportive and constructive, (2) equal talk time for all, (3) keep a practical focus, (4) avoid negative talk, and (5) respect confidentiality. Each ground rule is discussed individually and members are explicitly asked for their agreement to follow all of them.

The eight sessions following the orientation meeting share a consistent agenda: Homework is reviewed and discussed, new material is presented in a lecture by one of the leaders, there is a workshop to allow participants to begin to apply the new material under the supervision of the leaders, and homework is assigned for the next week. Fifteen minutes are reserved at the end of each session for completion of a quiz on that day's material and of "efficacy measures" (to be discussed below). Approximately halfway through each two-hour session participants take a 10-minute break, usually accompanied by coffee and a snack brought by one of the students or leaders.

The sequence of topics in the course is as follows: In Session 1, students hear a lecture on the topic of fluctuations in mood in response to environmental events and influences, and they are taught to monitor mood and life satisfaction on a daily basis. Session 2 focuses on the relationship between mood and key events, and students' daily mood data is perused for evidence and examples. Salient pleasant activities are identified using the Older Person's Pleasant Events Schedule (Hedlund, Gilewski, & Thompson, 1981), and a personalized list of 10 target pleasant events is developed for each student to keep track of daily. In Session 3, students learn to graph the relationship between mood and activity data, and correlations are discussed; lists of activities are revised to reflect the students' growing understanding of the events influential for their mood. At this point in the class, many students experience an "aha," realizing the mutual relationship between events and mood and the potential for personal influence on mood and satisfaction inherent in that relationship.

In session 4, after 2 weeks of data collection, students are ready to identify personal problem areas, and leaders help them to pinpoint a specific mood-related problem for change. In Sessions 5 and 6, self-change skills are taught, and each student designs and implements a behavioral self-change plan. Antecedents and consequences of target problems are identified, and strategies for overcoming "roadblocks to self-change" are developed. At this point, the leaders are able to focus on specific roadblocks frequently encountered by elders. A distinction is drawn between "internal" roadblocks (e.g., cognitions such as, "I'm too old to change"), and "external" roadblocks (e.g., constraints in resources or physical abilities), many of which can be overcome or bypassed with creative thought and effort. The final two sessions, Sessions 7 and 8, focus on revision of self-change plans, generation of new plans to systematically increase positive and satisfying activity in salient areas, and generalization of skills to other problem areas. During the eighth session, plans for maintaining positive mood and anticipating and coping with future difficulties are discussed. The 1-month and 6-month reunions serve to review salient points, check on and reinforce student progress, and further discuss generalized application of self-control skills.

ASSESSMENT

Two questions are of interest in our current evaluation of the Life Satisfaction course: (1) How effective is the course for improving mood and life satisfaction from pre- to posttreatment and continuing through follow-up, and (2) What factors mediate the effectiveness of the course?

Assessment to answer the first question involves the measures listed in the outline below, administered pretreatment, posttreatment, and at 1-month and 6-month follow-up. The main variables of interest with regard to outcome of the course are measures of depression, life satisfaction, morale, and perceived mastery. In addition, we are interested in students' expectations of change in these measures, and also in their sense of personal control over the domains measured by the instruments. Previous research with the Coping with Depression course has shown that expectations are significant predictors of outcome (Steinmetz et al., 1983), and that perceived control over the domain measured interacts significantly with expectations in predicting outcome (Steinmetz, Breckenridge, Thompson, & Gallagher, 1982).

Assessment: Comprehensive List of Measures
Screening
  Demographic information
  Health and medication information

Screening questions for depression, anxiety, other psychopathology
Folstein Mini-Mental State (Folstein, Folstein, & McHugh, 1975)
Beck Depression Inventory (Beck, Ward, Mendelson, Mock, & Erbaugh, 1961)
Pretreatment, Posttreatment, and Follow-up
Beck Depression Inventory (Beck et al., 1961)*
Affect Balance Scale (Bradburn, 1969)*
Life Satisfaction Index (Neugarten, Havighurst, & Tobin, 1961)*
Morale Questionnaire (Lawton, 1975)*
Mastery Questionnaire (Lewinsohn, Larson, & Muñoz, 1982)
Automatic Thoughts Questionnaire (Hollon & Kendall, 1980)
Andrus Attitudes and Expectations for Improvement Scale (Bisno & Gallagher, 1981)
Perceived Social Support: Family and Friends (Procidano & Heller, 1983)
Profile of Mood States (McNair, Lorr, & Droppleman, 1971)
Older Person's Pleasant Events Schedule (Hedlund, Gilewski, & Thompson, 1981)
*"Expected" ratings collected as well as current ratings.

The second question, that of factors mediating the success of the intervention, is addressed in three ways at each class session. The quiz administered at the end of each class provides information about how well each student understands the material presented that day. Thus, we are measuring assimilation of specific ideas presented in the sessions rather than assuming that students' presence at the class can be interpreted as their actually "receiving" the material presented. Students are clearly informed that the purpose of the quiz is to assess the leaders' success in communicating material to the class.

A second level of process assessment is addressed by having students complete three different kinds of expectation measures at the end of each session. The first of these is intended to assess students' efficacy expectations. Bandura (1977) has demonstrated that a person's judgments of how capable they are of performing tasks (in our case, carrying out homework assignments and bringing about change) are powerful predictors of self-initiated behavior. Thus, the first set of questions asks students to rate on a 100-point scale (0 = certain it is *not* true, 50 = not sure, 100 = certain it *is* true) their certainty that they *can* carry out aspects of the homework assignment (e.g., "Can you keep a complete and accurate daily record of your pleasant events?"). The second and third sets of questions are designed to assess on the same 100-point scale the students' expectations that they *will* carry out the assignments (e.g., "I will keep a complete and accurate daily record of my pleasant events."), and their judgments of how useful applying certain skills would be to them (e.g., "Keeping a complete and accurate daily record of pleasant events is a useful way to start thinking about how I can get more pleasure in my life."). The specific behaviors addressed by each set of questions are those targeted in that session's content and that require actions on the students' part to carry through and apply them before the next class session. As the end of the course draws near, students are asked to rate their perceptions of whether or not they will continue to use the self-monitoring and self-change skills in the future.

A third level of process assessment is provided by the weekly homework assignments. Students turn in their homework forms each week, and leaders record the data and return them the following week. Thus, on a weekly basis we have information about daily fluctuations in mood, life satisfaction and activity level; about the daily rate of the target behavior for change chosen by each student; and about the degree to which each student is completing the assigned homework and applying the skills taught in the class.

PRELIMINARY RESULTS

As of this writing, thirteen Life Satisfaction classes have been completed. Screening interviews have been conducted with 119 potential participants, 97 have enrolled in the classes, and 72 students have completed the entire Life Satisfaction course.

Although we are still in the process of evaluating the Life Satisfaction course, two preliminary reports have been presented at professional meetings (Breckenridge, Zeiss, Breckenridge, Thompson, & Gallagher, 1984; Zeiss, Steinmetz, Breckenridge, & Thompson, 1983). These results will be briefly summarized here.

Zeiss et al. (1983) postulated that in order for the Life Satisfaction course intervention to be maximally successful, students must (1) understand the material presented (as assessed by performance on the weekly quizzes), (2) attend the class sessions, and (3) apply the material presented (as assessed by completion of homework assignments). This study reported data concerning the relationship between quiz performance, attendance, and homework completion.

The sample for this analysis was the first 50 students enrolling in the course, 40 of whom completed the entire course. The students in this sample did very well on the quizzes, averaging one error out of 10 questions per quiz. Older students made more quiz errors; the correlation between age and mean number of errors was .25, $p < .05$. Better quiz performance was found to be associated with completing the sequence of classes. The mean number of quiz errors for those who dropped out of the class was 1.53, compared to a mean of .70 for those who completed the class, $t(49) = 1.93, p < .05$. There was a significantly greater probability of completing homework when no quiz errors were made ($t(38) = 5.43, p < .001$).

Zeiss et al. (1983) did not attempt to examine the postulated relationship between learning and application of the material presented in the Life Satisfaction course and eventual outcome. This study did demonstrate, however, the importance of assessing learning in psychological interventions for the elderly. The data indicate that elders *are* able to learn the material, and that those who have more difficulty grasping the course material are more likely to drop out. Complete grasp of the material is also a significant predictor of application of the ideas in students' lives.

The second study, Breckenridge et al. (1984), examined the relationship between quiz performance, homework completion, and course outcome. The first 52 subjects completing the entire Life Satisfaction course comprised the sample for this study.

Pretreatment scores on the four measures of mood and life satisfaction (BDI, LSI, ABS, and MQ) indicated that participants, on the average, were mildly depressed (mean BDI = 10.88, SD = 7.00) and had moderate life satisfaction (mean LSI = 14.58, SD = 6.49). Posttreatment scores indicated significant decreases in depression, $t(47) = 3.52, p < .001$, to a nondepressed level (mean posttreatment BDI = 7.47, SD = 6.94). Scores on the LSI, ABS, and MQ all increased significantly. Scores at pretreatment for each measure were highly correlated with each other; the mean intercorrelation of the measures was .655. A composite score was thus created which had high internal consistency at pretest (Cronbach's alpha = .78) and at posttest (Cronbach's alpha = .87), to be used as an omnibus measure in subsequent analyses.

None of the measures of mood or life satisfaction at pretreatment were related to homework completion during the course. Thus, participants who were relatively more depressed to begin with were just as able to follow through on assignments as those who began the class in a more positive state of mind.

Quiz performance was not found to be significantly related to outcome in this sample. However, note that Zeiss et al. (1983) found that those who did poorly on quizzes tended to drop out of the class. The present analyses included only those students who completed the course.

Homework completion was significantly related to positive outcome on the composite mood/life satisfaction measure, even after controlling for pretest scores, $F(1,49) = 4.18$, $p < .046$. Those who followed through on the assignments to apply the class material between sessions achieved the greatest improvements in mood and life satisfaction.

Analyses of the relationship of learning and utilization of course material to changes in mood and life satisfaction are crucial to this investigation. The psychoeducational approach taken argues that nonspecific factors which might lead to improvement, such as getting out of the house to go to the class or having social contacts, are of minor importance. More important, in this view, is that the participant is provided with new information and learns about skills which are relevant to improving day-to-day life, and that he or she practices these skills by following through on homework assignments. Only when participants understand the material and apply it in their own lives should improvement be expected. Thus, internal analyses are used to test the major hypotheses of this project, as opposed to comparing outcomes to those of a nontreated control group.

A more through analysis of the data will be initiated after more subjects have completed the course. Through explanatory modeling (discussed elsewhere in this volume by Dr. James Breckenridge), we intend to examine the relationship between understanding of course content, expectations about its usefulness and application, actual between-session application of the material, and changes assessed weekly and from pre- to posttreatment in mood and life satisfaction. We will be interested to see if the variables measured during the class will be predictive of students' use of skills and level of mood and life satisfaction through the follow-up period. We feel that the use of such efficacy and expectancy measures holds promise in prevention research.

FUTURE DIRECTIONS AND SUMMARY

The Life Satisfaction course as we have described it here has been a pilot project to develop an intervention to teach older adults specific behavioral skills for enhancing mood and life satisfaction, and for enhancing perceived efficacy for managing difficult life situations. We are guided by the hypothesis that teaching elders skills for controlling mood by planning and executing relevant self-change plans will be effective in preventing depressive reactions to life stress. We plan to follow our students for at least 6 months after the completion of each course to provide data on the continued progress of the elders who participated in the intervention.

In adapting Lewinsohn's Coping with Depression course for use with the elderly, we felt it necessary to delete a great amount of content in the interests of greater simplicity. Although the pace of the current Life Satisfaction course seems to be appropriate for the target population, we would like to be able to offer a broader range of coping strategies. We are currently considering the development of modules on relaxation, assertiveness, cognitive skills, and organization and time management to supplement the basic course. In addition, a module concerned with values and meaning is under consideration, to address the need expressed by our students to reassess and discuss such issues in a structured format.

We have had a number of requests to train other professionals working with the elderly to administer this course in their own settings. Based on the experience of Thompson et al. (1983), we believe it to be feasible for non-psychologist service providers to the elderly and for paraprofessionals to learn to administer the course. The structured nature of the class is important in this regard, and we agree with the guidelines suggested by Christensen, Miller, & Muñoz (1978), that paraprofessional therapists should be employed with well-specified treatment procedures under ongoing supervision, with clients who have been screened by professionals. Several service providers to the elderly have taken the course along with our regular students as a first step toward learning to teach it themselves, and to develop plans for adapting it for special populations, for example, the blind. Thus, it is our intention to make the course available to others who would find it useful and applicable in their work settings, and to provide training and supervision to maintain the quality of the intervention. The wider dissemination of the course made possible by this strategy certainly strengthens its preventive potential.

Although the Life Satisfaction course is still in its developing stages, we are pleased with the early results of evaluation efforts. We will be carefully observing the results of its application to other settings, and we look forward to executing our planned controlled evaluation of the course as an explicitly preventive intervention for depression. We feel that the psychoeducational model is an ideal one to apply to prevention of depression in the elderly. Lewinsohn's research (Brown & Lewinsohn, 1984; Steinmetz et al., 1983) demonstrates that it can be effective for treating depression, and the work of Thompson and his colleagues (e.g., Hedlund & Thompson, 1980) has proved its efficacy with clinically depressed elderly.

The psychoeducational model, as exemplified by these courses, has many features to make it attractive as a preventive intervention: The program can be brief and delivered to groups inexpensively; it can be administered by trained paraprofessionals with minimal supervision; it can be used for either primary or secondary prevention, and elders can enter the program without acquiring stigmatizing labels; and positive changes are attributed to participants' rather than leaders' efforts. Most importantly, the psychoeducational emphasis on acquisition, practice, and continued use of coping skills is expected to enable self-prevention of psychopathological response to future stresses.

REFERENCES

Bandura, A. (1977). Self-efficacy: Toward a unifying theory of behavior change. *Psychological Review, 84,* 191–215.

Beck, A. T., Ward, C. H., Mendelson, M. Mock, J. E., & Erbaugh, J. (1961). An inventory for measuring depression. *Archives of General Psychiatry, 4,* 561–571.

Bisno, B., & Gallagher, D. (1981). *The Andrus Attitudes and Expectancies for Improvement Scale.* Technical mimeograph, University of Southern California, Los Angeles, CA.

Blazer, D., & Williams, C. D. (1980). Epidemiology of dysphoria and depression in various adult age groups. *American Journal of Psychiatry, 137,* 439–444.

Bradburn, N. M. (1969). *The structure of psychological wellbeing.* Chicago, IL: Aldine.

Breckenridge, J. S., Zeiss, A. M., Breckenridge, J. N., Thompson, L. W., & Gallagher, D. E. (1984, November). Increasing life satisfaction in the elderly: Group intervention and research. In D. Upper and S. M. Ross (Chairs), *Innovations in behavioral group therapy.* Symposium conducted at the meeting of the Association for the Advancement of Behavior Therapy, Philadelphia, PA.

Brown, R. A., & Lewinsohn, P. M. (1984). A psychoeducational approach to the treatment of depression: A comparison of group, individual, and minimal contact procedures. *Journal of Consulting and Clinical Psychology, 52,* 774–783.

Christensen, A., Miller, W. R., & Muñoz, R. F. (1978). Paraprofessionals, partners, peers, paraphernalia, and print: Expanding mental health service delivery. *Professional Psychology, 33,* 249–270.

Feigenbaum, E. M. (1973). Ambulatory treatment of the elderly. In E. Pfeiffer & E. Busse (Eds.), *Mental illness in later life* (pp. 153–166). Washington, DC: American Psychiatric Association.

Folstein, M., Folstein, S., & McHugh, P. (1975). "Mini-mental State:" A practical method for grading the cognitive state of patients for the clinician. *Journal of Psychiatric Research, 12,* 189–198.

Gaitz, C. M. (1977). Depression in the elderly. In W. Fann, I. Karacan, A. Pokorny, & R. Williams (Eds.), *Phenomenology and treatment of depression* (pp. 153–166). New York: Spectrum.

George, L. K., & Bearon, L. B. (1980). *Quality of life in older persons.* New York: Human Sciences Press.

Gurland, B. (1976). The comparative frequency of depression in various adult age groups. *Journal of Gerontology, 31,* 283–292.

Hedlund, B., Gilewski, M., & Thompson, L. (1981). The Older Person's Pleasant Events Schedule. In D. Gallagher & L. Thompson, *Depression in the elderly: A behavioral treatment manual* (pp. 117–119). Los Angeles: University of Southern California Press.

Hedlund, B., & Thompson, L. W. (1980, August). *Teaching the elderly to control depression using an educational format.* Paper presented at the meeting of the American Psychological Association, Montreal.

Hollon, S., & Kendall, P. (1980). Cognitive self-statements in depression: Development of an Automatic Thoughts Questionnaire. *Cognitive Therapy and Research, 4,* 383–395.

Larson, R. (1978). Thirty years of research on the subjective well-being of older Americans. *Journal of Gerontology, 33,* 109–125.

Lawton, M. P. (1975). The Philadelphia Geriatric Center Morale Scale: A revision. *Journal of Gerontology, 30,* 85–89.

Lawton, M. P. (1982, August). *The varieties of wellbeing.* Distinguished Contribution Award address, Division 20, presented at the meeting of the American Psychological Association, Washington, DC.

Lewinsohn, P. M., Antonuccio, D. O., Steinmetz, J. L., & Teri, L. (1984). *The Coping with Depression Course: A psychoeducational intervention for unipolar depression.* Eugene, OR: Castalia.

Lewinsohn, P. M., Larson, D., & Muñoz, R. F. (1982). The measurement of expectancies and cognitions in depressed individuals. *Cognitive Therapy and Research, 6,* 437–446.

Lewinsohn, P. M., Muñoz, R. F., Youngren, M. A., & Zeiss, A. M. (1978). *Control your depression.* Englewood Cliffs, NJ: Prentice-Hall.

Lewinsohn, P. M., Youngren, M. A., & Grosscup, S. J. (1979). Reinforcement and depression. In R. A. Depue (Ed.), *The psychobiology of the depressive disorders: Implications for the effects of stress* (pp. 291–316). New York: Academic Press.

Lowenthal, M. F., & Berkman, R. L. (1967). *Aging and mental disorder.* San Francisco: Jossey-Bass.

McNair, D. M., Lorr, K., & Droppleman, L. F. (1971). *Manual for the Profile of Mood States.* San Diego, CA: Educational and Industrial Testing Service.

Neugarten, B. L., Havighurst, R. J., & Tobin, S. S. (1961). The measurement of life satisfaction. *Journal of Gerontology, 16,* 134–143.

Procidano, M. E., & Heller, K. (1983). Measures of perceived social support from friends and from family: Three validation studies. *American Journal of Community Psychology, 11,* 1–24.

Steinmetz, J. L., Breckenridge, J. N., Thompson, L. W., & Gallagher, D. (1982, November). The role of patient expectancy in predicting treatment outcome for young and old depressives. In D. Gallagher (Chair), *Factors influencing both assessment and response to psychological treatment in depressed older adults*. Symposium presented at the meeting of the Gerontological Society of America, Boston, MA.

Steinmetz, J. L., Lewinsohn, P. M., & Antonuccio, D. O. (1983). Client variables as predictors of outcome in a structured group treatment for depression. *Journal of Consulting and Clinical Psychology, 51*, 331–337.

Teri, L., & Lewinsohn, P. M. (1981, November). *Comparative efficacy of group vs. individual treatment of unipolar depression*. Paper presented at the meeting of the Association for Advancement of Behavior Therapy, Toronto.

Thompson, L. W., Gallagher, D., Nies, G., & Epstein, D. (1983). Evaluation of the effectiveness of professionals and non-professionals as instructors of "Coping with Depression" classes for elders. *The Gerontologist, 23*, 390–396.

Zeiss, A. M., Breckenridge, J. S., & Thompson, L. W. (1983, November). The Life Satisfaction Course: A psychoeducational program for elders. In B. Schwartz (Chair), *Education for aging: Models and methods of eldergogy for different needs*. Symposium conducted at the meeting of the Gerontological Society of America, San Francisco.

III

THE NEXT STEP: THE FIRST RANDOMIZED PREVENTION TRIALS

One of the continuing criticisms of prevention research is that it has not focused on clinical disorders, but rather on subclinical expressions of personal distress. Critics argue that run-of-the-mill problems in living are not in themselves reasonable targets for the mental health field. To answer this criticism, prevention advocates would like to provide documented evidence that interventions hypothesized to be preventive do in fact reduce the incidence of clinical depression.

In order to accomplish this goal, it will be necessary to carry out randomized, controlled prevention trials. As of this writing, results from such trials have not been published. However, there are two trials in progress which may be used to examine what such trials might involve.

The purpose of the two chapters in this section is to share with the field examples of ongoing randomized trials. The criteria for inclusion was an experimental design which explicitly identified cases of clinical depression. Such cases had to be screened out and referred for treatment in order to avoid becoming treatment outcome studies. In addition, identification of new cases at post and followup was also necessary to attempt to document the incidence rate of depression in the study sample, as well as in each of the experimental conditions.

The first randomized prevention trial presented is the San Francisco Depression Prevention Research Project. The intervention being evaluated focuses on teaching self-control oriented cognitive-behavioral skills, and it is being conducted in English, Spanish, and Chinese. The participants in the study are primarily low-income, minority, medical outpatients. In addition to documenting the appearance of new cases of clinical depression, depression levels, positive mental health variables, and medical utilization are also being assessed.

The second randomized prevention trial is the San Diego Hispanic Social Network Prevention Intervention Study. It uses epidemiological methodology to identify its sample, and two types of intervention: social support and social learning approaches. It focuses on Hispanic women.

Both studies highlight many of the important issues involved in prevention research: the need for representative samples of the community groups targeted, the need to include minorities in the sample, especially if the study is being done in major urban centers, the need to develop alternative ways to administer the intervention, the importance of being explicit regarding the theoretical framework from which the intervention stems, and of documenting changes in the mediating variables which are hypothesized to cause the preventive effect.

The first of the chapters also provides information that could be used to begin to establish norms for such elements as recruitment rates, acceptability, attrition, and retention during followups.

The time to begin depression prevention trials is now. It is my hope that these examples will be useful in deciding what to emulate and what to avoid in future trials.

12

The San Francisco Depression Prevention Research Project: A Randomized Trial with Medical Outpatients

Ricardo F. Muñoz, Yu Wen Ying, Regina Armas, Florentius Chan,
and Roberto Gurza
University of California, San Francisco

INTRODUCTION

The importance of developing prevention programs in the mental health area has been discussed extensively (Albee, 1982; Albee & Joffe, 1977; Bloom, 1979, 1981; Cowen, 1982; Kelly, 1968, 1977; Lemkau, 1955; Muñoz, 1976). Advocates of prevention programs argue that this is an area that the field must develop (Cowen, in press); critics hold that we do not yet know enough about prevention to justify the funding of such programs (Lamb & Zussman, 1981). In the area of depression, studies have not yet been carried out to determine whether the incidence of clinical episodes of depression can be reduced. The present chapter describes work in progress on the first (to our knowledge) randomized, controlled preventive trial focusing on clinical depression. It is our intention to share our experiences in the design and implementation of a randomized prevention trial. We will focus primarily on issues of identifying, recruiting, and retaining a representative sample of persons from a high risk population.

THEORETICAL ORIENTATION

The project described here was designed to test the hypothesis that depression can be prevented through the use of social learning, self-control methods.

Controlled studies in the psychotherapeutic treatment of depression have shown that cognitive (Rush, Beck, Kovacs, & Hollon, 1977; Murphy, Simons, Wetzel, & Lustman, 1984), behavioral (Lewinsohn, 1975; McLean & Hakstain, 1979), and social skill training approaches (Bellack, Hersen, & Himmelhoch, 1981), can be effective in reducing levels of depression in adults experiencing clinical levels of nonpsychotic, unipolar depression. This skill-training, or competency-building approach is theorized to produce its effect by changing 1) internal processes such as psychological factors (thinking patterns, beliefs, subjective probability estimates) and physiological factors (such as those that might result from the practice of relaxation and by increases in activity levels), and 2) external processes, such as the reaction of other persons in the social environment to newly-learned social skills. We hypothesize that the use of these techniques will counteract to some as-yet-undetermined extent the effects of other factors which influence the likelihood of suffering from depressive episodes.

There are many factors that have been implicated in the etiology of depression: heredity, biological factors, social and environmental history, life events, conscious and non-conscious psychological processes. Neither the main effects nor the interactions of these processes are adequately understood. Our project focuses on the modifiable factors which are primarily under the individual's control, in order to determine whether such a focus can produce a measurable preventive effect.

The cognitive and behavioral methods utilized in this study are based on social learning theory (Bandura, 1977). Behaviors, thoughts, and feelings are presumed to be subject to learning processes. The thoughts, behaviors, and feelings that are considered to be part of the depressive syndrome range on a continuum. At the "normal" end of the continuum, such thoughts, behaviors, and feelings are subject to the usual fluctuations brought upon by day-to-day occurrences, physical status (such as lack of sleep, overexertion, looking forward to exciting events, etc.), as well as longer lasting situations (such as low income, stressful environmental conditions, and so on.) Individual differences in reactions to similar events are explained by normal variations in the learned patterns of managing objective situations (such as interacting with other people) and subjective situations (such as judging one's worth or one's quality of life). In addition, differences in biochemical factors are assumed to moderate these reactions. As the depressive process becomes more severe, somatic factors often become more prominent. At the most severe levels, somatic interventions, such as antidepressant medications, may be particularly helpful. However, the well-documented therapeutic effects of psychological interventions which focus on changing thinking and behavioral patterns indicate that such interventions can reverse the depressive process. We were interested in determining whether the same interventions could prevent development of clinical depression among people at risk.

IDENTIFYING A HIGH–RISK GROUP

We decided to work with a medical outpatient sample for a number of reasons. First, a number of studies have shown that the prevalence of depression in ambulatory medical patients is higher than in the general population (Katon, 1982). Nielsen and Williams (1980), using as their criterion a score of 13 on the Beck Depression Inventory (BDI), report a 12.2% rate of depression in a private group medical practice population (n = 526) consisting of many healthy, upper- and middle-class persons. Hoeper, Nycz, Cleary, Regier, and Goldberg (1979) surveyed a primary care clinic using the Schedule for Affective Disorders and Schizophrenia—Lifetime Version (SADS–L) and Research Diagnostic Criteria (RDC) (Endicott & Spitzer, 1978; Spitzer, Endicott, & Robins, 1978). They found prevalence rates of 5.8% for major depression, 5.0% for intermittent depression, and 3.4% for minor depression.

Second, a number of studies have shown that providing psychotherapy to medical patients reduces medical utilization (Jones & Vischi, 1979). We were interested in finding out whether our preventive intervention might produce similar effects. If so, medical charts provide a rich source of data which can document the secondary effects of the intervention. The charts also serve as a more objective source of information, that is, one which is unlikely to be affected by such factors as response bias or desire to please the research team. The medical utilization data also allows us to perform cost offset and cost effectiveness analyses.

Finally, the targeted medical outpatient population is not a homogeneous group equally exposed to various risk factors. Users of primary care clinics in San Francisco include a large proportion of minority and non-English-speaking individuals. Many minority and non-English speaking individuals have the additional demographic characteristics of low levels of educational and occupational attainment. It has been argued that each of these social, economic and/or ethnic factors increases the risk for the development of depressive disorders (see chap. 3, this volume). For example, depression levels have been found to be higher for Blacks than for Whites (Comstock & Helsing, 1976) and this difference is more clearly present at the more severe end of the depressive continuum (Eaton & Kessler, 1981). Roberts (chap. 3, this volume) has consistently reported levels of depressive symptomatology to be higher among Mexican-Americans than among Anglo-Americans. He argues that this finding is primarily due to differences in socio-economic status indicators. In examining differences in depression level among groups of Hispanics, Vega, Warheit, Buhl-Auth, and Meinhardt (1984) found higher levels among non-English speaking Hispanics as compared to their English-speaking counterparts.

In addition to the issue of high risk status, the inclusion of ethnic and non-English speaking samples was necessary to achieve representativeness. San Francisco, like most major urban centers, is a socially, racially, and linguistically diverse city. Care was taken to establish liaisons with clinics which reflected the demographic characteristics of the city, and pilot studies were conducted early in the process to prepare to do the study in Spanish and Chinese. Pilot data on the Spanish language sample will be presented here. Pilot data on the Chinese language sample were not available at the time of this writing.

The inclusion of diverse ethnic groups and non-English speaking samples into our research design raised the further issue of comparability of research instrumentation and intervention. The study's cross-cultural design demanded that the data acquired from each of the samples be comparable in order to properly compare or pool findings across groups. Great attention was paid to the development of both linguistically and culturally appropriate translation of all research and intervention materials. Despite careful translation, however, certain elements of incomparability remain. Research and diagnostic instruments currently available were developed for and normed on mainstream populations. In the case of depression, for example, even if the general components of the disorder are similar across cultures, the specific symptomatology and the particular clustering of symptoms may vary (Marsella, Kinzie, & Gordon, 1973). In short, "perfect" translations do not assure conceptual or psychometric equivalence.

PROCEDURE

Overview

In order to carry out a true *prevention* trial, it was important to obtain a high-risk, but currently nondepressed sample. Therefore, a careful screening process was instituted. People were recruited into the study either by mail or through face-to-face contact. They were administered a diagnostic interview and requested to fill out a number of additional questionnaires. Eligible subjects were then randomized into the study conditions: class, videotape (information-only control), and no-intervention control. After the delivery of the interventions, post and followup assessments were conducted.

Screening

Adults between 18 and 69 years of age who had an appointment at participating primary-care clinics during the recruitment phase of the study and had a chart open for at least six months were contacted. They were informed about the Depression Prevention Research Project, and asked whether they would be interested in participating in the study. Those who agreed were further screened to determine that they were literate, not receiving mental health treatment, not terminally ill, and able to attend the classes at the predetermined times. Demographic information was obtained, and the Center for Epidemiologic Studies-Depression Scale (CES-D) (Radloff, 1977) was administered.

The second screening interview consisted of the Beck Depression Inventory (BDI) (Beck, Ward, Mendelsohn, Mock, & Erbaugh, 1961) and the NIMH Diagnostic Interview Schedule (DIS) (Robins, Helzer, Croughan, & Ratcliff, 1981). The latter produced DSM-III diagnoses on most major disorders, including Major Depression and Dysthymia. Participants were paid ten dollars for this interview.

Participants were also paid ten dollars for the third screening interview, which consisted of a number of paper and pencil and verbally administered measures which assess recent life events (Sarason, Johnson, & Siegel, 1978), social support information (based on Barrera, 1981), family history of psychological disorders, biculturality (for Blacks, Hispanics, and Asians), social desirability (Crowne & Marlowe, 1960), the Affect-Balance Scale (Bradburn, 1969), a measure of quality of life (Flanagan, 1978), and measures on the cognitive behavioral variables which the intervention is designed to influence: the Pleasant Activities Schedule, Social Activities Questionnaire, Assertion Questionnaire (Lewinsohn, Muñoz, Youngren, & Zeiss, 1986), the Personal Beliefs Inventory, Subjective Probability Questionnaire, and Cognitive Events Schedule (Muñoz, 1977).

A desirable by-product of our demanding screening procedure was that it identified individuals who were unwilling to participate in assessments, and thus would be unlikely to come to post and followup interviews. These individuals simply did not complete the screening process.

Persons who met criteria for a current (within the last six months) diagnosis of depression (major depression or dysthymia), mania, schizophrenia, drug or alcohol abuse or dependence, organic brain syndrome, or were judged to be in need of immediate treatment (e.g., suicidal) were not accepted into the study. This ensured that the randomized trial was a preventive trial and not a treatment trial. In addition, we felt that persons in need of treatment should be referred at once, rather than risking random assignment to a no-intervention control condition.

Randomization

Persons eligible for the study were assigned by chance to one of two conditions: half to the Class condition and half to the Control conditions. For English-speaking participants, the Control condition was divided into two equal groups:

one received a forty-minute videotape presentation which briefly covered the methods and ideas presented in the Class, and thus served as an "information-only" control, and the other was a no-intervention control group. The Spanish and Chinese pilot studies samples had only the no-intervention control conditions.

The Intervention

The Depression Prevention Course is an eight-week, two-hour per week intervention, in which groups of 8 to 10 persons are taught a number of social learning, self-control techniques of the type that are used in behavioral and cognitive therapies for depression. The course is based on *Control Your Depression* (Lewinsohn, Muñoz, Youngren, & Zeiss, 1986).

An instructor begins each class period by passing out an outline which covers the main points to be made. The previous class is reviewed, homework assignments are discussed, and then the outline is covered in detail, with questions, discussion, and comments encouraged. The class ends with the week's homework assignment, and the filling out of an evaluation of the day's class.

The topics covered include:

Class 1. Introduction: Depression, Social Learning Theory, and self-control approaches.
Class 2. How thoughts influence mood. Relaxation.
Class 3. Learning to change your thoughts.
Class 4. How activities affect mood.
Class 5. Increasing pleasant activities.
Class 6. How contacts with people affect mood.
Class 7. Increasing interpersonal activities.
Class 8. Planning for the future: Preventing depression.

Homework assignments focus on self-monitoring of mood through the eight weeks, and selective monitoring of thoughts, pleasant activities, and interpersonal activities. Self-change contracts are included in some of the homework assignments. Progressive deep muscular relaxation is taught, practiced during most sessions, and also assigned as homework.

Following the suggestions made by Zeiss, Lewinsohn, and Muñoz (1979), class participants are 1) given a rationale for the course as a whole and for each of the techniques; 2) taught specific skills which have been found to be effective in bringing about noticeable changes in mood; 3) encouraged to practice these skills "in real life," that is, outside of the class hours, and 4) told that the preventive effects are expected to come from continuing to utilize the techniques after the class is over (and not from just coming to the classes).

Post and Followup Assessments

All randomized participants were administered the outcome measures at post testing. Followups occurred at designated times from the pre (screening) assessments: At six months, the outcome measures were readministered. At twelve months, these measures plus the DIS were readministered. (This allows us to obtain one-year incidence data.)

PRELIMINARY RESULTS

Because this is a report of work in progress, final results are not available. Our emphasis will be on outlining some of the issues we consider important as randomized controlled prevention trials become more common. We will exemplify possible outcomes for such studies by presenting our findings 24 months into data collection. We will first address issues of recruitment and screening. Secondly, we will present data on how participants in the intervention reacted to the Depression Prevention Course. We will illustrate the types of differences that might result from working with culturally diverse populations by noting the results of both our main (English language) study and our pilot (Spanish language) study.

Sites of Recruitment

The subjects in our study were recruited from two sites. One is the University of California, San Francisco (UCSF) Medical Center, the other is San Francisco General Hospital (SFGH). UCSF is a teaching hospital of the University. It serves a lower middle class to middle class income population. SFGH is a county hospital affiliated with the University serving a population from a lower socioeconomic background. Table 1 shows the background characteristics of the participants who agreed to initial screening at the two sites. Some refused to continue with further screenings.

Recruitment and Screening

Our experience with the process of recruitment and screening for our prevention trial has made us keenly aware that most randomized studies have very selective samples. Participants must hear about the study, decide to participate, and meet both scientific and practical criteria to be able to take part in the study. Few such studies specify the potential pool of participants from which their randomized sample originated. It is fairly easy to give wildly different estimates for the proportion of persons from the sampled population which actually participated in the randomized trial.

In our study, the percentage of medical outpatients who agreed to participate in the randomized study after being found eligible by our screening process was 94% for the English-speaking (ES) sample and 100% for the Spanish-speaking (SS) sample. Compare this technically accurate statement with the percentage of medical outpatients who were randomized from all the patients who attended the clinics during our study, namely 1.6% for the ES and 3.6% for the SS. Clearly, neither of these figures is very helpful by itself. Table 2 presents the actual numbers of patients who took part in the recruitment and screening process. We utilized both face-to-face recruitment and mail recruitment. In the following paragraphs, we will suggest ways to derive meaningful figures which may be useful in comparing across outcome studies in the future.

The Maximum Inclusion Rate is defined by the number of eligible individuals divided by the sum of the eligibles plus the ineligibles. This rate sets the upper limit of generalizability of the findings for the population from which the sample is drawn. Eligibility is a function of the exclusion criteria set by the investigator. In our study, these criteria included literacy, an age range of 18 to 69 and a medical

Table 1 Background characteristics of English- and Spanish-speaking samples

	English-speaking		Spanish-speaking
	UCSF	SFGH	SFGH
	N = 340	N = 247	N = 121
Demographic characteristics	%	%	%
Ethnicity			
Black	10.6	44.1	
White	57.9	28.7	
Asian	9.7	12.6	
Latino	10.9	8.1	100.0
Other	10.9	6.5	
Sex			
Male	33.4	53.4	19.8
Female	66.6	46.6	80.2
Marital status			
Divorced	35.9	50.2	31.4
Married	32.9	28.7	53.7
Never married	31.2	21.1	14.9
Employment			
Unemployed	55.8	77.7	73.3
Employed	44.2	22.3	26.7
	Mean	*Mean*	*Mean*
Age	48.5	50.7	42.9
Education	13.2	11.3	8.4
Income[1]	16.2	7.2	9.0
CES–D[2]	19.8	19.0	23.3

[1]Annual household in thousands of dollars
[2]Center for Epidemiological Studies-Depression Scale

chart open for six months. Our Maximum Inclusion Rate can be calculated for our face-to-face recruitment. It was 60% for the ES and 63% for the SS. (ES: 1878/3125; SS: 389/619). Note that, had we not included a Spanish language pilot, there would have been an added exclusion criteria, namely, ability to speak English. This would have decreased the Maximum Inclusion Rate for the study from 61% (across both languages) to 50% (1878/3744).

The Initial Contact Rate is defined by the number of participants contacted divided by the number of eligible participants. The Initial Contact Rate is a function of the resources available to the investigator and the ease with which the population sampled can be contacted. In our study, the Initial Contact Rate can be calculated for our face-to-face recruitment by taking the number of eligibles interviewed and dividing by all eligibles. We find an Initial Contact Rate of 38.6 for the ES (725/1878) and 41.4% (161/389) for the SS. In our study, not all eligible patients could be contacted because of the ratio of appointments to interviewers. That is, as some patients were being interviewed, others were being seen by their physicians and leaving. In addition, many failed to show up for their appointments. As long as there is no systematic bias to the Initial Contact Rate, it can be considered merely a measure of the capacity of the research team to process all eligible potential participants. In our case, the sample contacted was not demographically different from the population of the clinic as a whole.

The Acceptance Rate is defined by the number of individuals who agree to participate divided by all individuals contacted. Our Acceptance Rate was 24.3% for the ES (176/725) and 46.6% for the SS (75/161) for our face-to-face recruitment. The Acceptance Rate for the mailing recruitment of the San Francisco General Hospital (SFGH) samples was 4.2% for the ES and 4.5% for the SS. At the University of California, San Francisco (UCSF) clinic the Acceptance Rate was 6.0%. It should be noted that what individuals were accepting at this stage is to enter the screening part of the study, knowing that the screening process was to determine whether they could participate in a year-long randomized trial. Participation in the trial would involve six two-hour interviews and possibly attendance at eight weekly two-hour classes. Thus, the Acceptance Rate may be different for a preventive intervention which is not embedded in a research project or for a study which requires a smaller time commitment.

After agreeing to participate in the screening process, individuals were excluded either for a priori reasons, such as needing treatment, or for practical reasons, such as missing their appointments. As we said above, those who completed the screening process and were eligible rarely refused randomization: 94% of the ES and 100% of the SS agreed to continue. However, there are other denominators which one could use to determine whether the randomized group represents an adequate proportion of the target group:

The Randomized Group as a Proportion of the Entire Population. This is the most strict proportion, defined by the number of randomized individuals divided by the entire population from which the sample is drawn. In our study, we can calculate these figures for the face-to-face samples: 1.6% for the ES (49/3125) and 3.6% for the SS (22/619).

The Randomized Group as a Proportion of the Eligibles in the Population. This proportion is defined by the number of randomized individuals divided by the total number of persons considered eligible according to initial criteria (such as age and literacy). From our face-to-face recruitment, we obtain 2.6% for the ES (49/1878) and 5.7% for the SS (22/389).

The Randomized Group as a Proportion of Those Contacted. This proportion is defined as the number of randomized individuals divided by those contacted. In our face-to-face recruitment, this proportion is 6.8% for the ES (49/725) and 13.7% for the SS (22/161). In our mail recruitment, the proportions are 3.1% for the UCSF sample (62/2000), 2.1% for the ES SFGH sample (11/527), and 1.3% for the SS SFGH sample (6/446).

The Randomized Group as a Proportion of Those who Agreed to Participate. This proportion is defined as the number of randomized individuals divided by those who agreed to take part in the study. In our face-to-face recruitment, we randomized 27.8% (49/176) of the ES and 29.3% (22/75) of the SS who agreed to be screened. In the mail recruitment, we randomized 41.9% (62/148) of the UCSF sample, 50.5% of the ES SFGH sample, and 30.0% of the SS SFGH sample who agreed to be screened.

The use of standard rates such as those detailed above helps to compare characteristics of prevention trials. It also helps to develop norms for what can be considered acceptable rates of participation. Obviously, specific studies might be justified in setting different Maximum Inclusion, Initial Contact, or Acceptance Rates, but at least such decisions should be made explicitly. The use of uniform ways of defining participation may allow the determination of differences across populations.

In our study, it appears that our exclusion criteria produced comparable Maximum Inclusion Rates in the ES and SS samples (60% and 63%, respectively). Our resources appear to have been used relatively evenly across both groups, as evidenced by the Initial Contact Rate (38.6% for the ES and 41.4% for the SS). But our project was more acceptable to the Spanish-speaking population. The Acceptance Rate was significantly greater for the SS (46.6%) than for the ES (24.3%).

The proportions based on a numerator of randomized individuals can also be helpful. The first two, based on denominators of all members of the population or on all eligible members of the population are least helpful. They define an unrealistic maximum based on individuals whom the investigator did not intend to contact for theoretical reasons or is not able to contact because of resource limitations. The latter two are more meaningful.

The proportion based on all those contacted gives an estimate of the arithmetic representativeness of the randomized sample. (Representativeness can be defined by many other factors, of course.) It can also be used to examine the differential effectiveness of different modes of recruitment in obtaining a randomized sample. In our study, for example, mail recruitment produces a markedly lower proportion of randomized-to-contacted participants. Looking at only the SFGH samples, for which we can compare mail to face-to-face recruitment, mail recruitment produced a proportion of 2.1% for the ES and 1.3% for the SS. (The UCSF ES rate is somewhat higher, namely 3.1%). Face-to-face recruitment produced a proportion of 6.8% for the ES and 13.7% for the SS. More importantly, the gain in effectiveness of face-to-face over mailing recruitment is clearly higher for the SS (a tenfold increase) than for the ES (a threefold increase). Even though mail recruitment is less expensive, it may still be more cost-effective to focus on face-to-face recruitment with the Spanish-speaking population.

The possibility that mail recruitment may be preferable for English-speaking samples is also supported by the proportion of randomized to those who agreed to participate. For the English-speaking, those who accepted in response to mail have a probability of being randomized of 50% versus 27.8% for those recruited face-to-face, an almost twofold gain. (In practical terms, this means half as many screening interviews need to be done for those recruited through the mail to arrive at the same number of randomized participants.) For the Spanish-speaking, the recruitment method makes little difference. The comparable proportions are 30% for mailing recruits, and 29.3% for face-to-face recruits.

Is our rate of recruitment into the randomized part of the study adequate? There are as yet no norms for randomized controlled depression prevention trials. Treatment outcome studies generally do not specify the course of recruitment in as much detail as we have done. Part of the reason for this is that treatment is generally a reactive service modality: individuals seek out treatment. Prevention, on the other hand, is a proactive modality: the focus is on reaching a high-risk population before they are in need of treatment.

Nevertheless, depression treatment outcome studies are the closest source of comparison we have. In one of the only studies to document screening data in its published report, Murphy, Simons, Wetzel, and Lustman (1984) report screening 263 patients for their study, and accepting 95 (36%) into the randomized trial. The comparable figures for our study are those who agreed to be in the study ("Accepted" in Table 2): 346 ES and 95 SS, for a total of 441; and those who were randomized: 122 ES and 28 SS, for a total of 150. The respective proportions,

Table 2 Recruitment for English- and Spanish-speaking samples

| Recruitment method | English-speaking | | Spanish-speaking |
	UCSF N	SFGH N	SFGH N
Mailing	2000	527	446
Responded	456	125	47
Interested	190	39	31
Accepted	148	22	20
Completed 2nd screening	110	18	15
Completed 3rd screening	87	14	10
Randomized	62	11	6
Face to face	N/A	3125	619
Ineligible		1247	230
Eligible, not approached		1153	228
Eligible, approached		725	161
Refused		445	76
Excluded		104	10
Accepted		176	75
Completed 2nd screening		109	40
Completed 3rd screening		91	32
Randomized		49	22

then are 35.3% for the ES, 29.5% for the SS, and 36% overall. The yield from those who start the screening process appears to be comparable at least across these two studies.

Participant Reaction to the Depression Prevention Course

Attrition

Attrition rates for comparative outcome studies of treatment of depression range from 20% to 47% of the original patient sample (Simons, Levine, Lustman, & Murphy, 1984). Most such studies are done with individual treatment modalities. In these studies, then, a missed appointment can merely be rescheduled, thus making a reduction in the attrition rate possible even if patients miss some appointments. In our study, once a participant missed a class session, the session could not be repeated. (In some cases, when we were holding concurrent courses at different times of the day, those who missed the earlier class were able to come to the class held later the same day.) Therefore, we expected our attrition rate to be higher than in individual treatment outcome studies. We also set an a priori criterion for what would constitute "having received the intervention." This criterion was attendance at half of the classes (4 two-hour sessions).

Twenty percent of those randomized to the class condition attended no classes. Another 17% attended at least one class, but less than our criterion of four classes. Our total attrition rate, therefore, is 37%.

The attrition for the videotape control condition was 9%. This involved coming to one one-hour session to view a series of videotaped segments which briefly covered the approach and some of the specific methods taught in the classes.

Ratings of the Class Sessions

At the end of each of the class sessions, participants are asked to rate the class on four five-point scales ranging from 1 (most negative) to 5 (most positive). The mean ratings across all subjects and all classes were:

Rating	ES	SS
Interesting	4.3	4.4
(1 = Very boring		
5 = Very interesting)		
Clear	4.2	4.5
(1 = Very confusing		
5 = Very clear)		
Practical	4.2	4.4
(1 = Very impractical		
5 = Very practical)		
Class made me feel better	4.1	4.6
(1 = Made me feel much worse		
5 = Made me feel much better)		

In addition, participants answered the following question: "Do you plan to try the techniques discussed today?"
They answered as follows:

Response	ES	SS
No	1.4%	0%
Don't know	9.0%	1.6%
Yes	89.6%	98.4%

These ratings are based only on those people who attended the classes, of course. Therefore, one expects a certain amount of positive bias. One possible source of bias is the desire to please the instructor. To reduce this source of bias, the ratings were collected and averaged by a teaching assistant. Participants were told that the instructor would not see their individual responses.

We consider these ratings to be a necessary (but not sufficient) element in evaluating the effectiveness of the intervention. Participants must experience the intervention as something positive and worthwhile in order for the intervention to have a chance to work. Our participants considered the classes interesting, clear, and practical. They reported that the classes made them feel better and they stated that they planned to try the techniques taught in the classes.

Ratings of the Specific Concepts and Methods Taught in the Course

At the end of the eighth session, participants were given a list of forty concepts and methods covered in the course and asked to report whether they remembered using them, and if so, "how helpful each technique was for you in helping you maintain a positive mood." Their responses (across all participants and all items):

Response	ES	SS
I don't remember using this one	7.5%	7.2%
Made me feel worse	0.6%	0
Made no difference	9.3%	4.7%
Helped a little	31.9%	31.3%
Helped a lot	50.7%	56.8%
Total	100.0%	100.0%

Participants report that over 80% of the material covered in the course was helpful in maintaining a positive mood. Almost none of the material was subjectively felt to have a negative impact on their mood.

Followup Rates

One of the greatest problems with longitudinal studies is the issue of losing participants. We are still in the process of gathering follow-up data. As of this writing, we have obtained a 92% completion rate at post, 90% at 6 months, and 92% at one year. In addition to regular refusals to continue in the study, some participants have died, been diagnosed with a terminal illness, or have moved out of the area.

Analyses in Progress

We plan to analyze the changes in the intermediate variables (such as thinking patterns, pleasant activity levels, interpersonal contacts, and so on). These are the elements which are theorized to have preventive effects. We predict that the class condition would have the largest effect in changing these variables.

The most interesting outcome, of course, is whether the intervention will produce a reduction in the frequency, intensity, and duration of depressive episodes and symptoms. This analysis must wait until a larger sample is collected. Our early findings will give us estimates of the incidence of depression in this population, and the size of the sample needed to obtain adequate power for this comparison.

DISCUSSION

Several issues we discussed in this chapter deserve careful consideration by prevention researchers.

Targeting a Prevalent and Severe Disorder

The incidence of the disorder targeted must be high enough to make it feasible to measure a reduction in incidence. For psychiatric diagnoses, the prevalence levels are not very high, and incidence levels are even smaller. Heller, Price, and Sher (1980) point out that in order to demonstrate a significant difference at the .05 level between experimental and control groups, one needs a very large number of participants. For example, with a very effective intervention which reduces new cases of the disorder to half of what is found in a control group, and with a disorder that has a relatively high incidence rate of 10% (so that the experimental group's incidence after intervention is 5%), one would need 151 participants per group. For a disorder with a lower incidence of 1%, such as schizophrenia, one would need 1611 participants in each group (Muñoz, 1983).

In our case, we chose depression as the target disorder because of the relatively high prevalence rate. The NIMH Epidemiological Catchment Area (ECA) project found lifetime prevalence rates ranging from 6% to 10% across its first three sites (Robins et al., 1984). Other epidemiological studies have shown even higher rates. For example, Weissman and Meyer (1978) reported a combined lifetime rate for major and/or minor depression of 26.7%. In addition, depression costs run an estimated $16.5 billion per year in this nation (Frank, Kamlet, & Stoudemire, 1985), not to mention the human suffering it costs.

Targeting High Risk Groups

It is important to target prevention research on high risk groups. In general, people with lower socioeconomic status report a greater prevalence of health problems. Since minority groups are overrepresented in the lower socioeconomic group, it is likely that they will have a higher incidence of the most common disorders. If one adds other factors such as number of life events (Dohrenwend & Dohrenwend, 1974) to the screening criteria, one can begin to identify high risk groups within high risk groups. Many Asians and Latinos, for instance, are recent immigrants, and thus have the added pressure of language and cultural adaptation.

In our study, we targeted ambulatory medical patients where the incidence of depression has been found to be higher than in the general population. The mean CES–D score in our sample of medical outpatients is 20.1 at pre-screening, as compared to the national mean of 8.7 (Sayetta & Johnson, 1980). The traditional cutoff score for significant levels of depression on the CES–D is 16. Others have documented that patients often seek medical service for psychological problems such as depression (see Katon, 1982).

In addition to targeting medical outpatients, we also selected sites which serve primarily low income patients (e.g., mean income of our San Francisco General Hospital respondents is $8,000 a year). We also have an ethnically diverse sample, which we believe has a higher probability of developing depression than the general white population. In fact, our screening data reveal that one-fourth of our sample met DIS/DSM III criteria for major depression.

Methods of Prevention

Chassin, Presson, and Sherman (1985) have argued for the importance of developing intervention grounded in knowledge about the target behavior and tailoring the intervention to specific subgroups. We chose an intervention that was found to be successful in the treatment of depression, i.e., the cognitive behavioral approach. At the outset of this chapter, we have presented the mechanisms hypothesized to mediate a person's mood level. We monitored these hypothesized mediating variables (e.g., types of thought, quantity and quality of pleasant activities) at pre, post and followup screenings to document if changes in these were in fact correlated with changes in mood level. Although this intervention has not yet been tried as a preventive measure, there was sufficient evidence in its therapeutic effects to justify testing its preventive effects.

The inclusion of diverse ethnic groups and non-English speaking samples raised the question of appropriateness of the intervention. In delivering the intervention across the language groups, we found that certain modifications were necessary for the Spanish and Chinese-speaking populations. U.S. culture focuses on the importance of the individual whereas Latin-American and Chinese cultures emphasize the importance of the family and role of the individual within the family system. Thus, instead of talking about what one can do to improve one's life and mood, we talked about this in the context of how these improvements would benefit a larger unit, i.e., the family as well. The concept of asserting one's needs may be considered impolite and needs to be discussed in terms of the context where it might be appropriate and comfortable for the participant. With the Spanish-speaking group, the term "self-control" was fund to be too constraining, and we chose instead to emphasize these methods as helping to increase one's freedom of action (Ying & Armas, 1985).

Reaching and Retaining the Target Group

Unlike treatment trials where the participant seeks out the researcher for help with a problem, prevention studies must interest the participant in a service which the participant does not need now and may not need in the future. Thus, recruitment and retention of subjects become important concerns facing the researcher. In working with participants from both a middle class and a lower socioeconomic background, we found that it was consistently more difficult to interest the latter group in our project and to maintain their interest for the period of the involvement. This is ironic since we hypothesized that it is precisely this group which is at higher risk for developing depression. A number of strategies have been found to be useful although we are not entirely satisfied with the result of our efforts.

Mailing vs. Face-to-Face Recruitment

Mailing is relatively inexpensive when compared to recruitment hours needed for face-to-face recruitment. It has the advantage of requiring active participation from the very start (i.e., respondent must contact the project). Subjects recruited through mailing were more successful in completing the screening process than the face-to-face recruitees. However, demographic data reveal that these participants also tended to be from the dominant culture and have higher income and education than subjects recruited face-to-face. For example, the proportion of contacted SS subjects who were randomized was ten times as high when contacted face-to-face than when contacted by mail. Once again it appears that there is no single superior method of recruitment but different methods may work better with different populations. Even though mail recruitment is inexpensive and less taxing on the research staff, it appears to be less effective in obtaining representative samples in low-income minority populations.

Relationship with Site of Recruitment

In face-to face recruitment, establishing a good relationship with the setting from which the participants will be recruited is crucial. In our case, liaison with the outpatient clinics and working with them in developing procedures convenient to them and us and maintaining a close working relationship was vital in our being able to access and elicit interest from the target population for our project.

Maintaining Contact with Participants

Once the participants are recruited, continued effort to keep them in the study is necessary. This may be in the form of letters and phone calls to remind them of their forthcoming interview or class session. It may also be advisable to circulate a newsletter about the progress of the project on a regular basis. Some of our subjects were unaware of the purpose of the project and did not understand the need for repeated interviews even at one year from the original contact. Despite verbal and written information that we disseminated at the initial contact, participants seem either to have never understood or to have forgotten what they were committing themselves to do when they joined the project. Clearly, a better understanding would allow not only truly informed consent but also engender greater involvement in the project.

Participant Payment

We found payment for the assessment interviews to be helpful in obtaining a better completion rate in some cases. Again, we found that payment was more important for participants from a lower socioeconomic background than for those from a middle class background. This reflects the real life situation of these participants and the need to increase their resources in tangible ways.

The field of prevention intervention is young and many imperfections exist. We believe that our understanding of depression is sufficient for the development and testing of preventive interventions, and have demonstrated how we conceptualized and implemented such a randomized controlled trial. Clearly, in working with a multiethnic, low-income group, we were confronted with the realization that the group which most needs the intervention and for whom the benefit is potentially the greatest may also be the most difficult one to reach and retain. This is partly because of the limited resources these individuals have available to them which diminishes their ability to join in a research venture. But, this also reflects the limitations of the tools we have developed thus far to work primarily with middle income, white populations. We believe that it is a challenge to researchers in general, and prevention researchers in particular, to develop methodologies and interventions for more needy and often neglected groups.

REFERENCES

Albee, G. W. (1982). Preventing psychopathology and promoting human potential. *American Psychologist, 37,* 1040–1050.

Albee, G. W., & Joffe, J. M. (Eds.). (1977). *The primary prevention of psychopathology: The issues.* Hanover, NH: University Press of New England.

Bandura, A. (1977). *Social learning theory.* Englewood Cliffs, New Jersey: Prentice-Hall.

Barrera, M. (1981). Social support in the adjustment of pregnant adolescents: Assessment issues. In B. Gottlieb (Ed.), *Social networks and social support.* Beverley Hills, CA: Sage Publications.

Beck, A. T., Ward, C. H., Mendelsohn, M., Mock, J., & Erbaugh, J. (1961). An inventory for measuring depression. *Archives of General Psychiatry, 4,* 561–571.

Bellack, A. S., Hersen, M., & Himmelhoch, J. (1981). Social skills training compared with psychotherapy in the treatment of unipolar depression. *American Journal of Psychiatry, 138,* 1562–1567.

Bloom, B. L. (1979). Prevention of mental disorders: Recent advances in theory and practice. *Community Mental Health Journal, 15,* 179–191.

Bloom, B. L. (1981). The logic and urgency of primary prevention. *Hospital and Community Psychiatry, 32,* 839–843.

Bradburn, N. (1969). *The structure of psychological wellbeing.* Chicago, IL: Aldine.

Chassin, L. A., Presson, C. C., Sherman, S. J. (1985). Stepping backward in order to step forward: An acquisition-oriented approach to primary prevention. *Journal of Consulting and Clinical Psychology, 53,* 612–623.

Comstock, G. W., & Helsing, K. J. (1976). Symptoms of depression in two communities. *Psychological Medicine, 6,* 551–563.

Cowen, E. L. (1982). Primary prevention research: Barriers, needs, and opportunities. *Journal of Primary Prevention, 2,* 131–137.

Cowen, E. L. (in press). Primary prevention in mental health: Ten years of retrospect and ten years of prospect. In M. Kessler & G. Albee (Eds.), *A decade of progress in primary prevention.* Hanover, NH: University Press of New England.

Crowne, D., & Marlowe, D. (1960). A new scale of social desirability independent of psychopathology. *Journal of Consulting and Clinical Psychology, 24,* 349–354.

Dohrenwend, B. S., & Dohrenwend, B. P. (1974). *Stressful life events: Their nature and effects.* New York: Wiley.

Eaton, W. W., & Kessler, L. G. (1981). Rates of symptoms of depression in a national sample. *American Journal of Epidemiology, 114,* 528–538.

Endicott, J., & Spitzer, R. L. (1978). A diagnostic interview: The schedule for Affective Disorders and Schizophrenia. *Archives of General Psychiatry, 35,* 837–844.

Flanagan, J. C. (1978). A research approach to improving our quality of life. *American Psychologist, 33,* 138–147.

Frank, R. G., Kamlet, M. S., & Stoudemire, A. (1985, May). The social cost of depression. In A. Stoudemire (Chair), *Perspectives in the prevention of depression.* Symposium conducted at the meeting of the American Psychiatric Association, Dallas.

Heller, K., Price, R. H., & Sher, K. J. (1980). Research and evaluation in primary prevention: Issues and guidelines. In R. H. Price, R. F. Ketterer, B. C. Bader, & J. Monahan (Eds.), *Prevention in mental health: Research, policy, and practice.* Beverly Hills: Sage.

Hoeper, E. W., Nycz, G. R., Cleary, P. D., Regier, D. A., & Goldberg, I. D. (1979). Estimated prevalence of RDC mental disorder in primary medical care. *International Journal of Mental Health, 8*(2), 6–15.

Jones, K. R., & Vischi, T. R. (1979). Impact of alcohol, drug abuse and mental health treatment on medical care utilization: A review of the research literature. *Medical Care, 17,* (Supplement), 1–82.

Katon, W. (1982). Depression: Somatic symptoms and medical disorders in primary care. *Comprehensive Psychiatry, 23,* 274–287.

Kelly, J. G. (1968). Towards an ecological conception of preventive interventions. In J. W. Carter (Ed.), *Research contributions from psychology to community mental health.* New York: Behavioral Publications.

Kelly, J. H. (1977). The search for ideas and deeds that work. In G. W. Albee & J. M. Joffe (Eds.), *Primary prevention of psychopathology: The issues.* Hanover, NH: University Press of New England.

Lamb, H. R., & Zussman, J. (1981). A new look at primary prevention. *Hospital and Community Psychiatry, 32,* 843–848.

Lemkau, P. V. (1955). *Mental hygiene in public health.* New York: McGraw-Hill.

Lewinsohn, P. M. (1975). The behavioral study and treatment of depression. In M. Hersen, R. M. Eisler, & P. M. Miller (Eds.), *Progress in behavior modification.* Vol. 1. New York: Academic Press.

Lewinsohn, P. M., Muñoz, R. M., Youngren, M. A., & Zeiss, A. M. (1986). *Control your depression* (Revised edition). New York: Prentice-Hall.

Marsella, A. J., Kinzie, D., & Gordon, P. (1973). Ethnocultural variations in the expression of depression. *Journal of Cross-Cultural Psychology, 4,* 435–458.

McLean, P. D., & Hakstain, A. R. (1979). Clinical depression: Comparative efficacy of outpatient treatments. *Journal of Consulting and Clinical Psychology, 47,* 818–836.

Multiple Risk Factor Intervention Trial Group. (1985). Baseline rest electrocardiographic abnormalities, antihypertensive treatment, and mortality in the multiple risk factor intervention trial. *The American Journal of Cardiology, 55,* 1-15.

Muñoz, R. F. (1976). The primary prevention of psychological problems: A review of the literature. *Community Mental Health Review, 1,* 1-15.

Muñoz, R. F. (1977). A cognitive approach to the assessment and treatment of depression (Doctoral dissertation, University of Oregon, 1977). *Dissertation Abstracts International, 38,* 2873B. (University Microfilms No. 7726, 505, 154).

Muñoz, R. F. (1983, February). *Prevention intervention research: A challenge to minority researchers.* Paper presented at the NIMH Technical Assistance Workshop on Prevention Intervention Research: Special Population Groups, Rockville, MD.

Murphy, G. E., Simons, A. D., Wetzel, R. D., & Lustman, P. J. (1984). Cognitive therapy and pharmacotherapy: Singly and together in the treatment of depression. *Archives of General Psychiatry, 41,* 33-41.

Nielsen, A. C., III, & Williams, T. A. (1980). Depression in ambulatory medical patients. *Archives of General Psychiatry, 37,* 999-1004.

Radloff, L. S. (1977). The CES-D scale: A self-report depression scale for research in the general population. *Applied Psychological Measurement, 1,* 385-401.

Robins, L. N., Helzer, J. E., Croughan, J., & Ratcliff, K. S. (1981). National Institute of Mental Health Diagnostic Interview Schedule: Its history, characteristics, and validity. *Archives of General Psychiatry, 38,* 381-389.

Rush, A. J., Beck, A. T., Kovacs, M., & Hollon, S. (1977). Comparative efficacy of cognitive therapy and pharmacotherapy in the treatment of depressed outpatients. *Cognitive Therapy and Research, 1,* 17-37.

Sarason, I., Johnson, J., & Siegel, J. (1978). Assessing the impact of life change: Development of the life experiences survey. *Journal of Consulting and Clinical Psychology, 46,* 932-946.

Sayetta, R. B., & Johnson, D. P. (1980). *Basic data on depressive symptomatology: United States, 1974-75. Vital and Health Statistics-Series 11,* Number 216. (DHEW Publication No. (PHS) 80-1666). Hyatsville, MD.: National Center for Health Statistics.

Simons, A. D., Levine, J. L., Lustman, P. J., & Murphy., E. E. (1984). Patient attrition in a comparative outcome study of depression: A follow-up report. *Journal of Affective Disorders, 6,* 163-173.

Spitzer, R. L., Endicott, J., & Robins, E. (1978). Research diagnostic criteria: Rationale and reliability. *Archives of General Psychiatry, 35,* 773-782.

Vega, W., Warheit, G., BuhlAuth, J., & Meinhardt, K. (1984). The prevalence of depressive symptoms among Mexican Americans and Anglos. *American Journal of Epidemiology, 120,* 592-607.

Ying, Y. W., & Armas, R. (1985, August). Implementing a prevention trial in English, Spanish and Chinese. In M. Barrera, Jr. (Chair), *Depression prevention research: Design, implementation, and analysis of randomized trials.* Symposium conducted at the meeting of the American Psychological Association, Los Angeles.

Zeiss, A. M., Lewinsohn, P. M., & Muñoz, R. F. (1979). Non-specific improvement effects in depression using interpersonal, cognitive, and pleasant events focused treatments. *Journal of Consulting and Clinical Psychology, 47,* 427-439.

13

The Hispanic Social Network Prevention Intervention Study: A Community-Based Randomized Trial

William A. Vega, Ramón Valle, Bohdan Kolody, and Richard Hough
San Diego State University, California

INTRODUCTION

This chapter briefly reviews the theoretical and design specifications for a community-based prospective preventive intervention study currently in process in San Diego, California. The study is funded by the National Institute of Mental Health as part of their program initiative to gain new knowledge about the feasibility and efficaciousness of conducting preventive interventions with a wide variety of sociodemographic groups. The goal of our project is to prevent the onset of depression and high levels of depressive symptoms among Mexican-American women between thirty-five and fifty years of age using a three-group design, including a control and two intervention groups. The research involves a large and carefully screened community sample drawn from a relatively homogenous ethnic subgroup (low income immigrants). By virtue of the careful design and sample, we believe that the study will provide an adequate test of contemporary concepts and methods in prevention research. The contents of this chapter include: (1) a rationale for target group selection; (2) a summary of the theoretical background underlying the research; (3) a description of the interventions; (4) a review of design features; and (5) a delineation of implications for the field of depression prevention.

SELECTION OF THE POPULATION

Recent epidemiological investigations carried out in California indicate that, despite significant underutilization of mental health providers, the true prevalence of depressive symptoms among Mexican Americans appears to be higher than corresponding rates in the general population. For example, Frerichs, Aneshensel, & Clark (1981), using the Center for Epidemiologic Studies-Depression measure (CES-D) (Radloff, 1977) with a caseness threshold of 16 or over, reported a prevalence rate of 27.4 for Hispanics and 15.6 for Anglos in Los Angeles County.

The Hispanic Social Network Prevention Intervention Study is supported in part by the Center for Prevention Research, National Institute of Mental Health (M.H. #38745, William A. Vega, P.I.), and housed at San Diego State University, San Diego, CA.

Vernon and Roberts (1982) used the CES–D in Alameda County and reported caseness rates of 28.9 for Mexican-Americans and 14.6 for Anglos. In a third urban study conducted in Santa Clara County, Vega, Warheit, Buhl-Auth, & Meinhardt (1984) report caseness rates of 27.1 for Spanish-speaking Mexican-Americans, 15.9 for English-speaking Mexican-Americans, and 12.0 for Anglos using the Florida Health Study depression measure (Schwab, Bell, Warheit, & Schwab, 1979).

The selection of the specific age-sex cohort for this study was based on the idiosyncratic distribution of symptoms found in the Los Angeles and Santa Clara surveys reported above, as well as a third survey conducted with Mexican-American farmworkers in Fresno County using the Health Opinion Survey (Vega, Warheit, & Palacio, 1985). These three studies all reported the highest age-specific rates of psychological symptoms for Hispanic women in middle life. This contrasts with epidemiological findings for general populations throughout the United States which have reported higher rates of depressive symptoms among young adults. In the Santa Clara survey, controlled analyses identified these high risk markers: gender (female), low socioeconomic status, immigrant status, Spanish monolinguality, disrupted marital statuses, and lower levels of available social support.

We suspect that the immigration process is a key element among the risk factors. Hispanics, in comparison to the general population, are disproportionately immigrants and experience the types of conflicts and strains described in the classic literature on immigration and subsequent adaptation (e.g., Thomas & Zaniecki, 1927). A more penetrating rationale, though, is required to explain why middle-aged women would be most symptomatic. Since descriptive point prevalence epidemiology is unsuited for producing such information, it was necessary to pursue clinical evidence.

A coherent profile of pathology is emerging from interviews with clinicians serving this population. As is being reported, low income Mexican-American women have the highest birthrate of any ethnic group in the United States. Since their advantage in childbearing carries well into the middle years of the life course, it is not uncommon to encounter middle aged Hispanic women in this cohort and their daughters both with children of the same age. Unfortunately, given the economic marginality and residential mobility of this population, many of the pregnancies are of a high risk nature and result in a variety of health problems for both the mother and the child (Boulette, 1980a).

Clinical evidence further indicates that role obligations often increase with age for these low income Mexican-American women, especially those who are immigrants, while at the same time their ability to cope with these burdens diminishes. The reasons for this diminution of coping ability are complex, but two factors appear to have primacy. First, many women in the cohort experience an almost absolute sense of powerlessness based upon lack of English language competence, little or no formal education, few if any marketable job skills, and a lack of familiarity with mainstream Anglo-American social and economic institutions. Second, the women in this group, at this point in their life course often begin to encounter circumstances wherein their marital partner's ability to provide instrumental and affective support also diminishes. This diminution of the marital partner's supportive capabilities is, in turn, nested in a variety of factors which include his own chronic and life threatening disorders or possible physical absence from the home. In the context of this increasing vulnerability, the onset of health anomalies as well as disruptive life events among family members can be seen to have greater impact on the low income Hispanic woman than at an earlier point in the life course.

A compounding factor is the fact that often the normative socialization and coping response patterns acquired by many low income Hispanic women resemble learned helplessness (Canino, 1982). For example, the head-of-household role obligations are ordinarily assigned to the male rather than to the female marital partners, even if for a variety of reasons they are unable to carry out these responsibilities. Moreover, since many women in this cohort marry men many years their senior, they are at higher risk for being widowed or acquiring additional caretaking burdens, in addition to their ongoing life course coping tasks, as the health of their marital partner deteriorates. Despite these circumstances, the women in this cohort are often found persisting in attempting to maintain the functional role of their spouse as "head-of-household" thereby only reinforcing their perception of being overwhelmed by environmental circumstances.

The psychological conflicts and feelings of powerlessness arising from these life situations are linked throughout the literature to somatic complaints and other symptoms of psychophysiological distress, including irritability, disturbed sleep and appetite patterns, negative affect, and a poor outlook toward the future (Link and Dohrenwend, 1980). When this attitudinal set is combined with other stressors such as the loss of expressive support, or even aggravated by spousal alcoholism or emotional and/or physical abuse, the risk of persistent and impairing depressive symptomatology is manifested.

In summary, women caught in this situation are not only faced with social isolation, moral conflicts and financial dilemmas, but also find themselves without sufficient or effective social support for confronting these stressors. We therefore believe, that within the current stage of development of prevention theory in mental health, the age-gender cohort selected for study is indeed a population at risk, and an appropriate target group for intervention. Our more specific methods for targeting the population are discussed in the "Principal Design Features" section below.

THEORETICAL BACKGROUND OF THE RESEARCH

Our intervention could be termed an early preventive intervention, since it encompasses both primary and limited secondary prevention objectives. We intend to prevent the onset of depressive symptoms in asymptomatic subjects and to prevent the exacerbation of existing symptomatology among those subjects already experiencing some depressive symptoms. In order to assure the appropriateness of the sample for a preventive intervention, a thorough two-stage screening, of the type suggested by Dohrenwend and Dohrenwend (1982), is being used to eliminate those respondents who are already seriously symptomatic, perhaps suffering from a preexisting psychiatric disorder, or who have a life-threatening illness.

The goal of the research are two-fold. First, we want to determine if changes in self concept (assessed with mastery, self esteem, and self-efficacy measures) can be introduced by increasing instrumental social support designed to extend the knowledge and skills of the subject concerning techniques for mediating environmental stressors. Second, we will examine whether depressive symptoms can be subsequently prevented or reduced by the improvement in self concept. Our premise is that enhancement of coping skills is directly related to self concept and in turn, to depressive symptoms. *It is important to note that self-efficacy, as operationalized in this study, is specific to the skills attainment targeted by the intervention, e.g., increased social competence.* These interventions will be conveyed by means of two discrete natural network modalities, which are explained below. The target malady is depressive symptoms which may be a precursor to clinical depression. There are important similarities between the affective and cognitive states that render the target group to be at-risk and the concept of demoralization as defined by Frank (1973), including lower self-esteem, states of helplessness-hopelessness, and feelings of sadness and anxiety.

Previous research has indicated that behavior which has produced poor outcomes can be changed by internalizing new performance standards providing that the appropriate conditions for successful actualization of goals are present. As Bandura (1982) states:

> *Inability to influence events and social conditions that significantly affect one's life can give rise to feelings of guilt and despondency as well as anxiety. Self-efficacy theory distinguishes between two judgmental sources of futility. People can give up trying because they seriously doubt that they can do what is required. Or they may be assured of their capabilities but give up trying because they expect their efforts to produce no results due to unresponsiveness, negative bias, or punitiveness of the environment. These two sources of futility have quite different causes and remedial implications. To change efficacy-based futility requires development of constituent competencies and strong percepts of self-efficacy (p. 40).*

Therefore, an intervention addressing this futility, which we believe is closely associated with depressive symptoms found among Mexican-American women, should address both perceptions of self-efficacy and outcomes.

Our two intervention modalities are based in social learning theory, especially in the four areas Bandura (1969, 1977) has linked to the development of personal efficacy, which include: (1) personal experience with a difficult task, (2) vicarious participation in problem solving, (3) verbal persuasion, and (4) the control of physiological reactions to a problem situation. Bandura has demonstrated that the perception of competence is more closely related to future activity than past performance, and that knowledge of the consequences of present behavior is a powerful mediator in reshaping behavior. Within the context of our intervention design, and based on Iscoe's (1974) work, we hypothesize that as knowledge of community resources increases along with cognitive and social skills for accessing them, the individual's sense of well being will also grow, and this will be reflected in the outcome measures. The structure and content of the interventions is discussed in the next section.

Two other key theoretical constructs that were central to the development of the preventive interventions used in this study are social support domains and valence. The seminal work of Pearlin and colleagues (1975, 1978) on social support domains has provided an important step forward in the conceptualization of social support, providing a finer gradient for assessing the structure of networks and the function of supportive roles. This work provides a more complete understanding of the interplay of life strain, life events, and coping responses within distinct domains of current life activity, e.g., parenting, marriage, work, etc. Within this framework, social support becomes synergistic with domain-specific stress and coping, and transcends the "stress buffering" assumptions associated with the previous generation of social support theory (Nuckolls, Cassel, & Kaplan, 1972). This implies that social support that is efficacious for offsetting stress in one domain may lack salience in another, or even in the same domain at a different stage in the life course, which calls into question whether a "universal coper" is attainable. Following this line of thought, we believe that our interventions may well have differential impact across domains and individuals. For a given individual, they may solve problems in one domain but leave other life course "compartments" relatively unaffected. We may also find that our intervention works differently for people in different circumstances. At the same time, we expect to use domain-specific information on stress and coping to better focus the interventions by depicting specific areas of widespread social dysfunction.

The theoretical issue of support valence (i.e., the positive or negative outcome of support) flows from the work of an increasing number of investigators, including Hammer (1981), Wellman (1981), Belle (1982) and Dean and Ensel (1983). One important conclusion of this body of work is that social support, even if available, is only helpful for problem solving and emotional nurturance under certain conditions. Unfortunately, it is the inadequacy rather than the unavailability of support that is too frequently encountered among the members of a demoralized group. In such a group social networks may in fact be very draining of limited emotional and material resources, thereby rendering members unable to provide the "lift" required to help each other overcome life's problems. This phenomenon has been described as a "high taker" (Goodman, 1980) relationship on the individual level and as an asymmetrical (Wellman, 1981) relationship at the systemic level. Also, it is patently obvious that many dense networks, such as those found among low income Hispanic populations, may be rife with expressive support which meets certain emotional needs of the network members, yet remain inadequate for a range of serious problems that require instrumental supportive activities. Although both instrumental and expressive support may be required for optional functioning, these two axes have discrete functions (Valle & Bensussen, in press). We are measuring the valence of instrumental and expressive support within life domains in order to identify the functional attributes of each axis, and their contributory role in producing global well being. Our intervention format is solidly anchored on the instrumental axis, although we recognize that elements of expressive and instrumental support are mutually reinforcing.

As frequently noted in the mental health literature, the search for single predisposing factors responsible for pathogenic outcomes is seductive and at times promising, but has not yet produced a solid body of knowledge upon which to base preventive interventions. Therefore, we must rely on prevention paradigms that specify multiple precipitating factors and multifactorial explanations (Bloom, 1981). In the absence of a careful specification of variable linkage among risk factors, mediators, and outcomes, it is impossible to establish the internal validity of the intervention effect. Price (1981) has set four criteria that facilitate the designing of prevention research, and provide a rational basis for measurement when modeling numerous variables. It would be useful to review these and illustrate their application in our research. They include:

1) *Solid evidence of risk, including marker variables and modifiable risk variables.* As indicated at the beginning of this chapter, epidemiological research iden-

tifies mid-life as a period of increased risk for depressive symptoms among low income Mexican-American women. Many of these women move into middle life often facing the prospect of learning new tasks as principal income providers and functional heads of households. Others have to adjust to transformations in marital roles. In addition, the demands of extended child rearing are often compounded by the needs of young adult children who are starting their own families under difficult circumstances, and who require additional social support. Many women will lack the personal and social coping resources to meet these multiple demands.

Further, we expect that the risk level is high among low income, middle age Mexican-American women irrespective of marital status. Among Hispanics, women who are separated, currently unmarried, or were never legally married, but who nevertheless have children, are much more common than single women. Finally, even single women in the Hispanic community will often be found in family settings and have considerable child rearing and family care responsibilities and therefore face many of the same mid-life transitional problems.

The modifiable risk factors for these women include cognitive and behavioral responses to stressors, as well as knowledge and ability to use extended support system resources for solving life course problems as experienced within the specific domains.

2) *A careful specification of the type of risk expressed by the study cohort in the broadest terms.* From a clinical perspective, the target group is at risk for experiencing impaired role performance at the personal, interpersonal, and structural level; including depressive symptomatology, anxiety, diffuse somatic complaints, and psychophysiological anomalies such as spontaneous episodes of weeping, extreme irritability, and disturbed eating and sleeping patterns. In the most extreme cases *una incapacidad nerviosa* (a "nervous breakdown") could occur, requiring the attention of health providers and medication. However, because of the screening criteria for selecting subjects, such signs and symptoms would not be widely prevalent in the prevention intervention sample.

3) *There should be a set of operational hypotheses that explain the relationship between factors and processes related to the perceived risk of the cohort.* In this context, the following operational hypotheses are related to risk in the study cohort:

1. In the presence of stressors of equal or increasing magnitude, those subjects with higher levels of mastery and self efficacy will have a lower prevalence of depressive symptoms;

2. In the presence of stressors of equal or increasing magnitude, those subjects with greater knowledge of support system resources, as well as access and use of instrumental network support, will have a lower prevalence of depressive symptoms and higher levels of mastery and self efficacy;

3. Mastery and self-efficacy will be inversely related to the frequency of stressful life events, the magnitude of role strain, and marginal acculturation;

4. Mastery and self-efficacy will be inversely related to maladaptive cognitive and behavioral responses to perceived stressors;

5. Maladaptive cognitive and behavioral responses to perceived stressors will be positively related to depressive symptoms, stressful life events and persistent life strain; and

6. Levels of reported health anomalies, medication usage, and use of health

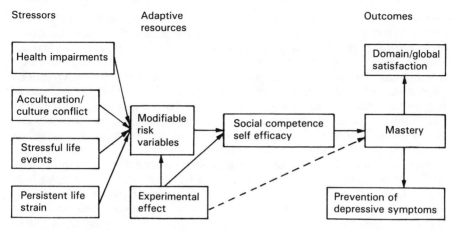

Figure 1 Prevention intervention variables.

providers will be positively related to depressive symptoms, stressful life events, persistent role strain, and maladaptive cognitive and behavioral responses to perceived stressors.

4) *There should be a theory of the intervention that can explain the effect of the intervention on the modifiable risk variables.* It is our view that the intervention should prevent onset of depressive symptoms by first increasing personal coping resources, including knowledge of networks and resources, thereby increasing perceived self-efficacy and mastery, and improving stress coping skills within specific domains. Figure 1 presents a simplified illustration of the expected linkage of major study variables and the intervention effect.

We anticipate both intervention formats to produce higher levels of *social competence,* self-efficacy, mastery, self-esteem, domain specific satisfaction, global satisfaction, positive affect, along with lower depressive symptoms, than will be found in the control group. Marginal acculturation is expected to have a positive association with persistent role strain, and experimental subjects who are marginally acculturated are expected to have the greatest change in the intended direction of the experimental effect.

DESCRIPTION OF THE INTERVENTIONS

The preventive interventions will be implemented in two distinct formats. The *linkperson* mode will feature one-on-one contacts initiated by a project-hired indigenous Hispanic natural helper known as the *servidora*. The second intervention mode will utilize a peer group format to be identified as the *merienda educativa* and similarly use the *servidora* natural helper as the group leader. Both prevention interventions will extend over a twelve month period. Each will begin with an intensive three month phase of interpersonal face-to-face contacts followed up by periodic booster contacts or sessions. For the *merienda educativa,* the initial intensive phase will include peer group sessions every two weeks, with sessions every six weeks for the remaining nine month booster contact period. Since both progress and relapses are anticipated among the participants, the booster contacts/ sessions are seen as essential to program maintenance. Since relapse is seen as a major factor impeding the long-term effects of the behavioral interventions (Marlatt & Park, 1982), the booster sessions will emphasize a gradual increase in responsibility for personal change on the part of the study subjects. At the same time, subjects will be assured that a certain amount of relapse occurs naturally and should not be a source of guilt (and resulting anxiety) for them, but rather an opportunity for reappraisal of gains made.

From a theoretical perspective, the preventive intervention has elements and goals similar to several strategies outlined in the literature. For example, it is similar to Albee's (1982) suggested strategy for enhancing coping skills, self esteem, and supportive interaction in order to decrease subject vulnerability; to Day's (1982) program to increase stress management capabilities; and to Gottlieb's (1983) training activities to "reinforce and enlarge the repertoire of interpersonal helping skills in ongoing social networks." We also regard Heller and Swindle's (1983) emphasis on learning appropriate network "appraisal" skills to be important in our study. While we have drawn on much previous work to develop our preventive intervention program, we have also been keenly aware that it must be relevant to the context of expressive and instrumental social support dynamics to be found among Hispanics.

The *linkperson* format is basically a one-to-one facilitative relationship grounded on the kind of reciprocity and exchange behaviors which typify natural helping networks in the Hispanic community (Valle & Mendoza, 1978; Mendoza, 1980; Valle & Mendoza, 1981). In the natural setting a servidora typically provides help to individuals in coping with a wide range of stressful life events and persistent strains by developing close personal rapport with individual "clients" and by linking them to the kinds of social resources (interpersonal and organizational) which can help with their problems. In the linkperson format, the project servidoras will recruit the assigned subjects into the intervention phase of the project and will help them develop, restore, maintain, and expand their coping abilities.

This will be accomplished by techniques generally stemming from social learning theory. For example, the subjects will be instructed as to the availability of community and interpersonal helping resources for addressing specific stressors and strains within major life domains; i.e., family problems, economic problems, work problems, health, etc., and encouraged to become assertive in their use of such resources. The primary focus will be on instrumental, problem solving techniques with the servidoras modeling appropriate coping strategies. The subject will be encouraged to role play such coping strategies and to experiment with them in real life situations with the close support of the servidoras. It is hypothesized that as coping skills improve, cognitive behavioral changes will occur in which the subject feels more self efficacy and personal empowerment. As a sense of competence emerges, the change in the subjects will become more self-directed and servidoras will concentrate more on developing self monitoring techniques and setting realistic goals.

The merienda educativa format is based upon group interaction dynamics widespread among Hispanics and is modeled after the work of Boulette (1980b). In addition to including the problem solving content found in the linkperson mode, the merienda educativa will provide for various peer group exchange and support experiences which are known within social learning theory to be powerful vehicles for behavior change. In addition to working with the subjects on the individual level as above, servidoras will use the groups to provide more formal instruction, modeling, role playing, and experiential guidance to deal with stressful life events and strains across the various life domains. The groups will allow the servidoras to provide for the development of coping repertoires and skills through encouragement of vicarious sharing in the experience of other group members with corresponding reinforcement of positive coping behaviors. As discussed with regard to the linkperson format, the three-month intensive intervention is followed by the nine-month maintenance period in order to consolidate and allow for the development of appropriate self-directed behavior.

On assignment, both the *linkperson servidora* and the *merienda educativa servidora* will contact the subjects, explaining in detail the mode of contact and its duration. It should be noted again that at this point in time subjects will have had several prior contacts with the project, and will have been informed of their inclusion in the study. In the linkperson format, intervention will take place in the context of the participant's home. For the merienda, the subjects will be contacted and invited to a "coffee clatch" session which will be held at a predetermined stationary location within the community. This will include church, school and community centers convenient for the subjects. The meeting places will have been secured by project staff prior to the implementation of the intervention. In some instances, as deemed appropriate, some meriendas will meet in private homes, but these will be the exception, as it is expected that few of the participants will have the living space or adequate environmental conditions to host the peer group structure on a sustained basis. A modest budget has been set aside for refreshments and for babysitting services. Subjects will receive no direct payment for attendance at these sessions.

A final important aspect of the research will be our documentation of what the servidoras actually do under the experimental conditions. Since the servidoras are an integral part of the research, every effort will be made throughout the intervention process to gather information on their functioning; this to be accomplished through a process of systematic debriefings by project staff. As Gottlieb (1983) indicates, it is of great importance to the field of prevention to understand the activities of persons in the community who are not trained mental health professionals but who are nevertheless involved in a great deal of informal counseling and lay-naturalistic referral work.

PRINCIPAL DESIGN FEATURES

The study design, summarized in the outline below, has four major stages. First, a screening-enumeration of respondents was used to identify the target population low income Mexican-American females age 35–50 who have lived in the United States a minimum of two years and who are not currently experiencing high levels of depressive symptoms. A county-wide sample was selected using a probability proportionate to size of stratified area sampling design. Current symptomatology was ascertained by the CES–D. At the second stage, respondents within the screening criteria on the CES–D (that is, a score of 16 or above) were given a baseline assessment which included a partial diagnostic protocol. Respondents not experiencing either a case-level psychiatric disorder or serious physical health problem were randomized into three groups, including a control and two experimental cohorts. These activities took place within the first year of the research. The third stage of the research is the intervention, which covers year two of the study and is to be followed by the terminal assessment in year three.

Operation Stages and General Study Design
1. Location, Screening, and Enlistment (year 1) - N = 2272
   A. Total enumeration and location of target population: low income Mexican American females age 35–50.
   B. Screening for early preventive intervention candidacy with CES–D and health probes.
   C. Enlistment for study participation of consenting eligibles
2. Second Stage Screening and Baseline Assessment (year 1) - N = 842 (expected)
   A. DIS and functionality screen to eliminate subjects with diagnosable disorders.
   B. Social network screen to eliminate subjects with *servidora* relationships.
   C. Baseline assessment on:
      1. Stressor variables
         a. Health impairments
         b. Acculturation, cultural conflict
         c. Stressful life events
         d. Persistent life strain
      2. Adaptive resource variables
         a. Knowledge of support resource availability and utilization
         b. Cognitive and behavioral responses
      3. Outcome variables
         a. Domain and global satisfaction
         b. Self concept (mastery, self esteem, self-efficacy)
         c. Depressive symptoms
3. Randomization of Eligibles into Three Modalities (year 2) - N = 600 (expected)
   A. Intervention through linkperson format (individual intervention)
   B. Intervention through *merienda* format (individual plus group intervention)
   C. Controls
4. Outcome Assessment on Items in IIC above (year 3) - N = 450 (expected)

Heavy respondent and subject mortality is anticipated at each stage of the research. We anticipate losing four out of every five women enumerated by the point of terminal assessment, resulting in 450 subjects (150 per group) available for analyses of outcome. Comparisons between those who complete the study and those who drop out will provide information about the generalizability of the study. Administration and evaluation of the interventions in this study are through a simple, randomized, three group pretest-posttest experimental design of the form:

Group		Number expected
E1	RO X$_1$ 0	200
E2	RO X$_2$ 0	200
C1	RO — 0	200

C1 is the control group, while E1 and E2 represent the "linkperson" and *"merienda"* intervention formats. This design was chosen for its simplicity as well as analytical power in facilitating examination of initial group differences, mortality, and change in both central tendency and variance. For example, we used statistical power estimates to determine sample sizes adequate to yield significance in tests for group differences of realistic, hence relatively small, changes in outcomes measures.

In order to find potential subjects, we conducted a total enumeration of all block groups in San Diego County with a proportion of Mexican-Americans of twenty percent or greater. Subject selection required calling on approximately 40,000 doors. Respondents were told at first contact about the study and informed that they could be recontacted. They were also asked to provide additional personal contacts to allow for subject tracking if they change residence, thereby lowering attrition.

The baseline assessment consists of scales and inventories that are too numerous to review here. However, it is important to note that a modified Diagnostic Interview Schedule (DIS) (Robins, Helzer, Croughan, & Ratcliff, 1981) was used to complete the subject screening process by excluding all respondents with case-level disorders. The protocol used includes current and lifetime depression and schizophrenia; and current anxiety, generalized anxiety, panic, phobia, obsessive compulsive disorder and dysthymia. The rest of the baseline interview schedule was designed around specific life domains in keeping with the logic of Pearlin's approach. In addition, we created a measure of *social competence* self efficacy that is task- and domain-specific. The outcome measurements incorporate all scales and inventories which are indicators of change on the study variables. We will also use the partial DIS to determine the rate of onset for case level depressive disorders among the three groups over the course of the research.

The enumeration and baseline assessment phases of the study constitute a serious field research burden as a consequence of the criteria for subject selection and the sheer numbers involved. Moreover, a referral process and clinical evaluation team had to be formulated in order to handle any respondents requiring immediate attention, including those who were found to be seriously disturbed. Despite its burdensome qualities, we opted for this design for three reasons. First, we felt the study population should be as representative as possible of the social demographic group from which it was drawn in order to enhance the external validity of the experiment. Second, the design had to anticipate heavy respondent and subject attrition at every stage of the research. Finally, two-stage screening efficiently identifies women who would be inappropriate for a preventive intervention because they already meet clinical diagnostic criteria.

In addition to changes in depressive symptomatology, the intervention aspires to experimentally induce changes in a number of objective and subjective areas, including: self-efficacy (operationally defined as perceived social competence), mastery, self esteem, and objective knowledge of community resources. Because most of the more abstract variables represent multidimensional constructs measured by sets of subscales, internal analyses ranging from simple discriminant and factor analyses to confirmatory factor analyses will be undertaken. Final outcome variables will be based upon these analyses. The analysis of outcomes will control for stressors, modifiable risk variables, and demographic characteristics. Examples of expected significant covariates include preintervention levels of knowledge of community resources, instrumental and expressive support and acculturation. Finding that such variables do not covary with outcomes would be as theoretically relevant as the opposite result.

Two fundamental strengths of the study design from the standpoint of addressing causation are that it is both experimental and longitudinal. This facilitates addressing the "stress-adaptive resources-outcomes" relationship (Hough, 1981) as a process. Causal questions may be dealt with directly. For example, we will be able to assess whether changes in modifiable risk factors buffer stress-outcome relationships or whether they have direct effects conditioned or not by other variables. A variety of multivariate techniques, including multivariate analysis of covariance, logistical regression, and linear structural modeling will be used to address our primary objectives of evaluating the intervention and modeling its underlying theory.

IMPLICATIONS FOR THE FIELD
OF PREVENTION

Large community based mental health studies are complex and expensive, and preventive intervention research is perhaps even more so. Readers familiar with prospective field studies in prevention can appreciate the complexity of design as well as practical issues that must be resolved in order to formulate an operational intervention. The shortage of a literature detailing outcomes of previous prevention studies among Hispanics, or any group for that matter, means that current researchers must proceed without definite "roadmaps" of the territory to be explored. The future of depression prevention obviously depends in great part on the structures that are created to support such research. At the same time, there does exist sufficient base of information, garnered from a number of subject areas, to mount prevention research which is feasible, with modest aims and measurable outcomes. We believe the Hispanic Social Network Prevention Intervention Study is an example of this.

A great deal of important new knowledge is forthcoming from prospective research of this type quite apart from that associated with the preventive intervention. For example, although the literature contains many speculative and impressionistic articles (Newton, Olmedo, & Padilla, 1982), little rigorous information is available about stressors and coping styles among low income Mexican-American women or the stress buffering capabilities of their natural network. Furthermore, this study incorporates measures and inventories which are also used in other major epidemiological, life course, and prevention studies, and this provides a clear set of comparisons of the mental health and related characteristics of our population in comparison to others.

In regard to the field of prevention, the expected contribution of this research will be in the beginning to answer two fundamental questions. The first can be stated as follow: *which population subgroups are willing to participate in prevention trials?* Given the novelty of large scale prevention research, acquiring new knowledge about subject recruitment and cohort maintenance is fundamental. We think it is important for us to document what kind of persons are attracted into prevention projects. This alone will reveal systematic biases that can help us focus future recruitment efforts. The field of prevention must also learn how to recognize subjects who are at high risk for attrition or noncompliance and about steps that can be taken to minimize these problems. Moreover, since the field lacks standards and nomenclature even for defining subject mortality, this project will help determine the feasibility of preventive interventions in general population settings and facilitate the growth of a new prevention technology. Because the characteristics of both the interventions and social demographic groups affected vary widely, it is important that the field of prevention research include from its inception a cross-cultural and multi-regional perspective.

The second question could be stated as follows: *How correct are we in our basic assumptions about how to produce preventive effects?* We think there are several ways through which this project can contribute knowledge to this issue. First, the project will provide accurate information on the interrelationship of factors and processes we believe to be associated with the target disorder. In this research, we have made several theoretical assumptions about etiology and the role of social support for ameliorating some of the pathogenic conditions experienced by our subjects. Although these derive from carefully conducted research and observation, they await confirmation. Second, it remains an empirical question whether natural support "adjuncts" are feasible and efficacious for preventing depressive symptoms. This research experience will help us determine if depressive symptoms in this population are amenable to this type of intervention, and to identify the risk factors that can be affected in this manner. Third, this project can contribute new knowledge about the adequacy of current psychological techniques for eliciting behavior change in ethnically diverse populations. Although social learning theory is widely used in a prevention research, there are no universal rules about: a) how to apply this knowledge for addressing a range of behaviors typically confronted in prevention research; or b) how social learning theory will be mediated by cultural expectations, thereby requiring variations in operationalization including the process and content of interventions. Finally, it will also provide insight into a number of other issues of traditional concern to investigators in the human services field, e.g., risks posed to human subjects, effects on health services utilization, time and parameters of prevention interventions, etc.

However, a word of caution is also appropriate. Since we are breaking new ground, we are wary of being overly optimistic concerning expected outcomes and we are prepared for quite mixed results, including major cohort mortality problems. In addition, since we have no definite knowledge on the length of time required for the intervention to "take," or how long the intervention effect will endure, we should also be prepared for long term follow-up of study cohorts. Admittedly, these conditions will test the perseverence of funding agencies and investigators in the field. Moreover, their disposition to follow through on such major issues as these could very will determine the future of community mental health.

REFERENCES

Albee, G. W. (1982). The politics of nature and nurture. *American Journal of Community Psychology, 10,* 4–30.

Bandura, A. (1969). *Principles of behavior modification.* New York: Holt, Rinehart and Winston.

Bandura, A. (1977). *Social learning theory.* New Jersey: Prentice-Hall.

Bandura, A. (1982). Self-efficacy mechanism in human agency. *American Psychologist, 37,* 122–147.

Belle, D. (1982). Social ties and social support. In D. Belle (Ed.), *Lives in stress* (pp. 133–144). Beverly Hills: Sage Publications.

Bloom, B. (1981). The logic and urgency of primary prevention. *Journal of Hospital and Community Psychiatry, 32,* 839–843.

Boulette, T. R. (1980a). Priority issues for mental health promotion among low income Chicanos-Mexicanos. In R. Valle & W. Vega (Eds.), *Hispanic natural support systems* (pp. 15–22). Sacramento: California Department of Mental Health.

Boulette, T. R. (1980b). Mass media and other mental health promotional strategies for low income Chicanos and Mexicanos. In R. Valle & W. Vega (Eds.), *Hispanic natural support systems* (pp. 97–102). Sacramento: California Department of Mental Health.

Canino, G. (1982). The Hispanic women: Sociocultural influences on diagnoses and treatment. In R. Becerra, M. Karno, & J. Escobar (Eds.), *Mental health and Hispanic Americans* (pp. 117–138). New York: Grune and Stratton.

Day, R. (1982). Research on the course and outcome of schizophrenia in traditional cultures: Some potential implications for psychiatry in developed countries. In M. J. Goldstein (Ed.), *Preventive intervention in schizophrenia* (pp. 17–219) (DHHS Publication No. ADM 82-1111). Washington, DC: U.S. Government Printing Office.

Dean, A., & Ensel, W. M. (1982). Modelling social support, life events, competence, and depression. *Journal of Community Psychology, 10,* 392–408.

Dohrenwend, B. P., & Dohrenwend, B. S. (1982). Perspectives on the past and future of psychiatric epidemiology. *American Journal of Public Health, 72,* 1271–1279.

Frank, J. D. (1973). *Persuasion and healing.* New York: Schocken Books.

Frerichs, R. R., Aneshensel, C. S., & Clark, V. A. (1981). Prevalence of depression in Los Angeles County. *American Journal of Epidemiology, 113,* 691–699.

Gottlieb, B. H. (1983). The nature of social support and its health impact. In B. H. Gottlieb (Ed.), *Social support strategies: Guidelines for mental health practice* (pp. 31–64). Beverly Hills: Sage Publications.

Goodman, C. (1980). *Natural helping among older adults.* Unpublished doctoral dissertation, University of California, Los Angeles.

Hammer, M. (1981). Social supports, social networks and schizophrenia. *Schizophrenia Bulletin, 7,* 45–57.

Heller, K., & Swindle, R. W. (1983). Social networks, perceived social support, and coping with stress. In R. Felner, L. Jason, J. Moritsugu, & S. Farber (Eds.), *Preventive psychology: Theory, research and practice* (pp. 87–103). New York: Pergamon Press.

Hough, R. (1981). Socio-cultural issues in research and clinical practice: Closing the gap. In E. Serafetinides (Ed.), *From research to practice: Biobehavioral contributions* (pp. 203–226). New York: Grune and Stratton.

Iscoe, I. (1974). Community psychology and the competent community. *American Psychologist, 29,* 607–613.

Link, B., & Dohrenwend, B. P. (1980). Formulation of hypotheses about the true prevalence of demoralization in the United States. In B. P. Dohrenwend, B. S. Dohrenwend, M. S. Gould, B. Link, R. Neugebauer, & R. Wunsch-Hitzig (Eds.), *Mental illness in the United States* (pp. 114–132). New York: Praeger Publishers.

Marlatt, G. A., & Park, G. (1982). Self-management of addictive behaviors. In P. Karoly & F. H. Kanfer (Eds.), *Self-management and behavior change: From theory to practice* (pp. 121–140). New York: Pergamon Press.

Mendoza, L. (1980). Hispanic social networks: Techniques of cultural support. In R. Valle & W. Vega (Eds.), *Hispanic natural support systems* (pp. 55–64). Sacramento: California Department of Mental Health.

Mendoza, L. (1981). *The servidor system: Policy implications for the elderly hispano.* San Diego: Center on Aging, San Diego State University.

Nuckolls, K. B., Cassel, J., & Kaplan, B. H. (1972). Psychosocial assets, life crisis and the prognosis of pregnancy. *American Journal of Epidemiology, 95,* 431–441.

Newton, F. C., Olmedo, E., & Padilla, A. (1982). *Hispanic mental health research.* Berkeley: University of California Press.

Pearlin, L. (1975). Sex roles and depression. In N. Datan & L. Ginsberg (Eds.), *Life span developmental psychology: Normative life crisis* (pp. 191–207). New York: Academic Press.

Pearlin, L., & Schooler, C. (1978). The structure of coping. *Journal of Health and Social Behavior, 19,* 2–21.

Price, R. (1982, July). Priorities for prevention research: Linking risk factors and intervention research. Paper presented to the National Institute of Mental Health, Rockville, MD.

Radloff, L. S. (1977). The CES-D scale: A self-report depression scale for research in the general population. *Applied Psychological Measurement 1,* 385–401.

Robins, L., Helzer, J., Croughan, J. & Ratcliff, K. S. (1981). National Institute of Mental Health Diagnostic Interview Schedule: Its history, characteristics, and validity. *Archives of General Psychiatry, 36,* 381–389.

Schwab, J., Bell, R., Warheit, G., & Schwab, R. (1979). *Social order and mental health.* New York: Bruner-Mazel.

Thomas, W., & Zaniecki, J. (1927). *The Polish peasant in Europe and the United States.* New York: Knopf.

Valle, R., & Mendoza, L. (1978). *The elder latino.* San Diego: Campanile Press.

Valle, R., & Martinez, C. (1981). Natural networks of elderly Hispanics of Mexican heritage: Implications for mental health. In M. Miranda, & R. A. Ruiz (Eds.), *Chicago Aging and Mental Health* (pp. 76–117) (DHHS Publication No. ADM 81-952). Washington, DC: U.S. Government Printing Office.

Valle, R., & Bensussen, G. E. (in press). Hispanic social networks, social support and mental health. In W. Vega & M. Miranda (Eds.), *Stress and Hispanic mental health.* Washington, DC: National Institute of Mental Health.

Vega, W., Warheit, G., Buhl-Auth, J., & Meinhardt, K. (1984). The prevalence of depressive symptoms among Mexican Americans and Anglos. *American Journal of Epidemiology, 120,* 592–607.

Vega, W., Warheit, G., & Palacio, R. (1985). Psychiatric symptomatology among Mexican American farmworkers. *Social Science and Medicine, 20,* 39–45.

Vernon, S. W., & Roberts, R. E. (1982). Prevalence of treated and untreated psychiatric disorders in three ethnic groups. *Social Science and Medicine, 16,* 1575–1582.

Wellman, B. (1981). Applying network analysis to the study of support. In B. H. Gottlieb (Ed.), *Social networks and social support* (pp. 171–200). Beverly Hills: Sage Publications.

IV

FUTURE DIRECTIONS
FOR DEPRESSION
PREVENTION RESEARCH

Depression prevention research has great promise. As we have seen in chapters past, the theoretical, empirical, and methodological advances that have taken place in the last two decades have set the stage for its development. However, there are also many obstacles in its way, and progress to date is very limited. Much work needs to be done, and the greatest advances in this field are still far off.

The three chapters that end the book focus on aspects of depression prevention research that are yet to be adequately addressed. Breckenridge develops an argument for the use of statistical techniques in depression prevention work which go beyond the commonly used statistical models. He points out that by using structural equation models, researchers can examine the evidence supporting hypothesized mechanisms of action of interventions being evaluated. Thus, approaches such as LISRL can go beyond mere group comparisons, and begin to shed light on how depression levels are influenced by multiple factors, including prevention programs. Although these methods require large sample sizes, Breckenridge reminds us that prevention research by its very nature requires such large sample sizes, and thus this is not as much of an added burden as it would be in research studies which traditionally use small samples.

Hagop Akiskal's chapter is a masterful overview of biological and behavioral factors that have been identified in the development of mood disorders. He argues that the evidence indicates that the many types of mood disorders appear to have common features, and that clear separations between, say unipolar and bipolar illness, may not be warranted. His observations are particularly important in that they blend psychological and biological theories. He thereby points out limitations of both approaches, as well as the benefits of complementing our study of depression by considering both sources of effects on the human organism. No prevention intervention studies to date have utilized biological approaches. The promise of such approaches is still to be tapped.

In the final chapter, I highlight the implications for depression prevention research of the information given in earlier chapters, list directions not already covered in the book, and speculate regarding promising new areas. I discuss why prevention in mental health has not been implemented and where we may find potential sources of support. I also bring up ethical issues related to prevention, and end by pointing out that the prevention of depression is a human goal that goes beyond the mental health arena and involves the gradual reduction of unnecessary suffering.

14

Structural Equation Models for Depression Prevention Research

James N. Breckenridge
Palo Alto Veterans Administration Medical Center
Palo Alto, California

INTRODUCTION

The purpose of this chapter is to show how recent developments in data analysis and hypothesis testing can help clarify whether an absence of depression can be attributed to having treated individuals who, albeit at "risk," were not originally depressed. These developments have been called part of "perhaps the most important and influencial statistical revolution to have occurred in the social sciences . . . the most influential since the adoption of analysis of variance," (Cliff, 1983, p. 115), techniques that may have "the greatest promise for psychological science," (Bentler, 1980, p. 420). Notwithstanding my own evident enthusiasm, however, this chapter offers no panacea for the difficult problems of evaluating prevention studies. Indeed, the examples discussed depict something of an ideal, suggesting much of what can be accomplished with foresight and substantial resources. Whether or not readers choose to apply these techniques to their own research, this discussion should illuminate some critical issues for the design and analysis of depression prevention research. In particular, I argue that the design and analysis of such research should seek to confirm, as explicitly as possible, the underlying rationale for the preventive intervention. Well-designed investigations allow a clear verification of a model specifying the supporting rationale or theory. If, ignoring such tests, we confine our attention to the results of a "horse race" (e.g., whether there are fewer depressed among the treated than among the controls), then it is very likely that positive outcomes will actually be overlooked or worse, be attributed to the wrong causes.

The following discussion is meant to be readily accessible to depression prevention researchers, who are not necessarily statistical specialists. Consequently, the presentation is essentially non-mathematical and less precise than many data analysts would prefer. This chapter briefly lists the types of questions that statistical analyses of prevention studies are asked to answer, reminds the reader of the limitations of the most commonly used methods, and describes at length the potential of a relatively new (for psychology) approach to data analysis which holds great promise for the field of depression prevention research, namely, structural equation modeling. Examples of issues faced by prevention studies will be used to illustrate the points made. It is hoped that the reader will use this chapter as a point of departure for examining in more detail the implications of the arguments presented here, and for delving into the details involved in structural equation models. To that end, references to primary sources will be liberally distributed throughout the chapter. Fortunately, covariance models have been a growing interest among social scientists, and many texts are now available. At the end of the chapter, suggested readings and a list of relevant computer software packages are provided.

The statistical/data analytic procedures discussed here have been variously referred to as "structural equation modeling" (Joreskog, 1977), "moment models" (Bentler & Weeks, 1979), "covariance models" (Browne, 1982), "causal modeling" (Kenny, 1979), or "mathematical modeling" (Horn & McArdle, 1980). I prefer the first three terms, simply because "causal" is too strong and "mathematical" is too broad. The models described in this chapter purport to explain the underlying structure of a matrix of correlations or covariances. (In the language of formal statistics, means, variances, and covariances are different "moments" of the data distribution; thus, "moment model" most broadly connotes structures on both means and covariations.) Covariance models encompass the linear regression and analysis of variance procedures familiar to social scientists, but can express much more complex hypotheses about the structure of the data. Recent developments have greatly extended the breadth of structural equation models and the ease with which they can be applied in practice.

The appraisal of preventive interventions presents some of the most troublesome difficulties encountered in the analysis of longitudinal multivariate data. Many of the assumptions fundamental to customary analyses are almost certainly violated in practice: As with all longitudinal group comparisons, the benefits of random assignment are seriously eroded by attrition. The use of statistical controls (e.g., analysis of covariance (ANCOVA)) to ensure group comparability is hampered by the fallibility of most clinical research measures; traditional analytical approaches do not distinguish between systematic and random error and thus are unable to estimate the effects of measurement error. Conventional procedures for longitudinal analyses (e.g., repeated measures analysis of variance and ANCOVA) make the unlikely assumption that error at one time of measurement is independent of later sources of error. When the influence of systematic error is unspecified, estimates of treatment effects can vary substantially across studies merely as a function of refinements in measurement. The analytical techniques reviewed in this chapter, however, can incorporate effects of both random and systematic error and express relationships among error terms. Thus, well-specified models can in a limited sense evaluate relationships among variables "independently" of measurement errors.

The thesis of this chapter is that evaluating a prevention study can be understood as a process of constructing analytical "models" that are hypothesized to explain the data in an explicit, detailed fashion. The level of specificity required is perhaps the most important advantage of this approach, because specification demands clear hypotheses and brings to the foreground relationships which are often passed over as mere "statistical assumptions."

Nevertheless, I urge the reader to keep in mind two cautions: First, the newness and complexity of this approach has spawned a fashionable, but far too uncritical acceptance of the results of analyses of "mathematical models." I once overheard a researcher claiming an ill-considered superiority for his work because "we're using models for our analysis—LISREL, you know." This is much like the nouveau riche character in the French play who is delighted to learn from his cultural tutor, at great expense, that he, the wealthy student, speaks prose. *All* investigations and their statistical analyses imply an underlying model. What the scientific evaluation of prevention studies needs is cogent analytical models that clearly link particular outcomes with specific aspects of the intervention. In view of the many potential confounds inherent in the design of prevention studies, such models are admittedly an ambitious undertaking. The data analytic techniques discussed in this chapter offer a useful, albeit incomplete solution.

Second, prevention designs are discussed with little attention to requirements of time or money—concerns of which I am painfully well aware. Of course, aspirations must always be tempered by the cost of reaching them. In this era of limited funding for social science, it is sobering to realize, to give but one example, that the number of subjects needed to evaluate complex relationships with adequate statistical power is often more than we can afford. Pragmatic concerns, however, must not encourage us to discount as "idealistic," methodological concerns that seriously limit interpretations of the data. I hope that this discussion will encourage prevention researchers to pool resources and pursue the most informative projects possible—no matter how idealistic they might seem.

This chapter will first consider the concept of covariance models and then the importance of models with latent variables. Next, elementary models contrasting intervention and control group outcomes are compared with more elaborate structures linking outcomes with the depression prevention factors, which are the intermediate goals of the intervention. More complex models are considered which further relate primary and intermediate outcomes with participant features and threats to validity, such as systematic measurement error and response-shift bias. Design implications and comparisons with more traditional analytical procedures are discussed throughout.

MODELS

Social sciences employ many kinds of formal models to express and evaluate theory. In this chapter, we will be concerned with models that purport to explain patterns of correlations and/or mean differences in terms of mathematically simple equations. Such models are often tacitly implied or suggested by procedures quite routine to depression research. Summing all the items on a depression inventory to yield a total score, for example, suggests a simple measurement model, e.g., that the correlations among items are a function of a single construct such as depression severity. Analysis of variance (ANOVA) and multiple regression analysis also imply data models. In the past, results have been discussed with an emphasis on significance levels and underlying models have been ignored or only vaguely stated. Most contemporary introduction to statistical methods now present data analysis as a process of model building (for a good example in the social sciences see Hanushek & Jackson, 1977).

Covariance models are systems of simultaneous equations representing hypothesized relationships among variables. A typical equation in a model explains one of the outcome dependent variables (e.g., severity of depression) in terms of other dependent variables (e.g., degree of coping skills acquired), further set of the explanatory variables (e.g., levels of self-efficacy, depression vulnerability, or perceived control), plus an "error" or "disturbance" term that represents chance or random variation. Thus, we might hypothesize that depression severity is a function of the level of coping skill acquired and that the level of coping skill is influenced by changes in self-efficacy and perceived control. These two "equations" are simultaneous, i.e., both are at once true and mutually influential. Each variable in the model is given a numerical weight expressing the size of its influence on the "explained" variable. These weights or parameters are estimated by computer programs implementing the LISREL model (Linear Structural Relations model, Joreskog, 1977). Usually, side conditions, such as the absence of correlations between error terms, are also specified for the model. Furthermore, it must be possible to estimate the correlation between any two variables given the model's equations, and each parameter in the model must be identified, such that for each parameter a single value uniquely satisfies the data. These identification requirements make possible unique estimates of the numerical weights in the model.

The data to be explained are usually in the form of a correlation matrix of all the directly measured variables. Parenthetically, a variance/covariance matrix (a non-standardized correlation matrix) is frequently employed, but for convenience we will use "correlation matrix" to stand for either alternative. If a model fits the data well, there will be little difference between the correlation matrix predicted by the equations and the matrix obtained from the actual data. Hence, the model equations "structure" the data.

For certain methods of estimating model parameters, statistical tests are available to determine the probability that the model fits the data by chance. In many cases a planned series of logically ordered tests can be performed to evaluate the degree to which model revisions represent a significant improvement over alternatives. We can, for example, compare models with and without an effect included; the difference in fit between models provides a test of whether the effect's inclusion represents a significant improvement. Model testing is at its best when the investigation is motivated by a comparison of clear alternatives, e.g., a test of whether changes in self-efficacy lead to or follow changes in coping skills. With some methods of estimating model parameters, standard errors for each estimate are generated. In addition, there are a variety of goodness-of-fit indices and other analytical procedures available to evaluate models and determine where things have "gone wrong." With the maximum likelihood and other methods of generating estimates of the parameters of a model, a chi-square test of the goodness-of-fit is available (see Bentler, 1980). Unfortunately, this statistic is highly sensitive to the sample size employed, and a variety of other indices should also be used to evaluate the fit. Judging a model's congruence with the data is always more than a statistical matter (Joreskog, 1977).

Covariance models are widespread in the social sciences, but the complete expression of familiar models are often treated as merely the tacit assumptions of a statistical test. Here is an example of a very simple model: Classical measurement theory hypothesizes that observed scores are equal to the variable's "true" score plus error. Thus,

$$\text{observed variable (A)} = \text{true score (C)} + \text{error 1}$$

$$\text{observed variable (B)} = \text{true score (D)} + \text{error 2}$$

This model predicts the correlation between the unobservable true scores. Assuming that the error terms are not correlated with each other or with the other model variables, then the correlation between C and D is given by the "correction for attentuation" (Lord & Novick, 1968)

$$r_{c,d} = \frac{rr_{a,b}}{(r_{aa} \cdot r_{bb})^{-1}}$$

where r_{aa} and r_{bb} are the reliabilities of A and B.

Multiple regression equations can also be construed as estimates of explanatory models. Suppose that X and Y are modeled as predictors of Y; (standardized) multiple regression gives the parameters of the equation

$$Y = \beta 1 X + \beta 2 Y + \text{error}$$

Ordinary least squares regression provides estimates of $\beta 1$ and $\beta 2$ which minimize the error term. There are many side conditions for such models which are often unrecognized by users of the statistical packages that readily generate their solution. In this instance, in addition to distributional assumptions, X and Y are assumed to be *perfectly* measured, i.e., error free. The methods for estimating equation systems discussed in this chapter can be used to test traditional analysis of variance or regression models, but their value lies in their capacity to evaluate much more complex relational systems, especially systems of relationships among unobserved or latent variables.

Models of simultaneous equations are commonly represented by path diagrams, a method first suggested by Wright (1934). Several formalisms exist, each with certain advantages, for representing explanatory models. Peter Bentler's (1982a) is perhaps the most comprehensive (also see McDonald, 1980), although we will follow Karl Joreskog's LISREL conventions (1977) since they are currently the most widely utilized. LISREL VI (Joreskog & Sorborm, 1981) is presently the most widely distributed computer software package available for the analysis of structural equation models with latent variables. Moreover, there has been much recent discussion of applications of LISREL to problems of the analysis of covariance (Sorborm, 1979a), the evaluation of quasi-experimental designs (Bentler & Woodward, 1978; Magidson, 1977); the assessment of multi-trait, multi-method matrices (Alwin, 1974); the analysis of longitudinal processes (Nesselroad & Baltes, & Grandy, 1979). Sturctural equation models have attracted the interest of psychologists, political scientists, sociologists, and economists, both in the U.S. and abroad, but have yet to be put to much use by those concerned with depression prevention research.

LATENT VARIABLES

Although structural equations can be used to model relationships among directly observed variables, latent variable models are particularly valuable to prevention researchers. Latent variables are hypothetical constructs that cannot be directly observed; the effects of latent variables are determined indirectly by attributing the influence of unobserved constructs to the variance shared among several observable measures. These latter variables are sometimes termed "multiple indicators," because their common variation references the same underlying construct.

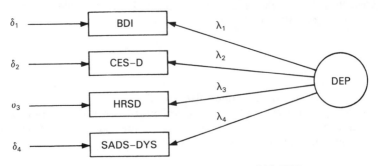

Figure 1 A simple measurement model for the latent variable DEP.

Differences in activity level, tearfulness, weight loss, and sleep can be construed, for example, as operational indices of "depression severity." Depression researchers frequently deal with unobservable constructs like "mood," "affect," and "anxiety," but they are by no means unique in this regard. Constructs such as "intelligence," "health," "ambition," and "desire" pervade the social sciences, and similarly elude direct measurement. That unobserved variables are ubiquitous in psychological research is not a consequence of a concern with "soft" concepts, nor of a focus on private mental events, but results from the level of abstraction entailed. "Metabolic arousal," inferred from direct, concrete biological measurements such as increased pulse and respiration, decreased electrodermal resistance, etc., nonetheless represents a higher order construct than any set of its indices. It is, therefore, only measured indirectly—no matter how tangible are the signs by which it is assessed. Moreover, investigators who employ structural equation models are free to adopt an agnostic stance toward the ontological status of latent variables. Whether they should be reified as true entities or construed as convenient fictions is a matter of interpretation and philosophy, not the result (or assumption) of any data analytic procedure discussed here.

Figure 1 is a path analytic illustration of a latent construct following the conventions of LISREL. Circled variables stand for variables under indirect observation. In this simple model, the latent variable "Depression Severity" (DEP) is hypothesized to account for the correlations among four directly observed or measured indicators: scores from two self-report scales (x_1, the Beck Depression Inventory (BDI), and x_2, the Center for Epidemiological Studies of Depression Scale (CESD)) and from two observor rating inventories (x_3, the Hamilton Rating Scale for Depression (HRSD)), and x_4, the Schedule for Affective Disorders and Schizophrenia (SADS)). The structural equations for each variable are

$$x_1 = \lambda_1 \, DEP + \delta_1$$

$$x_2 = \lambda_2 \, DEP + \delta_2$$

$$x_3 = \lambda_3 \, DEP + \delta_3$$

$$x_4 = \lambda_4 \, DEP + \delta_4$$

Thus, the model claims that the variance of each observed variable is a result of the underlying construct DEP and measurement error. These equations can be used to solve for the correlation between each pair of variables (see Kenny, 1979, pp. 110–120); the equation for the correlation between self-reports is

$$r_1 = \lambda_1 \cdot \lambda_2$$

The remaining correlations among the BDI, CESD, HRSD, and SADS scores can similarly be predicted from the model. If this set of "predicted" values is close to the actual correlations, the model fits the data. The predicted values can also be compared with subsequent data sets for cross-validation. Notice that a good fit implies only that the model is consistent with the data, not that no other model could apply equally well. Hence, the importance of comparing substantive alternatives, is a matter which depends, in this case, on depression theory, not statistics.

As Figure 1 illustrates, observed variables are enclosed within squares. Arrows indicate the direct influence of the underlying construct on the manifest variables. LISREL can accommodate models of influence among latent variables and/or the directly observed variables. One-headed arrows represent the immediate influence on the variable at which the arrow is directed; two-headed arrows signify a covariation between variables for which no explanatory (directional) hypothesis is specified. Subscripted lambdas associated with each arrow give the weight of this influence. Numerical estimates of these parameters will be expressed in the scale of the observed variable for which lambda has been set to 1. Since latent variables are unobserved, their scale is arbitrary and must be established either by equating their variance to some constant (typically 1.0) or adopting the scale of one of the observable indicators. Parameter estimates are usually generated through an iterative process by computers programs such as LISREL VI or several important alternatives.

The variance of the observed measures left unaccounted for by the underlying construct DEP is attributed to "error" in this example, signified by lower case deltas. These terms represent error in a broad sense, i.e., all the remaining variance not shared by the multiple indicators, thus denoting both random and systematic sources of variance uncorrelated with the underlying construct. Latent variable models necessarily require several observable variables for their measurement.

Figure 1 depicts a measurement model, familiar to psychometricians as a factor analysis model. Employed in a confirmatory fashion, structural equation models can avoid many of the problems that plagued traditional factor analysis by carefully examining the goodness-of-fit of hypothesized models (see Mulaik, 1975). Unobserved or latent variables are the simple structure "factors" of factor analysis. This shared versus unique variance understanding of latent variables is not the only approach possible. Wold's Partial Least Squares (1982) "pragmatic" approach differs significantly (in fact, it may not actually model latent variables, cf. Bentler (1980), p. 435). Latent variables may also be assumed to be categorical rather than continuous, as in latent class models (e.g., Lazerfeld & Henry, 1968). Latent variables are not necessary for structural equation modeling, but models with unobserved variables are well-suited to the analysis of longitudinal depression studies, because parameter estimates of relationships among latent variables should not be affected by changes in observed variable error. This is important since few variables of concern to social scientists are thought to be free of measurement error. Subsequent examples will illustrate these advantages.

The fundamental motivation for comparing the recipients of a preventive depression intervention with controls is to determine whether they differ significantly in levels of depression. This determination alone, however, constitutes an incomplete evaluation of a preventive intervention. We call analyses restricted to a comparison of outcome differences "minimal group comparison models." Structural equation models with latent variables do offer many substantial advantages over customary analyses of group comparisons, such as ANCOVA with pretreatment scores as covariates or repeated measures ANOVA. Nevertheless, preventive interventions presume a theoretical justification not addressed by such comparisons, since analyses restricted to outcome ignore the processes leading up to the final results.

A group at risk for depression will be hypothesized to avoid distress by ameliorating some risk factor or by developing an adaptive approach to the risk. An investigator might theorize, for instance, that patients suffering from intractible chronic disease will be less likely to become depressed if they are taught techniques to facilitate self-control and enhance self-efficacy. Prevention rationales clearly imply intermediate goals leading to the primary aim circumventing depression (cf., Heller et al. (1982) for a discussion of proximal and distal goals). Outcome differences in depression between intervention and control groups are not sufficient confirmation of the prevention rationale, especially when attrition and other biases common to longitudinal studies have occurred. For example, a proper evaluation of a psychoeducational intervention should assess the effectiveness of intermediate objectives: Do participants learn what is taught and does this learning lead to better coping, enhanced self-efficacy, or other changes that might diminish the chances of future depressions? If not, a failure to prevent depression would *not* contradict the underlying rationale for preventive intervention. Prevention may have occurred only among those for whom the intermediate goals were achieved. On the other hand, even when depression is less prevalent among the treated, a failure to accomplish intermediate aims (e.g., significant improvement in coping skills), contradicts the treatment rationale; such results—successful outcome, but failure at intermediate goals—lead to very different implications for subsequent policy and study.

Therefore, to fully evaluate preventive interventions we must establish not only the success of intermediate objectives, but determine whether their effects are *linked* with the ultimate outcome. Structural equation models are a powerful tool for estimating the strength of connections between method and outcome. They have appealed to sociologists, economists, and political scientists, because covariance models can simultaneously represent variable interactions which are difficult to investigate experimentally. Moreover, this approach can incorporate influence of confounding factors such as response bias, measurement error, and other persistent problems in clinical research.

In many cases, more familiar analytical methods can be employed to test the link between intermediate goals and final outcomes, as when ANCOVA finds outcome differences significant upon controlling differences in, say, acquired coping skills. However, structural equation models further permit the investigator to explore errors of measurement and to determine the extent to which variables measure the same construct in each group. Depression prevention research involves constructs which are difficult to measure precisely and are interrelated in complex ways. Structural equation models force the investigator to state explicitly the man-

Table 1 Percentage of observed variance explained by
depression constructs and measurement methods

Variable	Construct (%)	Method (%)
Disinterest		
SADS	26.81	13.09
HRSD	18.94	18.05
BDI	32.98	34.41
Dysphoria		
SADS	42.64	31.98
HRSD	19.77	25.94
BDI	14.76	22.28
Self-reproach		
SADS	84.82	10.75
HRSD	76.25	3.88
BDI	15.24	50.80
Suicidal ideation		
SADS	22.16	54.50
HRSD	36.13	48.74
BDI	37.60	20.05

Note The effects of sex in general and age on self-report
method variance in particular have been taken into account. This
model fit the data well ($X^2(49) = 59.10$, $p < .15$).

ner in which such constructs are measured and to specify the ways in which
variables are hypothesized to influence each other. *Whether or not the investigator
chooses to employ latent variable models, however, consideration of the issues
associated with their use should greatly facilitate the planning of prevention studies.*

Design Implications

Latent variable models cannot be constructed without several indicators of each
unobserved variable. Opinions differ concerning the optimal number required, but
two is the absolute minimum. The investigator should consider single measurements only when confident that the index measures what it purports to with negligible error (e.g., age, sex, etc.) and otherwise strive to include multiple measures
of abstract constructs such as self-concept, socioeconomic status, health, level of
functioning, and severity of depression.

This may be especially important with regard to the measurement of depressive
features. Table 1 shows the results of a multi-trait, multi-method study of three
methods (the Schedule for Affective Disorders and Schizophrenia; the Hamilton
Rating Scale for Depression, and the self-report Beck Depression Inventory) of
assessing aspects of depression (Breckenridge, 1983b). A structural equation
model was posited attributing the variance in each observed measure to three
sources: the underlying trait, the method of measurement, or random error. Estimates for method and trait variance were generated using LISREL VI. (Refer to
Alwin (1974) for a discussion of the use of structural equation models for evaluating multi-trait, multi-method models.) Inspection of Table 1 reveals a substantial

Table 2 Three-dimensional confirmatory factor analytic model of Beck
         Depression Inventory items

Variable	Factor 1	Factor 2	Factor 3
Irritability	.23		
Disinterest	.48		
Indecision	.54		
Work impairment	.61		
Fatigue	.55		
Somatic concern	.32		
Sexual disinterest	.26		
Dysphoria		.54	
Discouraged		.50	
Sense of failure		.64	
Self-dissatisfaction		.53	
Guilt		.56	
Self-punishment		.40	
Disappointment		.61	
Self-reproach		.52	
Suicidal ideation		.50	
Tearfulness		.37	
Feel unattractive		.31	
Insomnia			.32
Appetite loss			.98
Weight loss			.45

Note Model generated on 456 depressed (BDI 11) adults (mean age 41 years).
Goodness-of-fit index (Joreskog & Sorborm, 1982) equals .90 and root mean
square residual is .06 for this model. Age and sex differences controlled. Values
are for the standardized model.

range in the contribution of the method of measurement to the observed variance
of each feature. These findings suggest systematic differences in measurement
error and challenge the usual random error assumption.

Similarly, composite total scores for depression measures can obscure true differences in the underlying constructs measured. Table 2 shows the results of a
confirmatory factor analysis of the Beck Depression Inventory in several hundred
depressed individuals seeking treatment (Breckenridge, 1983a). This model fits the
data well and clearly identifies three distinct latent constructs accounting for the
structure among BDI correlations. Thus, identical total scores on the BDI may
result from very different underlying processes.

Before considering more complex models relating primary and intermediate
intervention objectives, we will present a latent variable model of depression outcome contrasted between two groups. Such models can not only "control" for
background differences in the usual way, but can evaluate quite specific hypotheses
regarding the effects of such differences.

THE MINIMAL GROUP COMPARISON MODEL

The measurement model in Figure 1 can be contrasted among several groups
and, provided that the same measurement model applies to each group, mean
differences on the latent variable can be directly compared (cf., Joreskog & Sor-

borm, 1981). Sorborm (1979a) has shown how between-groups comparisons of structural models provide a powerful alternative to the analysis of covariance, permitting error in both predictor and dependent variables without requiring randomized group assignment. Figure 2 illustrates an application of this approach to the evaluation of a preventive intervention. In this example, two factors are hypothesized to influence scores on the Depression Severity construct originally defined in Figure 1. The first factor represents differences in Socioeconomic Status (SES), and the second differences on a depression risk dimension—perceived social support (SUPPORT); obviously many more risk factors could be incorporated.

A variety of hypotheses concerning this three dimensional latent variable model can be evaluated. (The following issues are critical to group comparisons, but may be of less interest to those seeking a first acquaintance with this approach.) A typical sequence of hypothesis testing considers:

1. Are the treatment and control covariance matrices significantly different? Since the factors are meant to explain the covariance matrices, if the matrices themselves do not differ significantly, then neither does the factor structure. (Actually, although this logic is followed in practice (e.g., Joreskog, 1979, p. 199), it is inaccurate. Since a correlation matrix may be accounted for by several structures, identical matrices do not necessarily imply identical source structures. However, if the groups have identical matrices, they will always support the hypothesis that their structural equation models are identical.) In this case, only mean differences on the factor scores, assuming identical origins, are considered.

2. If the covariance matrices differ, the factor structure can nevertheless be identical for both groups. If the factor structure is not equivalent, the observed variables cannot be construed as measuring identical constructs, and this finding

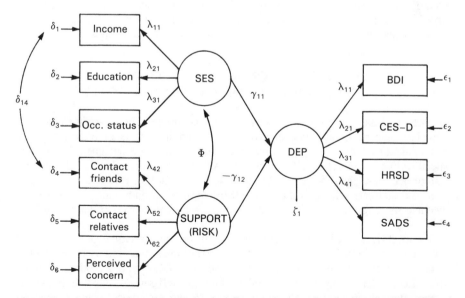

Figure 2 A latent variable model depicting the influence of two pre-intervention constructs, SES and SUPPORT, on DEP. Sophisticated between-groups comparisons of such equation systems are possible.

would have to be explored. The minimum test for factor invariance evaluates the fit of a model with equivalent factor loadings, but allows the relationships among factors and among error terms to differ between groups.

3. If the observed variables are measures of the same constructs, differences in the relationships among the three factors or latent variables can be examined. (Compare Alwin & Jackson's (1981) and Joreskog's (1979) discussions concerning differences in error variance prior to evaluating factor covariation.)

4. Once the relationships among latent variables is determined for each group, the groups can be contrasted for mean differences on the latent variables (Sorborm, 1979a).

The model depicted in Figure 2 further suggests the breadth of possibilities structural equation models can accommodate. In particular, latent variable models need not assume that all sources of error are independent of each other and can readily accommodate relationships among error terms. Notice the curved arrow between the error terms for reported income and reported number of close acquaintances. This signifies an association (represented by the letter phi) between the observed variables that is *not* explained by the relationship between the latent variables, SES and SUPPORT. This is an example of correlated error terms, a condition assumed to be absent, and thus ignored, in customary multivariate analyses. The correlated error in Figure 2 might be interpreted as reflecting response bias—a reluctance to report an undesirable or embarrassing lack of friends that has nothing to do with the SES/SUPPORT relationship. Perhaps those with greater incomes tend to claim more friendships both as a function of social desirability and the correlation between SUPPORT and SES. Correlated errors are especially troublesome when measurements are repeated over time, and usual ANOVA procedures simply assume they are not present in the data. Nevertheless, error at one time of measurement is likely to be correlated with that at another, since the measurements are made on the same individuals. Correlated errors over time can give a false appearance of measurement stability and attenuate estimates of the effects of earlier variables on those measured at later assessments.

DEPRESSION AS A FUNCTION
OF INTERMEDIATE INTERVENTION GOALS

The minimal group comparison model—no matter how sophisticated or complex—can be greatly improved by specifying the effects of intermediate or proximal objectives. The preventive intervention might be designed to enhance social support or increase self-esteem (cf., Albee, 1982), or, as in the life satisfaction project described in chapter 11, this volume, to bolster self-efficacy expectations and facilitate self-control of mood. Structural equation models can be used to evaluate the effect of such intermediate aims on post-intervention depression levels.

Figure 3 depicts a hypothetical evaluation of primary outcome as a function of secondary programmatic objectives. Again, the ultimate outcome is DEP, and the initial, pre-intervention variables are SES and SUPPORT. In this model perceived self-efficacy (EFFICACY), measured by multiple self-ratings, represents the intermediate goal of the preventive intervention. A series of model comparisons can be followed to evaluate this model. We can:

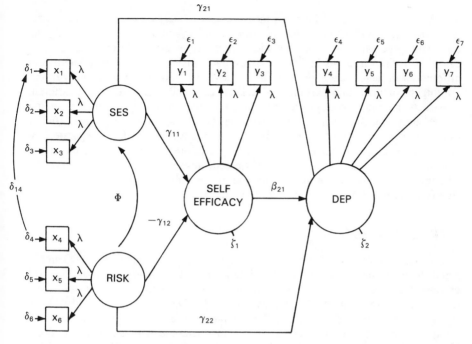

Figure 3 The previous model is elaborated to include the effects of an intermediate variable (SELF-EFFICACY), a construct critical to the outcome of a hypothetical depression prevention intervention. (The model is evaluated between-groups, although only a single group is illustrated.)

1. Determine whether the measurement model for EFFICACY is the same for both controls and intervention participants.

2. Test whether mean between-groups differences on EFFICACY are significant, *if* the measurement model is invariant.

3. Evaluate whether the effect of EFFICACY on DEP is significant in (a) the intervention group and (b) the control group.

4. If the EFFICACY/DEP link is significant in both groups, assess whether the effect differs significantly between-groups; and

5. Explore whether the model can be substantially improved by taking into account correlated errors.

The results at each stage of the analysis are much more informative than what is revealed by the minimal outcome model. Note that parameter estimates of effects relating DEP, SES, SUPPORT, and EFFICACY are modeled independently of error in the observed variables. Consequently, such estimates should be more stable on cross-validation than estimates based on only the observed variables.

There is much to consider at each stage of model evaluation. It may happen, for example, that things go wrong at step (2), e.g., the observed self-efficacy ratings do not appear to measure the same construct. What to do next is a matter of judgment, bolstered by expertise in self-efficacy theory and depression: As always, it is not strictly a statistical matter. It may be that measurement differences disappear when response biases are taken into account (see below). It is crucial that the goodness-of-fit of the equal measurement model be evaluated with respect to *several* criteria (Bentler & Bonnet, 1980; Hoelter, 1983). This is especially the case with large samples, since statistical comparisons are liable to reveal significant, but trivial variations in fit. The investigator may thus deem small significant differences in factor loadings clinically insubstantial. Alternatively, the investigator might conclude that participants' self-efficacy judgments represent different constructs in each group. Such a result should contribute to a deeper understanding of the study and does not rule out examination of the influence of self-efficacy (however it is measured) on outcome: Its impact can be modeled separately in either group. The investigator is always free to explore groups independently when comparability breaks down. It must be stressed, however, that differences in comparability (e.g., constructs are not measured equivalently between groups) may signify important findings in their own right.

Design Implications

Linkage models of this kind are predicated on research designs that have anticipated the need for measuring intermediate goals in both intervention and control groups. Are measures of both treatment goals and intermediate aims really necessary when group assignment is purely random? Of course! Without EFFICACY ratings for both groups, evaluating the complex interactions of self-efficacy with group assignment, background variables, and outcome would not be possible. Moreover, subject attrition in longitudinal clinical studies seems to be an unpleasant, but inescapable fact of life.

It is possible that a failure to establish a link between intermediate intervention goals and final levels of depression could result from poor design decisions. Model interpretations presume that intermediate effects have been measured correctly with sufficient replications at appropriate intervals. Only expertise with pertinent theory and data can determine how soon changes in intermediate objectives can be expected and how often they should be assessed.

INTERMEDIATE OBJECTIVES AS A FUNCTION OF PARTICIPATING IN THE INTERVENTION

Just as it is essential to establish a link between intermediate and ultimate goals of preventive interventions, so it is vital to examine the connection between intermediate objectives and participation in the prevention program. Our confidence that results are actually due to preventive intervention is strengthened by establishing that positive outcomes are associated with participatory factors such as comprehension of presented materials, attendance, ratings of participants' performance and motivation, therapist skill, and others. Some participatory variables might be comparably measured between groups when placebo control designs have been employed. If variables unique to the intervention are of primary interest, the model must be evaluated for that group alone.

Consider the psychoeducational depression preventive interventions described elsewhere in this volume. It is reasonable to suppose that better intermediate outcomes for psychoeducational programs are related to the degree to which participants both understand the principles taught and practice these principles through

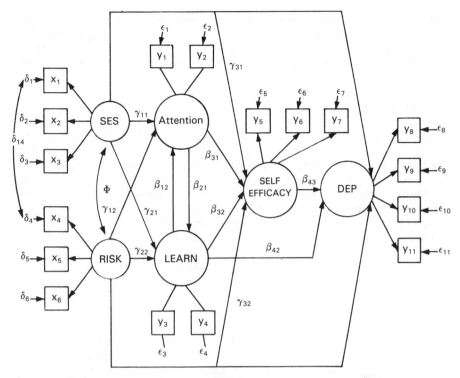

Figure 4 The model is further elaborated to include intermediate specific (LEARNING) and nonspecific (ATTENTION) participatory effects unique to the hypothetical psychoeducational intervention.

homework and other opportunities. Nonspecific features of the intervention program, such as the interest and concern participants judge they have received from those involved in the program, might also contribute to intermediate gains. Clearly, a comparison of the effects of specific and nonspecific program factors greatly illuminates interpretation of the data.

Figure 4 displays the previous model of intermediate and primary outcomes, amended to include the effects of a nonspecific factor (ATTENTION) and a specific skills acquisition factor (LEARNING). (As in prior examples, variables have been rather arbitrarily selected for illustrative purposes.) This model affords a test of whether specific or nonspecific participatory factors have an equal impact on the outcome of intervention. The extent to which specific variable effects can be contrasted between groups depends, of course, on whether the treatment of both groups is comparable with regard to each variable. Hence, certain participatory variables, such as attendance and homework completion can be evaluated when two preventive psychoeducational interventions are compared. Other factors, such as comprehension of unique program concepts, can be examined meaningfully in a single group.

The effects of participatory variables can be examined throughout follow-up periods. Two competing models, sampling variables at several intervals, could be compared to determine whether negative affect, for example, preceded a decline in the use of target skills or whether a deterioration in skills preceded the development of depression (see Rogosa, 1980, and Kessler & Greenberg, 1981, pp. 59–76, for a discussion of the use of structural equation modeling for panel and cross-lagged panel analysis.) This approach should be particularly useful in modeling the interaction of postintervention life stress with the use of acquired prevention skills.

Design Implications

Ethical and other considerations may occasionally prohibit the use of control groups in some prevention studies. Can structural equation models like Figure 4 be used to show that an intervention prevented depression without employing a control group? Suppose, that without reference to a control group an investigator establishes a significant link between program participation and outcome depression. Can we thus put measurements of what we cannot control to good use? That a model linking participation to outcome in a single group fits the data bolsters our confidence in attributing the outcome to the intervention. This is not a substitute for a controlled evaluation, but it does constitute a major improvement over a simple pre-post comparison. The evidence would be especially strong if the influence of specific factors exceeded the contribution of non-specific variables. Failure to link positive outcomes with specific participatory features challenges attributions of effects to the intervention, or, at the least, the theoretical motivation for the intervention.

There is simply no sufficient substitute, however, for experimental control. Much greater caution must be exercised in interpreting nonsignificant effects in models like Figure 4 than is the case for true experiments. The absence of participatory-outcome effects can result from a variety of benign, yet potentially misleading circumstances. Homework, for example, may in fact substantially influence outcome, but participants in the study happen to vary little in the amount or quality of homework completed. Restricted variances could thus limit correlations with outcome.

In that case, the causal relationship between homework and outcome can be expressed in counterfactual form: Participants *would* have had poorer outcomes *if* they had not performed as well as they did on their homework. Structural equation models, however, are only models of "factual" conditions—the actual means and correlations observed. Covariance models are no better than the parameters or statistics they represent. An uncritical acceptance of a well-fitting model may be avoided by careful inspection of the original correlation matrix. Is the pattern of correlations initially plausible? There is a "garbage in, gospel out" danger inherent in all new analytical techniques. Structural equation models attempt to account for variations within the group examined, not the uniform characteristics that define the sample. Because they cannot express counterfactual causal relationships and represent particular data sets only, "causal" modeling is clearly misleading language with regard to structural equation models.

Structural equation models must therefore be interpreted within the context of each particular data set. The presence or absence of significant effects may be more a result of sampling limitations than a consequence of a true functional relationship. This applies to any analytical procedure, however, and highlights the importance of cross-validation. Bentler (1980) and Cudeck and Browne (1983) present a powerful set of strategies for interpretation and cross-validation of latent variable models, strategies which may be especially useful for evaluating prevention studies.

The series of examples just reviewed illustrate the utility of modeling immediate, intermediate, and long-term consequences of preventive interventions, linking program outcome to both participant and participatory variables, additional comparison groups, and more complex relational patterns. The influence of potentially confounding factors can also be incorporated.

INCORPORATING THREATS TO VALIDITY

Graff and Schmidt (1982) have recently shown how restrictions implicit to LISREL models can be relaxed to permit a wide range of models (see also Rindskopf, 1984). In their approach the basic LISREL structure is extended to accommodate non-recursive relationships (i.e., with reciprocal feedback loops) among the observed variables. They demonstrate how confounding effects of repeated testing in longitudinal designs (such as increased familiarity with repeated testing materials at the conclusion of an intervention) can be controlled (better, "estimated") without experimental manipulation.

Many other internal or external threats to validity can be modeled without modification of ordinary LISREL restrictions. As a brief example of the use of covariance models in this regard, consider the problem of response-shift bias with self-report measures (Howard, 1980; Howard, Ralph, Gulanick, Maxwell, Nance, & Gerber, 1979). Response-shift bias occurs when, over the course of an intervention, subjects change their criteria or standard for their self-report of the outcome variable. Even true experimental designs using self-report alone cannot provide unbiased estimates of intervention effects when response-shift bias occurs (Howard et al., 1979). Since depression prevention studies repeatedly assess participants on the same self-report measures, response-shift bias may seriously distort the interpretation of results.

After frequently encountering questions concerning depressive features, subjects may differentially revise their standards: Some may view their dysphoria as more intense than they had believed prior to the intervention, even though they judge no true pre/post change to have taken place. More severe outcome ratings for these subjects would reflect a change in standards, not a failure of the intervention. Howard et al. suggest that pre/post changes be compared with the difference between posttest ratings and subjects' retrospective ratings at posttest of their symptoms as they recall them having been prior to intervention. Although this substitutes one bias for another (differential memory effects), interpretation of the influence of such effects can be facilitated via appropriate structural models.

The effects of participant and participatory factors on retrospective ratings of EFFICACY and DEP can be incorporated in previous examples. Thus, difference scores between pre-intervention and retrospective ratings of self-efficacy could be included as a new variable, and its influence on post EFFICACY could be evaluated. A significant effect would indicate a mean response-shift. This process could be replicated over repeated retrospective ratings of earlier assessments, and the stability of response-shifts (the paths between the new difference scores at each time of measurement) could be determined. Alternatively, preintervention and retrospective self-efficacy ratings could be modeled as indicators of the same latent variable. A negative correlation between error terms could be construed as an index of response shift bias. These models could be elaborated by accounting for the influence of postintervention mood on retrospective ratings.

Design Implications

Modeling the effects of such confounding influences requires careful consideration of the number of repeated assessments and the lag-time planned to occur between them. This is no trivial matter and demands the knowledge of the depression specialist, not the data analyst. The data analyst's role remains nonetheless critical, since as models grow in complexity, identification issues and interpretive problems are likely to become much more complex. There is an "algebra" of rules for decomposing correlations into structural equations among variables (see Kenny, 1979, pp. 13–44, for an introduction.) It is by these rules that LISREL VI and other programs "predict" a correlation matrix from the model to be compared with the actual correlations yielded by the data. These rules impose certain conditions on the kinds of models that can be tested against a given set of correlations, e.g., there must be at least as many correlations as there are parameters in the models. Often, considerable ingenuity and craft is required of the data analyst to arrange a test of the investigator's hypothesized model. Such problems are not associated with ordinary multiple regression models simply because they do not evaluate such sophisticated models. Although for brevity's sake we have omitted identification from our discussion of the examples in this chapter, the reader must remember that not every model that can be imagined, can be tested. There are few general guidelines for identification, and models must be examined on a case by case basis. An introduction to identification issues can be found in Duncan (1975); for more extensive discussions see Geraci (1976), Robinson (1974), Werts, Joreskog, and Linn (1973), and Wiley (1973).

To summarize thus far, evaluating a preventive intervention can be understood as a process of model building: Primary outcomes are compared between control and target groups, preferably taking the contribution of systematic error and relationships among error terms into account by utilizing latent variables. Links between primary and intermediate goals are examined with attention to the role of three dimensions: participant features (depression risk factors, background and other individual differences), specific participatory variables (such as attendance, compliance, skill acquisition, etc.), and nonspecific participatory factors (e.g., variations in the attention and concern of those who provide the intervention). The extent to which each dimension can be compared between-groups depends upon the comparability of active and control interventions; in many cases, participatory variables will be examined only within the intervention group. An explicit model of participant and participatory factors for the active intervention should facilitate the design of the control procedure and ensure that all factors are adequately (and, perhaps, repeatedly) measured. Sufficient methodological foresight also permits elaborating designs to include evaluation of potential threats to internal or external validity.

The design of preventive interventions is constrained by practical limitations in resources and participants' patience. To take advantage of latent covariance models, large (i.e., expensive) sample sizes and multiple (i.e., time-consuming) measures are required. Moreover, quite explicit hypotheses about the cause and effect of outcomes must guide the specification of each model evaluated. This does not mean that merely the rich get richer, and the profits of structural equation techniques are accrued only in ideal circumstances. In many cases, the link between program and outcome can be inferred through customary analyses. Nevertheless, modeling relationships among intervention components with structural equations does highlight the limitations of shotgun studies and is a useful heuristic for planning and evaluating depression prevention studies. Furthermore, many of the disadvantages of LISREL and other approaches to evaluating covariance models are shared, to some degree, with more familiar data-analytic strategies.

CAUTIONS, CONCERNS, AND COMPARISONS

Sample Size

According to current wisdom, sample sizes of *at least* 200 (better, 300) subjects per group are needed to reliably estimate the parameters of a structural equation model (Bearden, Sharma, & Teel, 1982; Boomsma, 1982). Empirical studies of the effects of sample size have considered only simple models, and complex models with many variables almost surely require greater numbers. Although this may seem a burdensome demand to researchers in many areas, this should present no special limitation to depression prevention projects.

Suppose that an investigator expects that depression among those receiving the intervention should occur at half the rate observed in the control group. If this study employs "normals" with a depression point prevalence of 4.5% (e.g., Roberts & Vernon, 1982) then at least 686 participants *per group* would be required to detect this difference at the .01 level with .80 power. Even samples whose risk for depression is 3 times greater than normal would require 193 subjects per group to detect a 50% difference with comparable power. The need for adequate sample size sometimes seems to go unrecognized in prevention research. Thus, Polak et al. (1975) concluded that their controlled evaluation of a preventive intervention did not significantly reduce the risk for psychiatric illness among families who had experienced the sudden death of a family member. The investigators compared an intervention group of 39 families with two control groups of 66 and 56 families. Even if 80% of the largest control group had been depressed, 90 subjects per group would have been needed to find a 20% difference significant at the .05 level with a .80 power. On the other hand, success in small samples should also be cautiously appraised. Raphael (1977) compared 31 experimentals and 33 controls at risk for postbereavement morbidity and concluded that the preventive intervention significantly ($p < .02$) benefited the experimental group. In view of the importance of depression prevention and its relatively short history as an area of interest among social science researchers, no finding can be ignored. However, small sample findings offer little promise of replication. We should not be deceived that with a little luck or a very powerful intervention a few subjects will do.

Satorra and Saris (1985) have recently developed a technique for determining the power of the usual significant test for evaluating covariance models. This will enable investigators to determine whether wrong models can be rejected in small samples and if small, trivial errors can lead to rejection of acceptable models in large samples.

Many strategies have been suggested for reducing sample sizes. Size requirements might be reduced by accepting a higher probability of Type I errors and targeting samples greatly at risk for depression, but it seems unlikely that many serious depression prevention studies will avoid the use of large samples. If Type I errors are deemed less serious (e.g., an alpha of .10), say because the results are to be taken only as an indication for further research (cf., Fleiss, 1981), fewer subjects would be required for a single group comparison. As the series of examples in this chapter illustrates, however, a full evaluation of preventive interventions entails many variables and many statistical tests and comparisons. Since the investigation-wide Type I error rate increases incrementally with every test performed, the overall error rate will be large indeed—especially if liberal levels are set for each test.

Prevention researchers have also stressed the need for targeting populations with high base rates to achieve more power with fewer subjects (e.g., Heller, Price, & Sher, 1980). Unfortunately, although it may be ethically desirable to focus on such groups (Cowen, 1973), their greater risk may also make them more resistant to preventive efforts and actually do little to reduce the number of participants needed: Prevention interventions are perhaps less likely to be as effective with more difficult populations, and therefore, greater power to significantly detect potentially small indifferences must once again be sought, quite probably by increasing sample size. Populations at high risk for depression could also require proportionately more complex, multifaceted interventions, which cannot be adequately evaluated by a few simple analyses on a small sample of subjects. Of course, higher initial depression scores, greater motivation, and other factors might make groups at high risk for depression more amenable to change. These factors, however, are also likely to influence comparable control groups, and thus proportionately greater power will be required to significantly detect between-groups differences. This task is greatly facilitated when careful measurements of depression severity, motivational factors, and other differences are incorporated into the analysis of outcome differences. A comprehensive evaluation, to reiterate a central theme of this chapter, demands careful scrutiny of the associations among intervention components, participant characteristics, and outcomes at every stage of the program. Large samples may be required to tease out the many critical interrelationships among the components and consequences with suitable power.

Distributional Assumptions

There are several ways to estimate the parameters of a structural equation model. Maximum-likelihood (ML) estimation has been employed most often because it yields parameters with good statistical properties and provides standard errors for each parameter and a significance test for the overall goodness-of-fit (refer to any of the introductions to this area cited below). Unfortunately, ML estimation makes the strong assumption that the underlying distribution of the data is multivariate normal, and violations of this assumption can seriously distort results and their interpretation. It is questionable whether multivariate normality is a reasonable assumption for practical applications. In response to this concern, some investigators have analyzed their data twice, once with ML estimates and once using parameter estimates that do not entail strong distributional assumptions (e.g., unweighted least squares (ULS)). The ML and ULS parameters are then correlated, and a high positive correlation is interpreted as discounting distributional problems.

This approach is not likely to be as helpful as it might appear: First, examining global correlations alone can obscure important differences between a few parameters; consequently, meaningful subsets of estimates should be compared. Second, ML parameter estimates are more robust to distributional violations than are their standard errors and overall significance tests (Browne, 1982). It is these latter statistics, however, that have the most interpretive value. Methods for obtaining asymptomatic standard errors for least squares estimates have only recently been developed (Browne, 1974; Joreskog, 1983). Since in a sample of adequate size, ML, ULS, and other estimates may not differ appreciably due to nonnormal distributions, their correspondence provides little support for the ML significance tests.

Fortunately, recent refinements now enable researchers to employ structural equation models in a confirmatory fashion under a variety of less restrictive distributional assumptions. Building on work by Browne (1982), Bentler's (1982b) computer program EQS provides several types of parameter estimates with correct standard errors and significance tests but without the stringent assumption of multivariate normality. Indeed, the two-stage asymptotically distribution free estimates computed by EQS have good statistical properties in large samples no matter what the underlying distribution happens to be (Bentler, 1983a, 1983b). Although EQS has only recently become available, its flexibility is bound to facilitate the use of latent variable models in most branches of the social sciences.

Parameter estimators for continuous data do not directly apply to dichotomous and categorical data. Here too recent developments are very promising. Muthen (1983, 1984) has developed a system for evaluating covariance models for ordered and nonordered categorical data which can be used to test a very wide variety of models (see Muthen (1984) for an example of a longitudinal probit model). Muthen's approach allows the investigator to model continuous latent variables that are measured by categorical observations. If the latent variables are construed as categorical, the data can be analyzed as an instance of latent class model (Andersen, 1983; Clogg, 1979, 1982; Lazerfield & Henry, 1968). Estimates of latent structures for this type of model can be found with Clogg's MLLSA program (Clogg, 1977).

No matter what distributional assumptions are made or which estimating procedure is employed, model comparisons should be preceded by a careful examination of the data. Variable transformations may be needed to justify the focus on linear relationships (i.e., the attempt to model a correlation matrix). Turkey's (1977) exploratory data analytic approach is useful in this regard. The search for outliers and influential observations is essential if stable, generalizable findings are to be achieved. A small number of subjects in a very large sample can seriously distort relationships among variables and suggest very different interpretations than would be apparent had aberrant cases been detected from the analysis. Practical multivariate techniques for screening the data prior to further analysis are given in Cook and Weisberg (1982), Gnanadesikan (1977), and Hicks (1981).

Whereas nonlinear relationships among observed variables can often be eliminated by transformation of the data, to date there is no practical procedure available to model nonlinear relationships among the latent variables. This is the major limitation to latent variable models, and alternatives should be selected if curvilinear relationships are of central concern. Confirmatory methods for nonlinear measurement models are available (e.g., McDonald, 1983), suggesting that an approach to more complex models may soon be possible.

Outcome: Depression Level or Depressive Disorder?

The outcome of depression prevention studies can be expressed in three forms: *level* of depression (the degree to which participants differ in the number and intensity of depressive features); clinical *state* (whether or not participants meet criteria for a depressive disorder); and *time* to target state (the length of the interval between intervention and some outcome condition or critical event). The last approach is most familiar in situations where the outcome is very likely and it is more critical how soon the event occurs. Thus, one might evaluate an attempt to prevent rapid deterioration in a lethal form of cancer. The principal statistical approach to this form of data is survival analysis or life table analysis (Klabfleisch & Prentice, 1979; for an introduction, see Anderson et al., 1980, pp. 199–231). This approach has been taken in studying relapse among individuals with treated depressive disorders (e.g., Keller et al., 1982). Few populations are so at risk for depression, however, for the total time at risk to have been a major concern among prevention researchers; depression simply does not appear inevitable for any population. In any case, the structural equation models described earlier are not appropriate for this kind of outcome data. It is difficult to see how latent variable models of outcome can be readily applied to period data, although Muthen's (1984) approach might serve for single-variable outcomes.

For depression prevention studies, the level of depression or the presence depressive disorders will be of greatest interest. The sequence of model-testing examples discussed in this chapter represented outcome as a function of average differences in the level of depression severity. Although prevention studies have often utilized continuous outcome variables, prevention theories are commonly framed in terms of relative risks and the odds ratio of the probability of depressive disorders in the intervention group versus the controls. Many sophisticated procedures have been developed to compare group outcomes on categorical variables and relate both interval and categorical data to such dependent measures. Discussion of these statistical approaches, such loglinear models for contingency tables and logistic regression, is beyond the scope of this chapter. Very accessible introductions for social science and biomedical readers can be found in Anderson et al. (1980), Fienberg (1980), Fliess (1981), and Kennedy (1983). These techniques are only appropriate to observed variables which may be subject to measurement error, however. When observed categorical variables are employed in such analyses, no provision for measurement is made.

Structural equation models for this type of observed data are possible (see pp. 120–139, Fienberg, 1980), but the recency of approaches like Muthen's to latent variable models of categorical data, which might incorporate correlated error terms as above, has not yet permitted sufficient experience with multiple clinical measures of diagnoses. Should (or could) the common variance of judges' diagnostic ratings be construed as indicating a latent continuous diagnostic construct (i.e., appropriate to Muthen's general model) or representing a latent categorical variable (i.e., appropriate to the latent class model)? Clearly, this is not simply a statistical issue. In any case, the extension of structural equation models to categorical data should allow investigators to evaluate sophisticated hypotheses about differences in the proportion of depressed observed following preventive intervention.

What is more important to stress, however, is that prevention researchers should not choose between the study of level or state, but incorporate both into their protocol. Each type of outcome answers a different concern, and results of one kind amplify the interpretation of the other. We cannot assume that two groups differ in mean levels of depression, because there are more depressions in one group, or vice versa. (This is especially the case for small samples.) If we find, for example, that there are fewer depressed in the intervention group, but only a small between-groups difference in the average number and intensity of depressive features, our interpretation would necessarily be more cautious than it might have been given only the diagnostic results. The diagnostic criteria for depression employed might have been too extreme; alternatively, a smaller than anticipated difference in depression levels might signal that the number of depressions among the treated will not be maintained—more depressions appear likely on subsequent follow-ups. There are good reasons, then, for including both types of outcome in prevention protocols whether or not structural equation models are utilized.

Latent Variable Models and Traditional Analyses

The reader may agree with the appeal for prevention research linking outcome, participant, and participatory variables, but question whether sophisticated structural equation model analyses are worth the effort. This chapter aims to raise that question in the minds of every researcher planning a depression prevention study. Each response should reflect both the priorities among research goals and the investigator's willingness to make certain assumptions. A major consideration is whether the investigator judges relationships to be so strong that error will have a relatively negligible effect. Structural equation models with latent variables permit the researcher to investigate the effects of measurement error, errors correlated over time, and certain confounding factors, as well as to specify "causal" relationships among the independent variables that are considerably more complex than those that can be represented by the usual main effects and interactions of traditional linear models.

I have argued that the analytical capabilities of covariance models are a close match with many characteristics of depression prevention research: Concepts pertinent to the prevention of depression, such as self-efficacy, perceived support, social skill, and self-esteem, are clearly influenced by the way they are measured and warrant the use of multiple, overlapping indicators to reflect the indirect, imprecise assessment and abstract character of these constructs. As with all longitudinal designs, especially those subject to attrition, randomized group assignment is not likely to eliminate systematic dependencies among error terms. Measurement error (or other systematic error) at one assessment time is liable to be related to that of another, if only because measurements are made on the same individuals.

Finally, although there is always the danger with model-fitting techniques that sufficient tinkering with the model will yield a statistically acceptable fit (Cliff, 1983), such dangers are minimal when verifying models motivated by strong, explicit theory. Structural equation models are especially appropriate for prevention studies, because preventive intervention entails a clear and specific rationale. I believe that the crucial distinction between treatment and prevention research is the extra theoretical assumptions the latter presumes: One must hypothesize not only the means by which depression can be prevented, but the manner in which it is expected to originate in the first place. Therefore, kept close to the studies' theoretical underpinnings, structural equation models for prevention research can offer much more than the results of a fishing expedition, gilded with attractive diagrams that tempt us to "suspend our critical faculties," (Cliff, 1980). Indeed, they provide an elegant analytical framework capable of supporting the complex hypothesis-testing characterizing prevention research.

Multivariate analysis of variance, multiple regression, and other instances of the general linear model can be employed to evaluate many of the hypotheses expressed in latent variable models. For instance, factor scores (used to minimize the influence of error in the observed variables) comprised of several depression measures can serve as dependent variables in a intervention vs. control MANOVA. The effect of self-efficacy on outcome could be inferred from a comparison of MANOVA results with a MANCOVA employing self-efficacy factor scores as covariates. A series of "stepdown tests" could suggest the degree of outcome due to a sequence of factors. Regretably, there are many difficulties with this approach when there are several covariates or when measures are repeated over time. Relationships among "covariates" must be separately assessed, correlations among sources of error in the dependent variables cannot be specified, and varying relationships between covariates and dependent variables at different times are difficult to incorporate into the repeated measures MANOVA. The use of factor scores provides some data reduction, but sample sizes must nevertheless be sufficiently large to yield stable factors. In some cases, trying to account for these difficulties with a variety of analyses is tantamount to a piecemeal estimation of a simultaneous structural equation model with or without latent variables—much like the classic estimation of recursive models in path analysis.

Much current depression prevention research, however, will be preliminary to larger, more comprehensive projects. Measurement error and other biases may be of lesser interest, and hypotheses may be more focused and restricted at this stage of research. Complex structural equation models may be less desirable at this point.

WHERE TO GO FROM HERE

A brief, well referenced introduction to latent variable models is given by Bentler (1980). More elaborate introductory texts are James, Mulaik, and Brett (1982), and Kenny (1979). The LISREL approach for longitudinal models is discussed in detail in Joreskog (1979). Many of the seminal papers concerning LISREL are in Joreskog and Sorborm (1979). Journals such as *Journal of Econometrics, Multivariate Behavioral Research, Psychometrika, Psychological Bulletin,* and *Sociological Methods and Research* are regular sources of refinements and developments in this area. Anyone serious about mastering this area should make a point of studying Peter Bentler's and Michael Browne's work referenced in the bibliography.

There are several computer software packages available for structural equation modeling. The SAS Econometric and Time-Series Library (ETS, SAS Institute, 1982), although not applicable to simultaneous latent variables, provides estimates for structural equations with observed measures. LISREL VI (Joreskog & Sorborm, 1981) provides maximum likelihood and several least squares parameter estimates of latent variable models. This is currently the most widely available package and is also distributed as part of the SPSS X library (SPSS, 1983). COSAN is a program for computing ML and least squares estimates of McDonald's general model (1980); information regarding this package can be obtained from the Department of Measurement, Evaluation and Computer Applications, The Ontario Institute for Studies in Education, 252 Bloor Street West, Toronto, Ontario, Canada M5S1V66. Bentler's EQS package (Bentler, 1982b) provides the ML, least squares, and asymptotically distribution free estimates to models which are specified in a very simple fashion (the user does not need to know the matrix algebra expression required to use alternative packages.) By the time this volume is in print, this package should be distributed by BMD in both mainframe and microcomputer versions. The most flexible program for estimating latent class models is MLLSA (Clogg, 1977). Finally, it is my understanding that the distributors of LISREL will soon make available a program by Muthen called LISCOMP, which will implement Muthen's approach to latent variable models for categorical data.

Progress in science is quite often a function of a change in the way we calculate the consequences of theory. In many branches of the social sciences, research has been conceptualized in terms of the main effects and interactions of a simple linear model, so well suited to the circumstances of experimental methodology. Multivariate extensions have been a practical reality only since the advent of digital computers. Modern computer capacities and increasingly efficient computational algorithms now enable social scientists to explore relationships among factors they can never hope to control experimentally. Perhaps, the future progress of our science will be to a large extent attributable to this liberation from the limitations of earlier analytical models.

Yet sophistication and breadth of expression demand a dear price: A minimum of large-scale, longitudinal projects using carefully constructed multiple measurements, replicated at appropriate intervals. It is difficult to imagine fully adequate depression prevention research on this scale without considering collaborative projects coordinated among several research centers. Whether depression prevention is sufficiently high among the priorities of the public and the scientific community to justify such expense remains to be seen. I hope that the advantages of covariance models for depression prevention research will inspire investigators to employ all their ingenuity to garner the resources to put them into practice. As a review of methodological considerations makes uncomfortably clear, depression prevention research is not for those unwilling to tackle demanding tasks.

REFERENCES

Albee, G. W. (1982). Preventing psychopathology and promoting human potential. *American Psychologist, 37,* 1043–1050.

Alwin, D. F. (1974). Approaches to the interpretation of relationships in the multitrait, multimethod matrix. In H. L. Costner (Ed.), *Sociological methodology* (pp. 79–105). San Francisco: Jossey-Bass.

Alwin, D. F., & Jackson, D. J. (1981). Applications of simultaneous factor analysis to issues of factorial invariance. In D. J. Jackson & E. F. Borgatta (Eds.), *Factor analysis and measurement in sociological research: A multi-dimensional perspective* (pp. 249–280). Beverly Hills, California: Sage Publications.

Anderson, E. B. (1983). A general latent structure model for contingency table data. In H. Wainer &

S. Messick (Eds.), *Principals of modern psychological measurement* (pp. 117–138). Hillsdale, NJ: Lawrence Erlbaum Associates.

Anderson, S., Auquier, A., Hauck, W. W., Oakes, D., Vandaele, W., & Weisberg, H. I. (1980). *Statistical methods for comparative studies.* New York: Wiley.

Beardon, W. O., Sharma, S., & Teel, J. E. (1982). Sample size effects on chi square and other statistics used in causal modeling. *Journal of Marketing Research, 19,* 425–430.

Bentler, P. M. (1980). Multivariate analysis with latent variables: Causal modeling. *Annual Review of Psychology, 31,* 419–456.

Bentler, P. M. (1982a). Linear systems with multiple levels and types of latent variables. In K. G. Joreskog, & H. Wold (Eds.), *Systems under indirect observation (Part 1)* (pp. 101–131). Amsterdam: North Holland Publishing.

Bentler, P. M. (1982b). *Theory and implementation of EQS: A structural equation program.* Los Angeles: University of California, Technical Report.

Bentler, P. M. (1983a). Simultaneous equation systems as moment structure models. *Journal of Econometrics, 22,* 13–42.

Bentler, P. M. (1983b). Some contributions to efficient statistics in structural models: Specification and estimation of moment statistics. *Psychometrika, 48,* 493–517.

Bentler, P. M., & Bonett, D. G. (1980). Significance tests and goodness of fit in the analysis of covariance structures. *Psychological Bulletin, 88,* 588–606.

Bentler, P. M., & Weeks, D. G. (1979). Interrelations among models for the analysis of moment structures. *Multivariate Behavioral Research, 1979, 14,* 169–186.

Bentler, P. M., & Woodward, J. A. (1980). A Head Start reevaluation: Positive effects are not yet demonstrable. *Evaluation Quarterly, 2,* 493–510.

Boomsma, A. (1982). The robustness of LISREL against small sample sizes in factor analysis models. In K. G. Joreskog, & H. Wold (Eds.), *Systems under indirect observation (Part 1)* (pp. 1499–174). Amsterdam: North Holland Publishing.

Breckenridge, J. N. (August, 1983a). *Structural equation modeling for evaluating treatments for depressed elderly.* Paper presented at the Annual Convention of the American Psychological Association, Los Angeles, CA.

Breckenridge, J. N. (December, 1983b). *A multi-trait, multi-method study of the assessment of depressive disorders: Age and gender effects.* Paper presented to annual meeting of the Association for the Advancement of Behavior Therapy, Washington, D.C.

Browne, M. W. (1974). Generalized least-squares estimation in the analysis of covariance structures. *South African Statistical Journal, 8,* 1–24.

Browne, M. W. (1982). Covariance structures. In D. M. Hawkins (Ed.), *Topics in applied multivariate analysis* (pp. 72–141). London: Cambridge University Press.

Browne, M. W. (1984). Asymptotically distribution-free methods for the analysis fo covariance structures. *British Journal of Mathematical and Statistical Psychology, 37,* 62–83.

Cook, R. D., & Weisberg, S. (1982). *Residuals and influence in regression.* New York: Chapman & Hall.

Cliff, N. (March, 1980). *Some cautions concerning the application of causal modeling methods.* Paper presented to the National Institute for Justice Workshop on Research Methodology, Baltimore.

Cliff, N. (1983). Some cautions concerning the application of causal modeling methods. *Multivariate Behavioral Research, 18,* 115–1266.

Clogg, C. (1977). *Unrestricted and restricted maximum likelihood latent structure analysis: A manual for users.* University Park, Pennsylvania: Population Issues Research Office, Working Papers.

Clogg, C. (1979). Some latent structure models for the analysis of Likert-type data. *Social Science Research, 8,* 287–301.

Clogg, C. (1981). New developments in latent structure analysis. In D. J. Jackson & E. F. Borgatta (Eds.), *Factor analysis and measurement in sociological research: A multi-dimensional perspective* (pp. 215–248). Beverly Hills, California: Sage Publications.

Cook, R. D., & Weisberg, S. (1982). *Residual and influence in regression.* New York: Chapman & Hall.

Cowen, E. L. (1973). Social and community interventions. *Annual Review of Psychology, 24,* 423–472.

Cudeck, R., & Browne, M. W. (1983). Crossvalidation of covariance structures. *Multivariate Behavioral Research, 18,* 147–167.

Duncan, O. T. (1975). *Introduction to structural equation models.* New York: Academic Press.

Fienberg, S. E. (1980). *The analysis of cross-classified data.* Cambridge, Mass.: The MIT Press.

Fleiss, J. L. (1981). *Statistical methods for rates and proportions.* New York: Wiley.

Geraci, V. J. (1976). Identification of simultaneous equation models with measurement error. *Journal of Econometrics, 4,* 2663–283.

Gnanadesikan, R. (1977). *Methods for statistical data analysis of multivariate observations.* New York: Wiley.

Graff, J., & Schmidt, P. (1982). A general model for decomposition of effects. In K. G. Joreskog, & H. Wold (Eds.), *Systems under indirect observation (Part 1)* (pp. 131–148). Amsterdam: North Holland Publishing.

Hanushek, E. A., & Jackson, J. E. *Statistical methods for social scientists.* New York: Academic Press, 1977.

Heller, K., Price, R. H., & Sher, K. J. (1980). Research and evaluation in primary prevention: Issues and guidelines. In R. H. Price and Associates (Eds.) *Prevention in mental health: Research, policy, and practice* (pp. 285–313). Beverly Hills, California: Sage Publications.

Hoelter, J. W. (1983). The analysis of covariance structures: Goodness-of-fit indices. *Sociological Methods and Research, 11,* 325–344.

Horn, J. L., & McArdle, J. J. Perspectives on mathematical/statistical model building (MASMOB) in research on aging. In L. W. Poon (Ed.), *Aging in the 1980's* (pp. 503–541). Washington, D.C.: American Psychological Association.

Howard, G. S. (1980). Response-shift bias: A problem in evaluating interventions with pre/post self-reports. *Evaluation Review, 4,* 93–106.

Howard, G. S., Ralph, K. M., Gulanick, N. A., Maxwell, S. E., Nance, D. W., & Gerber, S. K. (1979). Internal invalidity in pretest-posttest self-report evaluations and a re-evaluation of retrospective pretests. *Applied Psychological Measurement, 1,* 1–23.

James, L. R., Mulaik, S. A., & Brett, J. M. (1982). *Causal analysis: Assumptions, models, and data.* Beverly Hills, California: Sage Publications.

Joreskog, K. G. (1977). Structural equation models for the social sciences. In P. R. Krishnaiah (Ed.), *Applications of statistics* (pp. 213–312). Amsterdam: North Holland Press.

Joreskog, K. G. (1979). Simultaneous factor analysis in several populations. In K. G. Joreskog & D. Sorborm (Eds.), *Advances in factor analysis and structural equation models* (pp. 189–206). Cambridge, MASS: Abt Books.

Joreskog, K. G. (1983). Factor analysis as an errors-in-variables model. In H. Wainer & S. Messick (Eds.), *Principals of modern psychological measurement* (pp. 185–196). Hillsdale, NJ: Lawrence Erlbaum Associates.

Joreskog, K. G. & Sorborm, D. (1979) *Advances in factor analysis and structural equation models.* Cambridge, MASS: Abt Books.

Joreskog, K. G., & Sorborm, D. (1981). *LISREL VI, Analysis of linear structural relationships by the method of maximum likelihood and least squares: A user's guide.* Chicago: National Educational Resources.

Joreskog, K. G., & Sorborm, D. (1982). Recent developments in structural equation modeling. *Journal of Marketing Research, 19,* 404–416.

Keller, M. B., Shapiro, R. W., Lavori, P. W., & Wolfe, N. (1982). Recovery in major depressive disorder. *Archives of General Psychiatry, 39,* 905–910.

Keller, M. B., Shapiro, R. W., Lavori, P. W., & Wolfe, N. (1982). Relapse in major depressive disorder. *Archives of General Psychiatry, 39,* 911–915.

Kennedy, J. J. (1983). *Analyzing qualitative data: An introductory log-linear analysis for behavioral research.* New York: Praeger Publishers.

Kenny, D. A. (1979). *Correlation and causality,* New York: Wiley.

Kessler, R. C., & Greenberg, D. F. (1981). *Linear panel analysis: Models of quantitative change.* New York: Academic Press.

Kiabfleisch, J. D., & Prentice, R. L. (1979). *The statistical analysis of failure time data.* New York: Wiley.

Lawrence, R. J., Mulaik, S. A., & Brett, J. M. (1982). *Causal analysis: Assumptions, models, and data.* Beverly Hills, CA: Sage Publications.

Lazerfeld, P. F., & Henry, N. W. (1968). *Latent structure analysis.* Boston: Houghton Mifflin.

Lord, F. M., & Novick, M. R. (1968). *Statistical theories of mental test scores.* Reading, MA: Addison-Wesley.

Magidson, J. (1977). Toward a causal model approach for adjusting for preexisting differences in nonequivalent control group situation: A general alternative to ANCOVA. *Evaluation Quarterly, 3,* 399–420.

McDonald, R. P. (1980). A simple comprehensive model for the analysis of covariance structures: Some remarks on applications. *British Journal of Mathematical Statistics in Psychology, 33,* 161–183.

McDonald, R. P. (1983). Exploratory and confirmatory nonlinear factor analysis. In H. Wainer and S. Messick (Eds.), *Principals of modern psychological measurement* (pp. 197–214). Hillsdale, New Jersey: Lawrence Erlbaum.

Mulaik, S. A. (1975). Confirmatory factor analysis. In D. J. Amick & H. J. Walberg (Eds.), *Introductory multivariate analysis for educational, psychological and social research* (pp. 170–207). Berkeley, CA: McCutchan.

Muthen, B. (1983). Latent variable structural equation modeling with categorical data. *Journal of Econometrics, 22,* 43–65.

Muthen, B. (1984). A general structural equation model with dichotomous, ordered categorical, and continuous latent variable indicators. *Psychometrika, 49,* 115–132.

Nesselroade, J. R., & Baltes, P. B. (1979). *Longitudinal research in human development: Design and analysis.* New York: Academic Press.

Polak, P. R., Egan, D., Vandenbergh, R., & Williams, W. V. (1975). Prevention in mental health: A controlled study. *American Journal of Psychiatry, 132,* 146–148.

Raphael, B. (1977). Preventive intervention with the recently bereaved. *Archives of General Psychiatry, 34,* 1450–1454.

Roberts, R. E., & Vernon, S. W. (1982). Depression n the community. *Archives of General Psychiatry, 39,* 1407–1409.

Robinson, P. M. (1974). Identification, estimation, and large-sample theory for regression containing unobservable variables. *International Economic Review, 15,* 680–692.

Rindskopf, D. (1984). Using phantom and imaginary variables to parameterize constraints in linear structural models. *Psychometrika, 49,* 37–47.

Satorra, A., & Saris, W. E. (1985). Power of the likelihood ratio test in covariance structure analysis. *Psychometrika, 50,* 83–90.

SAS Institute Inc. (1982). *SAS/ETS User's Guide: Econometric and time-series library.* Cary, North Carolina: SAS Institute.

Sorborm, D. (1979a). An alternative to the methodology for analysis of covariance. *Psychometrika, 43,* 381–396.

Sorborm, D. (1979b). A general method for studying differences in factor means and factor structure between groups. In K. G. Joreskog & D. Sorborm (Eds.), *Advances in factor analysis and structural equation models* (pp. 207–218). Cambridge, Mass.: Abt Books.

SPSS Inc. (1983). *SPSS X: A user's guide.* New York: McGraw Hill.

Tukey, J. W. (1977). *Exploratory data analysis.* Reading, Mass.: Addison-Wesley, 1977.

Werts, C. E., Joreskog, K. G., & Linn, R. L. (1973). Identification and estimation in path analysis with unmeasured variables. *American Journal of Sociology, 78,* 1469–1484.

Werts, C. E., Rock, D. A., & Grady, J. (1979). Confirmatory factor analysis applications: Missing data problems and comparison of path models between populations. *Multivariate Behavioral Research, 14,* 199–213.

Wiley, D. E. (1973). The identification problem for structural equation models with unmeasured variables. In A. S. Goldberger & O. D. Duncan (Eds.), *Structural equation models in the social sciences.* New York: Seminar.

Wright, S. (1934). The method of path coefficients. *Annals of Mathematical Statistics, 5,* 161–215.

Wold, H. (1982). Soft modeling: The basic design and some extensions. In K. G. Joreskog, & H. Wold (Eds.), *Systems under indirect observation (Part 2)* (pp. 1–54). Amsterdam: North Holland Publishing, 1982.

15

Overview of Biobehavioral Factors in the Prevention of Mood Disorders

Hagop S. Akiskal
University of Tennessee College of Medicine,
Memphis, Tennessee

INTRODUCTION

Prevention efforts in depressive disorders can be focused on individuals at risk for such disorders (primary prevention), on arresting the progression of minor to major, single to recurrent, or unipolar to bipolar episodes (secondary prevention), and on preventing chronic outcomes or minimizing the suffering and social complications in chronic depression and forestalling suicidal outcome (tertiary prevention). This review will assess the feasibility of such preventive efforts from a multicausal perspective.

In previous work, the author and his associates (Akiskal & McKinney, 1973, 1975; Akiskal, 1979; Akiskal & Tashjian, 1983; Akiskal, 1985) have formulated a unified psychobiologic model of depression which is based on the joint contribution of psychosocial and biological pathogenetic factors (see Figure 1). This model hypothesizes that remote or predisposing risk factors lower the threshold for depressive decompensation under the influence of proximate stressors. Predisposing factors include heredity, developmental experiences, personality, and certain demographic characteristics; stressors can be psychosocial or biologic (e.g., loss or major illness). Within the framework of this model, this chapter reviews recent biobehavioral findings from research on depression, that may be relevant to prevention efforts.

THE RISK PROFILE FOR MOOD DISORDERS

At the primary level, the goal is to prevent the occurrence of clinical episodes of illness. Ideally, such efforts would reduce or eliminate risk factors predisposing to clinical depressions. Unfortunately, most of these factors appear to be traits or remote psychosocial events that cannot readily be modified. Nevertheless, an understanding of these predisposing factors is useful for developing a risk profile. By focusing on individuals who fit such profiles, it may be possible to identify those who are most likely to develop depression when faced with major stressors. Pri-

Parts of this Chapter appeared earlier in *Psychopharmacology Bulletin*, 22, 579–586, 1986.

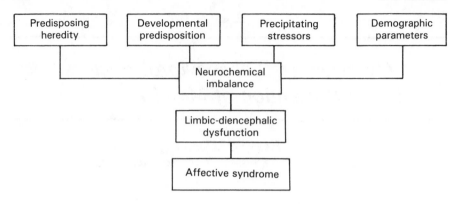

Figure 1 Multicausal scheme for the development of depression and mania.

mary prevention efforts then might be most profitably pursued by attempting to reduce *exposure* to such stressors, or by improving coping behavior or introducing "protective" factors that would buffer the impact of stressors in individuals at risk. I shall return to this topic following a discussion of the various risk factors, which can be categorized under the headings of heredofamilial predisposition, early home environment, temperament and character, precipitating circumstances, and demographic parameters. As discussed below, these risk factors often interact in complex fashions.

Heredofamilial Predisposition

Individuals who have a first-degree biological relative with an affective disorder are at increased risk for developing clinical depression (see Table 1). This risk is highest in the relatives of "schizoaffective" bipolars, followed by those of bipolar I and bipolar II (Gershon, Hamovit, Guroff, Dibble, Leckman, Sceery, Targum, Nurnberger, Goldin, & Bunney, 1982).* According to current estimates, heredity may contribute 50% of the variance in the pathogenesis of *recurrent* affective

---

*Bipolar II refers to manic-depressives with a predominantly depressive course punctuated by mild hypomanic periods. Bipolar I patients experience full-blown mania, in addition to depressive episodes, though such episodes may be absent or infrequent in some. Schizoaffective disorder is characterized by severe psychotic affective episodes with mood-incongruent (i.e., Schneiderian) symptomatology.

Table 1 Morbidity risk (given in percentages) in first-degree relatives of affective probands

Probands	Schizoaffective	Bipolar I	Bipolar II	Unipolar	Total
Schizoaffective	6.1	10.7	6.1	14.7	38
Bipolar I	1.1	4.5	4.1	14.0	24
Bipolar II	0.6	2.6	4.5	17.3	25
Unipolar	0.7	1.5	1.5	16.6	20
Normal	0.5	0	0.5	5.8	7

Note Summarized from Gershon et al. (1982).

disorders (Gershon, Dunner, & Goodwin, 1983). Although the risk for depression is relatively modest in the relatives of unipolar depressives (those who do not experience excited periods), many recurrent depressives come from families with bipolar illness. This is best interpreted to mean that some apparently "unipolar" depressions are in fact less penetrant forms of bipolar illness. These depressions typically have early onset, are hypersomnic-retarded in symptom pattern, may exhibit brief switches to hypomania when treated with heterocyclic antidepressants, monoamine oxidase inhibitors, electroconvulsive therapy, or sleep deprivation, and may show preferential responses to lithium carbonate (Akiskal, 1983b; Akiskal, Walker, Puzantian, King, Rosenthal, & Dranon, 1983).

The heredofamilial risk factor in depression is most dramatically illustrated by comparing the risk for the offspring of unaffected parents with that of individuals who have one affected parent ("single matings") or both parents affected ("dual matings"). The risk is tripled from population baselines for single matings and increased at least 10-fold for dual matings (Gershon et al., 1982).

Increased familial risk of course is not synonymous with increased genetic risk. Definite evidence for genetic contributions has come principally from adoption studies and monozygotic-dizygotic differences in concordance rates. Adoption studies (e.g., Mendelwicz & Rainer, 1977; Cadoret, 1978; Kety, 1985) have demonstrated increased risk for affective illness in subjects born to parents with such disorders but raised by normal adoptive parents. However, these findings appear more relevant to recurrent bipolar, rather than unipolar, mood disorders (Von Knorrig, Cloninger, Bohman, & Sigvardsson, 1983; Cadoret, O'Gorman, Heywood, & Troughton, 1985). The wide difference in monozygotic-dizygotic concordance also indicates a strong genetic component (Bertlessen, Harvald, & Hauge, 1977); concordance is the same for monozygotic pairs regardless of whether they are reared apart from birth (Price, 1968). It is of great theoretical interest that where monozygotic pairs are discordant for affective breakdowns, the unaffected twin almost always exhibits cyclothymic or dysthymic tendencies (Bertlessen et al.). This suggests that affective illness may not be inherited as such, but may be transmitted in the form of temperamental deviations.

The fact that the concordance rate is less than 100% even in the most genetic (bipolar) forms of affective illness suggests that nongenetic familial and other environmental factors are of importance in the predisposition to affective episodes. Furthermore, genetic factors, appear neither necessary nor sufficient for the production of depression. Thus, many nongenetic forms of affective—especially unipolar—disorder do exist. Finally, the recurrent nature of the illness suggests that factors other than heredity are involved in provoking the onset of individual episodes.

Early Home Environment

Although heredity seems to account for a major portion of the variance in the pathogenesis of recurrent affective disorders, non-genetic familial factors appear to modify the actual clinical *expression* of the disorder. The child reared in a family where one parent suffers from primary affective illness is exposed to a dual disadvantage: genetic vulnerability to affective illness, as well as separation experiences during childhood through parental illness, suicide, divorce or more subtle forms of emotional deprivation secondary to conflictual interaction between parents. Such conflict is often aggravated by the fact that the other parent frequently exhibits psychiatric disturbance (assortative mating), ranging from personality and affective disorders to alcoholism (Gershon, Dunner & Sfert, 1973).

Psychoanalytic theory has long traced adult depressions to early deprivations that preclude adequate mastery of loss situations. According to a specific version of this viewpoint, formulated by Bowlby (1961), the failure to successfully mourn major losses during childhood provides the behavioral sensitization to adult depressions. This notion has found partial support in the high rates of depression in women who have been maternally bereaved in childhood or adolescence (Brown & Harris, 1978). However, the cumulative retrospective evidence has been generally inconclusive regarding the specificity of childhood loss to adult affective disorder (Lloyd, 1980a). Accordingly, in his latest writings, Bowlby (1977) has broadened his formulation to include in the consequences of early loss a large spectrum of adult personality disturbances characterized by dysphoric acting out.

While failing to specifically relate adult depression to childhood object loss, the available research evidence does suggest several interesting links in line with Bowlby's formulations. For instance, we now know from the work of Perris (1966) that unipolar depressives who experienced developmental object loss have an illness onset 10 years earlier than those depressives without such loss. Others (Levi, Fales, Stein & Sharp, 1966; Hill, 1969) have reported that suicide attempts are more common in depressed subjects who have sustained early separations. Finally, work conducted at the University of Tennessee (Akiskal, Bitar, Puzantian, Rosenthal & Walker, 1978; Rosenthal T. L., Akiskal, Scott-Strauss, Rosenthal R. H., & David, 1981) has shown that early losses are associated with the adult occurrence of "unstable" characterologic attributes, such as immaturity, hostile dependency, manipulativeness, impulsiveness and low threshold for alcohol and drug abuse rather than frank affective disorders. These findings illustrate how breaks in early object relations could be relevant to certain clinical aspects of depressive illness. While not causing depressive illness, developmental object loss seems to modify the clinical expression of the adult disorder. The characterologic propensity toward hostile dependency may prepare a fertile soil of interpersonal friction that facilitates a depressive onset earlier than that determined by innate genetic factors. Such friction may actually create the life events that trigger the depression.

Another possible mechanism whereby early losses can influence the occurrence of adult depression is by creating conditions favorable to the development of character traits associated with what Seligman (1975) refers to as "learned helplessness," or with the self-denigrating depressive mental schemata described by Beck (1967). It is reasonable to assume that situations wherein the individual has failed to master a series of tasks can lead to subsequent helplessness when faced with similar situations. Although they have not been documented in research in humans, these approaches are concordant with classical work at the Wisconsin Primate Laboratory (Harlow, 1975), which demonstrated that coping skills are developed in the context of the contact comfort provided by caring and loving parental objects. Conversely, the loss of this contact comfort often precludes the development of environmental exploration and of coping skills in general. Thus, early separations from parent(s), without adequate substitutes, may prevent the emergence of a sense of mastery of the environment. Such children may become insecure adults who feel unable to face the challenge of new situations. It should be noted that the mere presence of parents, however, does not immunize against the trait of helplessness; developing a sense of mastery requires suitable role models and the opportunity to cope with a series of life events of increasing complexity. Such formulations, while plausible, need verification in prospective designs in clinical populations.

Arguing against the proposed relationship between childhood loss and depression is the fact that history of such loss is not present in two-thirds of adult depressives (Lloyd, 1980a). Furthermore, childhood parental deprivation does not appear to exert *specific* formative influence on depressive illness.

Temperament and Character

It is widely believed that affective episodes often arise from predisposing personality attributes. This position was most directly articulated by Kretschmer (1936), who believed that "the endogenous psychoses are nothing but accentuation of normal types of temperament." While Kretschmer, as a faithful follower of the Kraepelinian tenets (1921), emphasized constitutionally determined temperamental contributions, much of current theorizing has focused on learned characterologic attributes believed to be a legacy from developmental vicissitudes.

Ideally the study of personality in a given patient should begin prior to the first onset of affective episodes; assessing personality during an episode of illness is unsatisfactory because affective states may bias or even mask the patient's personality profile. Even when the affectively ill are examined during a euthymic period, the illness episodes, or the treatments provided for them could have altered significantly personality structure. For these reasons, very few studies have succeeded in prospectively assessing the contribution of personality to affective illness. Despite such thorny methodologic barriers, many interesting findings on the relevance of enduring personality characteristics to affective illness have been formulated (Akiskal, Hirschfeld & Yerevanian, 1983).

Kraepelin (1921) postulated that the various forms of manic-depressive illness often arose from their respective temperamental foundations. For instance, it is fairly well established that certain temperamental disorders—the dysthymic, the hyperthymic, and the cyclothymic—are the precursors of the more serious affective episodes (Akiskal, Djenderedjian, Rosenthal & Khani, 1977; Akiskal, Rosenthal T. L., Haykal, Lemmi, Rosenthal R. H., Scott-Strauss, 1980; Depue, Slater, Wolfstetter-Kausch, Klein, Goplerud, & Farr, 1981). In these temperaments, the genetic potential for affective episodes is considered to be subclinically active at all times and to be easily triggered into clinical illness by environmental challenge. Table 2 summarizes the types of episodes seen during prospective observations on cyclothymic and dysthymic individuals compared with nonaffective personalities. It is interesting to note both temperaments are at highest risk to develop depression; the risk for hypomania is augmented by exposure to tricyclic antidepressant. Recent Italian work (Kukopulos, Reginaldi, Laddomada, Floris, Serra, & Tondo, 1980) has shown that tricyclic antidepressants may actually *accelerate* the inherent cyclicity of mood disorders in hyperthymic and cyclothymic individuals. It would therefore appear that certain "affective personalities" are at high risk for developing depressive states under conditions of environmental challenge; they are also prone to hypomanic and manic states under pharmacologic challenge, as well as under other reactive conditions (to be discussed below under precipitating stres-

Table 2 Rate of affective episodes (given in percentages) in affective temperaments and controls during prospective observation of 1–4 years

Episode	(N)	Major depression	Hypomanic/mania (spontaneous)	Tricylic-hypomania
Cyclothymic	(46)	24	22	35
Subaffective dysthymic	(20)	55	0	33
Nonaffective personality controls	(50)	4	0	0

Note Summarized from Akiskal et al. (1977 & 1980). Experimental groups significantly higher than controls (p < .02).

sors). In other words, one mechanism whereby genetic factors may produce affective episodes is by preparing a fertile soil of affective liability in the form of affective personalities. This viewpoint is strengthened by the recent demonstration of shortened REM latency in individuals with dysthymic (Akiskal, 1983a) and hypomanic (Akiskal, 1984) temperaments, very much like the findings in individuals experiencing major full-blown depressions (Akiskal, Lemmi, Yerevanian, King, & Belluomini, 1982; Kupfer & Thase, 1983.)* This sleep neurophysiologic abnormality seems to behave like a trait marker of vulnerability and is not merely a nonspecific stress reaction or a correlate of anxiety (Akiskal, Lemmi, Dickson, King, Yerevanian & VanValkenburg, 1984). Overall the sleep findings in affective temperaments suggest that biologic abnormalities precede full-blown affective episodes.

Temperamental contributions appear to have greater relevance in the recurrent and cyclic forms of affective disorder (Akiskal et al., 1983). In the more purely depressive forms of affective illness, dependency and obsessionalism have long been hypothesized as predisposing factors (Chodoff, 1972); more recent formulations have focused on cognitive-behavioral factors (Lewinsohn, 1974; Kovacks & Beck, 1978). These formulations, which have been developed through retrospective reconstruction of the premorbid characteristics of already depressed subjects, have been based on small clinical populations, have not taken the heterogeneity of affective disorders into consideration, have not used reliable personality measures and, most seriously, have generally tended to confuse state and trait. A recent study (Hirschfeld, Klerman, Clayton, & Keller, 1983), which—except for being retrospective—was methodologically superior to earlier attempts, reported that introversion, lack of social adroitness, and dependency are the major attributes of recovered depressives. These findings are more consistent with behavioral formulations and suggest the existence of enduring measurable deficits in social skills. Prospective studies are now needed for the more definitive clarification of the characterologic contributions in affective illness. Despite this limitation, clinical experience suggests mechanisms whereby the postulated characterologic disturbances contribute to major affective episodes. Individuals who are introverted and lack social adroitness do not possess an adequate behavioral repertoire for eliciting rewarding interactions with other people. In particular, they may lack the requisite skills to develop and maintain the supportive relationships that are widely believed to provide a buffer against the depressant impact of aversive life situations (Akiskal, 1979). Passive-dependent individuals can easily exhaust the tolerance of

*Although dysthymics and hyperthymics appear to be clinical opposites, their compulsive dedication to work constitutes a fundamental shared characteristic.

their spouses or lovers and thereby prepare the ground for marital or romantic break-ups. In other words, they may contribute to the very life situations which bring about their depressive breakdowns. Once they become depressed, their dependency needs grow, providing further opportunities for alienating the supportive individuals in their lives.*

In summary, the individual prone to develop affective episodes is no longer portrayed just in terms of the temperamental traits of cyclothymia, hyperthymia, and dysthymia, but those of related characterologic attributes such as dependency, introversion, and a relative lack of social assertiveness. Given the heterogeneous nature of the depressive disorders, it is conceivable that varied mixtures of these temperamental and characterological traits predispose to different clinical subtypes of affective disorder.

Precipitating Circumstances

Affective episodes are often temporally related to external and internal circumstances. The preceding discussion suggests that in vulnerable individuals affective disturbance is present subclinically—and that it is activated into overt clinical episodes by environmental challenge. Environmental circumstances may determine the precipitation of the initial episode and, perhaps, the timing of subsequent recurrences. These circumstances are extremely varied and include psychosocial, biologic, and seasonal factors.

Although the majority of individuals exposed to losses and other aversive life circumstances do not sink into morbid despair, those predisposed to affective illness may do so at such times. The lifetime risk for melancholia is about 15% (Helgason, 1979), yet no more than 5% of those exposed to "exit"-type life events decompensate into clinical depression (Paykel, 1976; Clayton, 1979; Lloyd, 1980b). Even predisposed individuals do not develop affective episodes in the face of a major loss; rather, other concurrent or antecedent events seem to mediate the effect of such events. What then are the factors that augment or diminish the depressant impact of life events? More specifically, what is the impact of losses, the most common psychosocial antecedent of clinical depression? Research evidence (reviewed in Akiskal, 1979) favors the view that the depressant impact of loss is considerably amplified by the concomitant presence of other life events. It would appear that a series of life events may cumulatively threaten psychobiologic homeostasis. The occurrence of "success depressions," however, suggests that the stressful impact of a life event may additionally reside in the adaptive demands imposed on individuals as they attempt to cope with any significant departures from routine, whether positive or negative.

Absence of social support also appears to be an important factor in mediating the depressive response to loss. Interpersonal support can be viewed as a protective emotional buffer that, to a considerable degree, neutralizes the noxious effect

---

*The relationship between personality and affective illness, however, is not always etiological (Akiskal, Hirschfeld and Yerevanian, 1983). Personality may favor the appearance of certain *symptoms* if and when an affective episode does occur, it may modify the apparent severity of the depressive state and, in many instances, results from recurrently incapacitating episodes of illness (Cassano, Maggini, and Akiskal, 1983).

of stressful events (Rabkin & Struening, 1976). It is striking that in a well-controlled study on conjugal bereavement (Clayton, Halikas, & Maurice, 1972), the occurrence of depression was related less to the presence of heredofamilial factors than to the unavailability of adult children who could provide emotional support for the widows during the first few months after bereavement. Likewise, it is now known that the syndrome of "anaclitic depression" described by Rene Spitz (1942) occurs in only 15% of children permanently separated from their mothers, because adequate substitute mothering is often effective in preventing (or reversing) the syndrome.

Early experience is widely believed to be yet another factor in mediating the response to adult losses (reviewed in Akiskal & McKinney, 1975; Lloyd, 1980a). The cumulative evidence suggests that sensitivity to loss and rejection, especially to romantic disappointment, is more characteristic of a group of personality disorders than of primary affective illness *per se*. It is further conceivable that prior exposure to loss—successfully "metabolized" by the psyche—may even "immunize" against future losses. This is perhaps one reason why older individuals cope better with bereavement than do younger individuals (Clayton, 1979). It has also been hypothesized that the insensitivity of certain sociopathic personalities to interpersonal losses is an extreme and pathologic version of the "immunity" imparted by permanent early losses (Halleck, 1966).

The impact of life events on the overall life-style of the individual, or the symbolic meaning of these events, is another potent force in determining whether a depressive outcome will occur (Akiskal, 1979). For instance, a young man whose life dream was to become a plastic surgeon may be permanently crippled as a result of early rheumatoid arthritis afflicting his hands. Similarly, the individual who is promoted may find himself in the threatening position of being unprotected by his earlier and more "secure" dependent position.

Whether losses will lead to helpless despair may, in the final analysis, depend on the individual's overall social skills. Those who possess a narrow repertoire of social and vocational activities may find themselves unable to engage in activities that would provide sources of substitute gratification (Lewinsohn, 1974). In behavioral terms, such individuals will find themselves on prolonged extinction schedules because they are unable to emit behaviors that can be reinforced by the environment. In the presence of significant personality disturbance, the sick or depressed "role" may become a way of life—a way of ensuring attention, sympathy, and interpersonal support.

In the endogenous-reactive dichotomy, some depressions are viewed as arising in the absence of life stress, while others are defined by their presence. In the extreme, it is believed that innate constitutional factors determine the onset of the former, and environmental challenge plays a formative influence on the latter. However, Hirschfeld (1981) found that endogenous depressions were as likely to be precipitated as other types of depression. Furthermore, Thomson and Hendrie (1972) failed to show an inverse relationship between life stress scores and family history for affective illness (taken as an indirect measure for the presence of a genetic constitution). It would appear that genetic predisposition may actually *lower* the threshold for depressive responses to life events. Nevertheless, psychosocial precipitants are not always apparent in melancholic depressions—especially in the bipolar forms; furthermore, in recurrent depressions, the importance of psychosocial precipitants seems to diminish after the first few episodes (Kraepelin,

1921). Indeed, Warheit (1979) has shown that the variance contributed by proximate psychosocial factors in predicting new episodes is negligible and that remote factors—including the fact of having past episodes—are the most powerful predictors of depressive recurrences.

The mechanism whereby life events interact with the neurophysiologic substrates of depression is unknown. However, studies in experimental animals (reviewed in Akiskal and McKinney, 1975) have shown that stressful situations induce increments in tyrosine hydroxylase and dopamine-beta-hydroxylase—enzymes that are involved in the biosynthesis of norepinephrine. Coping with stress calls for the ability to increase biogenic amines at critical synapses in the hypothalamus. A genetic deficiency that interferes with the organism's ability to induce enzymes under environmental challenge can lead to insufficient mobilization of biogenic amines. Alternatively, the postsynaptic receptor may be relatively insensitive to norepinephrine as a result of a genetic defect in the structure of the receptor molecules; the end result is the same as with insufficient mobilization of norepinephrine. Conceivably, chronic stress—and the chronic overproduction of norepinephrine—may "exhaust" the postsynaptic receptor, especially in the presence of thyroid deficits in thyroid hormones that are necessary for the optimal functioning of the noradrenergic receptor.

The mechanism of action of the somatic contributions (Hendrie, 1978) to affective illness is equally uncertain. The fact that clinically significant depression occurs, on the average, in about 15% of the medically ill (Cavanaugh, 1983)—which represents the lifetime risk for melancholia—is an indication that medical contributions to depression are in the nature of precipitant rather than cause. Essentially, any debilitating chronic illness can produce depression because of serious limitations imposed on the person's life-style. We are here more concerned with those illnesses (listed below) in which somatic effects on the brain are likely.

Medical conditions and pharmacologic agents commonly associated with onset of pathologic mood states.

Depression	*Elation*
Medical	
Influenza; viral pneumonia	Influenza
Infectious mononucleosis	Q fever
Viral hepatitis	St. Louis encephalitis
Tertiary syphilis	Tertiary syphilis
Multiple sclerosis	Multiple sclerosis
Stroke	Stroke
Cerebral tumor	Diencephalic and IIIrd ventricular tumors
Head injury	Head injury
Temporal lobe epilepsy	Temporal lobe epilepsy
Alzheimer's Disease	Huntington's chorea
Avitaminoses (pellagra)	Liver cirrhosis
Systemic lupus erythematosus	Systemic lupus erythematosus
Rheumatoid arthritis	Rheumatic chorea
Hypo- and hyperthyroidism	Hyperthyroidism
Hypo- and hyperparathyroidism	
Cushing's Disease	
Addison's disease	
Sleep apnea	
Pharmacologic	
Steroidal hormones (including oral contraceptives)	Steroidal hormones

L-dopa	L-dopa
Reserpine; α-methyldopa Propranolol	Bromocriptine
Indomethacin	Cocaine
Cimetidine	Tricyclic antidepressants
Sulphonamides	Monoamine oxidase inhibitors
Anticholinesterase insecticides	
Alcohol/Barbiturates	
Vincristine; Vinblastine	
Mercury; Thallium	
Cycloserine	

In conditions like systemic lupus erythematosus, the occurrence of depressive manifestations—as well as other psychiatric symptoms—largely depends on brain involvement by the disease process (Guze, 1966). However, heredofamilial predisposition seems operative in other conditions. This is particularly true for reserpine-induced depressions (Goodwin and Bunney, 1971), which occur in 15% of hypertensive individuals on 0.5 mg/d or higher doses of the drug; this drug works by depleting the brain stores of all three of the biogenic amines. Yet, a closer look reveals that two-thirds of these represent "pseudodepressions" secondary to the sedative side effects of the drug, which reverse as the latter medication is discontinued; melancholia persisting in an autonomous fashion despite withdrawal of the offending chemical—occurs in the remaining third (i.e., not more than 5% of the total). Such findings suggest that the risk of developing a "true" depression on reserpine is actually less than the 15% lifetime risk for affective illness in the general population and is largely limited to individuals with heredofamilial predisposition. These considerations are extremely important for the pathogenesis of affective disorders as they imply that the mere depletion of biogenic amines is not a sufficient cause for depressive illness. This conclusion is further supported by the Mendels and Frazer (1974) study that failed to induce a full depressive syndrome by the administration of alpha-methylparatyrosine, a selective inhibitor of norepinephrine synthesis, and para-chlorphenylalamine, a selective inhibitor of serotonin synthesis. Thus, neither life events nor chemical events appear to be *sufficient* causes for the occurrence of clinical depression: They seem to exert a depressant influence in the presence of predisposing factors.

Obviously, chemical and psychosocial stressors may occur simultaneously. Conceivably, bereaved individuals on reserpine would be more likely to develop depression because they would be unable to mobilize the biogenic amines necessary to cope with the stress of their loss. This possibility, although never formally tested in the human for obvious ethical reasons, has been demonstrated experimentally in the Wisconsin Primate Laboratory (Kraemer and McKinney, 1979): Juvenile monkeys exposed to separation paradigm that had not previously produced depressive behavior succumbed to depression with the concomitant administration of the catecholamine-depleting alpha-methylparatyrosine.

We know even less about the precipitation of hypomania or mania. The relevance of life events is suggested by a study (Ambelas, 1979) that carefully excluded life events that could in any way be construed as resulting from the illness; an excess of such life events, compared to control subjects, was shown to precede manic episodes. Psychoanalytic theory has long held the view that mania is a mask for depression—a defensive attempt to ward off the pain of loss (Recamier and Blanchard, 1957). Thus, in "maniacal grief"—also known as "funerary mania"—

the widow exhibits inappropriate elation, hyperactivity, expansive behavior, and lack of insight. More systematic studies of this subject are indicated. The best known precipitants of hypomania—and to a lesser extent of mania—are drugs and physiological procedures that increase the central level of catecholamines (Vogel, 1975; Bunney, 1978; Kukopulos et al., 1980). These include the noradrenergic tricyclics, the monoamine-oxidase inhibitors, ephedrine, L-dopa, cocaine, amphetamine-like drugs, REM-deprivation, and total sleep deprivation. However, these factors are more consistent in producing a switch from depression to hypomania than from euthymia to hypomania. Thus, the pharmacological switch is largely limited to individuals with a bipolar diathesis—measured as a function of personal or family history of mania (Akiskal, 1983b). The same, incidentally, applies generally to postpartum affective episodes, whether manic, mixed, or retarded depressive. As for the somatic illnesses listed above, the evidence to date suggests that heredofamilial background may not be necessary in the production of such "secondary" manias (Krauthammer and Klerman, 1978).

A class of precipitating circumstances that has received recent attention is seasonality (Rosenthal, Sack, Gillin, Lewy, Goodwin, Davenport, Mueller, Newsome, Wehr, 1984). This is largely relevant to bipolar II disorder in which depressive episodes tend to largely cluster between October and April, with a peak in early winter. The relevant factor here seems to be the shortening of photoperiods, i.e., the total hours of daylight.

To summarize, this discussion on precipitating circumstances in affective illness suggests that the onset of affective episodes is most commonly associated with an interaction between triggering and predisposing factors. However, certain classes of environmental challenge, especially somatic processes may, on occasion, play more than a triggering role and can be considered to have a formative influence on affective episodes.

Demographic Parameters

Age and gender are the most important demographic correlates of depression (Boyd and Weissman, 1981). Although the incidence of depression does not increase during senescence, in recurrent illness the intervals between episodes tend to shorten and in bipolar disorder, the frequency of depressive attacks increases with age. (Angst, Felder, Frey, 1979). Despite some recent disclaimers, there is broad consensus that the incidence of mood disturbances is higher among women. Gender differences are most pronounced for nonsyndromal mood changes and tend to disappear in bipolar disorder (Boyd and Weissman, 1981).

It is customary to ascribe these age and gender differences to social and psychological factors. For instance, it is argued that elderly individuals are overexposed to losses and experience overall decrease in environmental opportunities, and that women are more likely to sink into helpless states of despair because of greater passive-dependence and powerlessness as compared with men. However, there are no controlled studies to show that such factors indeed account for the major variance in the occurrence or recurrence of depressions in women and elderly subjects. By contrast, several lines of evidence suggest that the biology of womanhood and senescence may be highly relevant to the increased vulnerability of women to depression and that of the elderly to depressive recurrences.

Monoamine neurotransmitters concentrated in the hypothalamus are an important component of the organism's response to stress. Experimental studies in the infrahuman species have shown increased turnover rates of these neurohumors under conditions of successful coping, and depletion of neurohumors when adaptation to stress was hampered (Anisman and Zacharko, 1982). It is therefore highly relevant to our discussion of the mediating influence of age and gender in depression that the enzyme monoamine-oxidase—which normally degrades the biogenic amines—has been shown to increase with age and to have higher concentrations in women across all ages (Robinson, Davis, Nies, Ravaris and Sylvester, 1971). This means that elderly subjects and women will have less aminergic neurotransmitters available for coping with stress and may easily break down under even ordinary stresses in the presence of predisposing heredity and personality variables. The elderly are further handicapped by the fact that the biosynthesizing enzymes involved in the production of these monoamine transmitters decline with age.

Although profound depression is common in hypothyroid states, hyperthyroidism in its entire range appears to give "immunity" against depressive decompensation. Indeed, at the turn of the century, mania was sometimes treated surgically by thyroidectomy. Even subclinical hypothyroidism is known to produce subtle cognitive and affective changes. The relevance of these findings to a discussion of sex differences in rates of depression is quite apparent in light of the fact that the hypothalamothyroid axis in women is more susceptible to dysfunction under environmentally stressful conditions. Furthermore, 10% of women with unipolar depression have been shown to be mildly hypothyroid (Gold, Potash, Mueller & Extein, 1981). As expected, the addition of small doses of thyroid hormone in this group accelerates recovery from depression treated with tricyclic antidepressants (Prange, Wilson, Wabon, & Lipton, 1969). Evidence of this kind may partially explain the pathophysiology of melancholia in women. Since synaptic function is jointly determined by presynaptic and postsynaptic events, and the effects of noradrenaline on the postsynaptic membrane are mediated by thyroid hormone, women would be at higher risk for monoamine dysfunction because of their generally more precarious thyroid status. Compensatory increase in monoamines may suffice for a while, but monoamines can be easily exhausted under continued environmental challenge.

The postpartum premenstrual phases are high risk periods for bipolar affective episodes (Winokur, 1981). The biochemical factors involved are not well understood at this time. The same is true for the occurrence of unipolar depressions in women using steroidal contraceptives (Kane, 1977). One thing is clear: premenstrual, postpartum and contraceptive-induced affective states are most prevalent in women with a familial or personal history of affective illness.

To summarize, in addition to psychological factors, the biology of womanhood and of senescence appear to be potentially important determinants of the response to stress in and resulting risk of affective episodes in these demographic groups.

SUMMARY OF RISK FACTORS
FOR AFFECTIVE EPISODES

Based on the preceding review of the literature and research conducted in the author's affective disorders program, the risk profile that emerges for affective episodes is as follows:

- Positive family history for affective illness, especially "loaded" pedigrees in three consecutive generations;
- Hyperthymic, cyclothymic and dysthymic temperaments;
- Dependent and introverted personality types and related deficits in social skills;
- Exposure to depressed parents during childhood and/or early breaks in attachment bonds without adequate parenting substitutes;
- Disabling physical illnesses and/or drug treatment of such, especially those affecting the central nervous system;
- Life events—especially losses and those beyond the individual's control—in an individual with few supportive social ties;
- Female gender;
- Use of contraceptive steroids;
- Hypothyroidism, even when levels of circulating thyroid hormones are in the borderline range.

Additional risk factors particularly relevant for bipolar episodes include:
- Treatment with or abuse of catecholaminergic drugs;
- Sleep deprivation;
- The premenstrual phase;
- The postpartum period;
- Seasonal changes in photoperiods.

PREVENTION STRATEGIES

Prevention efforts for affective disorders are in an embryonic state of development. Nevertheless, the available knowledge on risk factors may help in delineating the most promising areas of intervention. As empirical research in this area is just beginning, the discussion of prevention strategies will necessarily be brief.

Primary Prevention

Positive family history—especially when "loaded"—is the most unambiguous major risk factor for affective illness. The risk for offspring is highest when both parents are ill; the risk is also high for the monozygotic co-twin of an affected individual. Many of those individuals will exhibit cyclothymic or dysthymic tendencies. Given the long-term adverse effects of lithium carbonate, it would not be advisable at this stage to prescribe prophylactic lithium to this at-risk group. However, in cyclothymic women with loaded bipolar family history, it would be logical to prescribe lithium for few months immediately postpartum. Also, cyclothymic and hyperthymic members of bipolar families should be educated to avoid sleep deprivation as well as catecholaminergic drugs—e.g., caffeine, other CNS stimulants, antidepressants, certain cold and anti-asthmatic medications.

Education of primary care physicians on the risks of prescribing certain depressant drugs (e.g. contraceptives, nondiuretic antihypertensives) to those with positive family history would perhaps be the major practical approach to a primary prevention strategy at this stage of our knowledge.

Secondary Prevention

Here the aim is to prevent affective recurrences. Avoiding the prescription of depressant drugs would be even more cogent for an individual who has already developed an episode. The most logical group to focus on would be those who are at risk by virtue of family history and have developed a mild (first) episode. Improving social skills and providing vocational counseling might also be useful here. Such counseling might be beneficial in the cyclothymic and related personalities who seem to achieve optimum psychobiologic homeostasis if engaged in jobs that best fit their temperamental propensities (Kretschmer, 1936). For instance, dysthymic individuals may do best in jobs that require loyalty, attention to detail, and self-sacrifice (e.g., civil service, secretarial jobs, bookkeeping, etc.).

Whether traditional psychodynamic or more recent psychotherapeutic approaches such as cognitive therapy can *prevent* affective recurrences is uncertain at this time.

Prevention of major recurrences is best accomplished with lithium carbonate or heterocyclic antidepressants. Considerable supportive psychotherapeutic efforts is obviously necessary here to ensure compliance with medication regimens (Jamison and Akiskal, 1983).

Preventing the switch from unipolar to bipolar illness can be accomplished by: 1) instructing the patient to avoid the use of stimulant drugs; 2) educating the patient about the risk of sleep deprivation and treating insomnia promptly with a short-term course of a sedating phenothiazine; 3) avoiding the prescription of catecholaminergic heterocyclic antidepressants or limiting their use to small doses and to short periods.

In those with seasonal illness, lithium prophylaxis during vulnerable periods (e.g., September through May) is a clinically proven strategy. In such patients depression can also be reduced by exposure to bright white light at home during months when they are at highest risk, as determined by past history of periodicity. This latter strategy, however, carries the risk of inducing hypomania.

Tertiary Prevention

The effort here is to minimize or avert complications. These include substance abuse, social (especially marital) dysfunction, symptomatic chronicity, and suicide.

With respect to substance abuse, it is necessary to continue efforts to educate primary care physicians—and medical students—about the risks of sedative hypnotics. The residual symptoms of affective episodes—which may linger on for many months—should be vigorously treated with thymoleptic agents; anxiolytic and hypnotic agents are rarely indicated, and should they be prescribed at all, their use should not extend beyond a few weeks. Unfortunately, relatively little can be done to reduce abuse of ethanol—so readily available—which patients tend to use to treat their insomnia.

Social complications can best be prevented by vigorous chemotherapy for acute episodes, combined with interpersonal psychotherapy (Weissman and Akiskal, 1984). As for symptomatic chronicity, continued thymoleptic chemotherapy, avoidance of depressant medical drugs, and supportive social measures are extremely important. Rates of chronic depression are especially high among those with severe disabling and long-lasting medical illness. Such individuals should constitute a priority in prevention efforts. Group therapy and education of families or significant others could enhance these supportive measures.

Since two-thirds of completed suicides come from the ranks of mood disorders, vigorous treatment of these disorders should lead to decreases in suicide rates. However, despite promising data from mood disorders clinics (Khuri & Akiskal, 1983), this ideal has not been reached at a community or national level. Murphy's data (1975) suggest that many primary care physicians not only under-diagnose mood disorders but provide patients with lethal supplies of sedative drugs given as hypnotic agents. It would appear that no significant prevention of suicidal behavior can occur until all physicians are educated in the diagnosis and appropriate management of mood disorders. However, recent developments in effective approaches for the management of coma resulting from overdose of various psychoactive drugs may have reduced the actual *mortality* of suicide attempts. An increasing number of suicide victims are using violent methods such as firearms, so gun control legislation may also eventually prove useful in reducing suicidal mortality. Asberg's recent claim that lowered cerebrospinal fluid levels of 5-hydroxy-indoleacetic acid—an index of brain serotonin turnover—are predictive of violent suicidal acts, raises the provocative (but hitherto unattained) possibility of treating such individuals with thymoleptic agents that normalize central serotonergic homeostasis.

In all suicide prevention efforts, it is obviously necessary not only to treat the mood disorder vigorously, but also to institute an individualized psychotherapeutic approach, emphasizing round the clock vigilance or availability of help by the clinician and significant others. It is also necessary in hospitalized patients to avoid early discharge—an effort contrary to current third-party payer policies. Since Kraepelin's time, it has been known that improvement in psychomotor retardation precedes mood changes, and removes the inertia that may have prevented the patient's acting on suicidal urges.

SUMMARY

Sufficient data have now accumulated on the course of mood disorders to make preventive efforts—at least at the secondary and tertiary level—thinkable. Clinical psychologists, social workers, educators, clergymen, and primary care physicians bear a major responsibility in this regard because they are usually the first to be consulted during early and milder episodes of depression. Given the fact that most psychiatrists typically see patients during more severe episodes and later stages of illness, their role will be more germane to secondary prevention efforts which emphasize energetic treatments of severe illness and tertiary prevention of bipolar switches as well as prevention of complications.

REFERENCES

Akiskal, H. S. (1979). A biobehavioral approach to depression. In R. Depue (Ed.), *The psychobiology of depressive disorders: Implications for the effects of stress* (pp. 409–437). New York: Academic Press.

Akiskal, H. S. (1983a). Dysthymic disorder: Psychopathology of proposed chronic depressive subtypes. *American Journal of Psychiatry, 140,* 11–20.

Akiskal, H. S. (1983b). The bipolar spectrum: New concepts in classification in diagnosis. In

L. Grinspoon (Ed.), *Psychiatry update: The American Psychiatric Association annual review* (pp. 271–292). Washington, DC: American Psychiatric Press.

Akiskal, H. S. (1984). Commentary (Critical and unresolved issues of borderline personality). *Integrative Psychiatry, 2,* 181–182.

Akiskal, H. S. (1985). Interaction of biologic and psychologic factors in the origin of depressive disorders. *Acta Psychiatrica Scandinavica, 71,* 131–139.

Akiskal, H. S., Bitar, A. H., Puzantian, V. R., Rosenthal, T. L., & Walker, P. W. (1978). The nosological status of neurotic depression: A prospective three-to-four year examination in light of the primary-secondary and unipolar-bipolar dichotomies. *Archives of General Psychiatry, 35,* 756–766.

Akiskal, H. S., Djenderedjian, A. H., Rosenthal, R. H. & Khani, M. D. (1977). Cyclothymic disorder: Validating criteria for inclusion in the bipolar affective group. *American Journal of Psychiatry, 134,* 1227–1233.

Akiskal, H. S., Hirschfeld, R. M. A., & Yerevanian, B. I. (1983). The relationship of personality to affective disorders: A critical review. *Archives of General Psychiatry, 40,* 801–810.

Akiskal, H. S., Lemmi, H., Dickson, H., King, D., Yerevanian, B. I., & VanValkenburg, C. (1984). Chronic depressions: Part 2. Sleep EEG differentiation of primary dysthymic disorders from anxious depressions. *Journal of Affective Disorders, 6,* 287–297.

Akiskal, H. S., Lemmi, H., Yerevanian, B. I., King, D., & Belluomini, J. (1982). The utility of the REM latency test in psychiatric diagnosis: A study of 81 depressed outpatients. *Psychiatry Research, 7,* 101–110.

Akiskal, H. S. & McKinney, W. T., Jr. (1973). Depressive disorders: Toward a unified hypothesis. *Science, 1982,* 20–28.

Akiskal, H. S. & McKinney, W. T., Jr. (1975). Overview of recent research in depression: Integration of ten conceptual models into a comprehensive clinical frame. *Archives of General Psychiatry, 32,* 28–305.

Akiskal, H. S., Rosenthal, T. L., Haykal, R. F., Lemmi, H., Rosenthal, R. H., & Scott-Strauss, A. (1980). Characterological depressions: Clinical and sleep EEG findings separating "subaffective dysthymias" from "character-spectrum" disorders. *Archives of General Psychology, 37,* 777–783.

Akiskal, H. S., & Tashjian, R. (1983). Affective disorders: Part II. Recent advances in laboratory and pathogenetic approaches. *Hospital and Community Psychiatry, 34,* 822–830.

Akiskal, H. S., Walker, P. W., Puzantian, V. R., King, D., Rosenthal, T. L., & Dranon, M. (1983). Bipolar outcome in the course of depressive illness: Phenomenologic, familial and pharmacologic predictors. *Journal of Affective Disorders, 5,* 115–128.

Ambelas, A. (1979). Psychologically stressful events in the precipitation of manic episodes. *British Journal of Psychiatry, 135,* 15–21.

Angst, J., Felder, W., & Frey, R. (1979). The course of unipolar and bipolar affective disorders. In M. Schou and E. Stromgren (Eds.), *Origin, prevention and treatment of affective disorders* (pp. 215–226). London, Academic Press.

Anisman, H., & Zacharko, R. K. (1982). The predisposing influence of stress. *Behavioral and Brain Sciences, 5,* 89–137.

Asberg, M., Schalling, D., Rydin, E., & Traskman-Bendz, L. (1983). Suicide and serotonin. In J. P. Soubrier & J. Vedrinne (Eds.), *Depression and suicide* (367–404). New York: Pergamon Press.

Beck, A. T. (1967). *Depression—Causes and treatment.* Philadelphia: University of Pennsylvania Press.

Bertlessen, A., Harvald, B., & Hauge, M. (1977). A Danish study of manic-depressive disorders. *British Journal of Psychiatry, 130,* 338–351.

Bowlby, J. (1961). Childhood mourning and its implications for child psychiatry. *American Journal of Psychiatry, 118,* 481–498.

Bowlby, J. (1977). The making and breaking of affectional bonds II: Aetiology and psychopathology in the light of attachment theory. *British Journal of Psychiatry, 130,* 201–210.

Boyd, H. G., & Weissman, M. M. (1981). Epidemiology of affective disorders: A re-examination and future directions. *Archives of General Psychiatry, 38,* 1039–1046.

Brown, G. S., & Harris, T. (1978). *Social origins of depression.* London: Tavistock Publications, 1978.

Bunney, W. E. (1978). Psychopharmacology of the switch process in affective illness. In M. A. Lipton, A. Dimasco, & K. F. Killam (Eds.), *Psychopharmacology: A generation of progress* (pp. 1249–1259). New York: Raven Press.

Cadoret, R. J. (1978). Psychopathology in adopted-away offspring of biologic parents with antisocial behavior. *Archives of General Psychiatry, 25,* 1–15.

Cadoret, R. J., O'Gorman, T. W., Heywood, E., & Troughton, E. (1985). Genetic and environmental factors in major depression. *Journal of Affective Disorders, 9,* 155–164.

Cassano, G. B., Maggini, C., & Akiskal, H. S. (1983). Short-term subchronic and chronic sequelae of affective disorders. *Psychiatric Clinics of North America, 6,* 55–67.

Cavanaugh, S. (1983). The prevalence of emotional and cognitive dysfunction in a medical population. *General Hospital Psychiatry, 5,* 15–24.

Chodoff, P. (1972). The depressive personality: A critical review. *Archives of General Psychiatry, 27,* 666–673.

Clayton, P. J. (1979). The sequelae and nonsequelae of conjugal bereavement. *American Journal of Psychiatry, 136,* 1530–1534.

Clayton, P., Halikas, J., & Maurice, W. (1972). The depression of widowhood. *British Journal of Psychiatry, 120,* 71–77.

Depue, R. A., Slater, J. F., Wolfstetter-Kausch, H., Klein, D., Goplerud, E., & Farr, D. (1981). A behavioral paradigm for identifying persons at risk for bipolar depressive disorders: A conceptual framework and five validation studies. *Journal of Abnormal Psychology, 90,* (suppl.), 381–438.

Gershon, E. S., Dunner, D. L., & Goodwin, F. K. (1971). Toward a biology of affective disorders. *Archives of General Psychiatry, 25,* 1–15.

Gershon, E. S., Dunner, D. L., & Sfert, L. (1973). Assortative mating in the affective disorders. *Biological Psychiatry, 7,* 63–74.

Gershon, E. S., Hamovit, J., Guroff, J. J., Dibble, E., Leckman, J. F., Sceery, W., Targum, S. D., Nurnberger, J. I., Goldin, L. R., & Bunney, W. (1982). A family study of schizoaffective, bipolar I, bipolar II, unipolar and normal control probands. *Archives of General Psychiatry, 39,* 1157–1167.

Gold, M. S., Pottash, A. C., Mueller, E. A., & Extein, I. (1981). Grades of thyroid failure in 100 depressed and anergic psychiatric inpatients. *American Journal of Psychiatry, 138,* 253–255.

Goodwin, F., & Bunney, W. E., Jr. (1971). Depression following reserpine: A re-evaluation. *Seminars in Psychiatry, 3,* 19–53.

Guze, S. B. (1967). The occurrence of psychiatric illness in systemic lupus erythematosus. *American Journal of Psychiatry, 123,* 1562–1570.

Harlow, H. F. (1974). *Learning to Love.* New York: Jason Aronson.

Helgason, T. (1979). Epidemiological investigations concerning affective disorders. In M. Schou & E. Stromgren (Eds.), *Origin, prevention and treatment of affective disorders* (pp. 241–255). London: Academic Press.

Hendrie, H. C. (1978). Organic brain disorders: Classification, the "symptomatic" psychoses, misdiagnosis. *Psychiatric Clinics of North America, 1,* 3–19.

Hill, O. (1969). The association of childhood bereavement with suicide attempt in depressive illness. *British Journal of Psychiatry, 115,* 301–334.

Hirschfeld, R. M. (1981). Situational depression: Validity of the concept. *British Journal of Psychiatry, 139,* 297–305.

Hirschfeld, R. M., Klerman, G., Clayton, P., & Keller, M. (1983). Personality and depression: Empirical findings. *Archives of General Psychiatry, 40,* 993–998.

Kane, F. (1977). Iatrogenic depression in women. In W. E. Farn, I. Karacan, A. D. Pokorny, & R. L. Williams (Eds.), *Phenomenology and treatment of depression* (pp. 69–80). New York: Spectrum Publications.

Kety, S. S. (1985). Interactions between stress and genetic processes. In M. R. Zales (Ed.), *Stress in Health and Disease.* New York: Brunner/Mazel.

Khuri, R., & Akiskal, H. S. (1983). Suicide prevention: The necessity of treating contributory psychiatric disorders. *Psychiatric Clinics of North America, 6,* 193–207.

Kovacs, M. & Beck, A. T. (1978). Maladaptive cognitive structure in depression. *American Journal of Psychiatry, 135,* 525–533.

Kramer, G. W., & McKinney, W. T. (1979). Interaction of pharmacologic agents which alter biogenic amine metabolism in depression. *Journal of Affective Disorders, 1,* 33–54.

Kraepelin, E. (1921). *Manic-depressive insanity and paranoia.* Edinburgh: Livingstone.

Kretschmer, E. (1936). *Physique and character* (E. Miller, trans). London: Kegan Paule, Trench, Trubner and Co., Ltd.

Krauthammer, C., & Klerman, G. L. (1978). Secondary mania: Manic syndromes associated with antecedent physical illness or drugs. *Archives of General Psychiatry, 35,* 1333–1339.

Kukopulos, A., Reginaldi, D., Laddomada, P., Floris, G., Serra, G., & Tondo, L. (1980). Course of the manic-depressive cycle and changes caused by treatments. *Pharmacopsychiatria, 13,* 156–167.

Kupfer, D. J., & Thase, M. E. (1983). The use of the sleep laboratory in the diagnosis of affective disorders. In H. S. Akiskal (Ed.), Diagnosis and treatment of affective disorders, *The Psychiatric Clinics of North America*, 3–25.

Levi, D. L., Fales, C. L., Stein, M., & Sharp, V. H. (1966). Separation and attempted suicide. *Archives of General Psychiatry, 15,* 158–164.

Lewinsohn, P. M. (1974). A behavioral approach to depression. In R. J. Friedman & M. M. Katz (Eds.), *The psychology of depression: Contemporary theory and research.* New York: Halstead.

Lloyd, C. (1980a). Life events and depressive disorder reviewed, I: Events as predisposing factors. *Archives of General Psychiatry, 32,* 285–305.

Lloyd, C. (1980b). Life events and depressive disorder reviewed, II: Events are precipitating factors. *Archives of General Psychiatry, 37,* 541–548.

Mendels, J., & Frazer, A. (1974). Brain biogenic amine depletion and mood. *Archives of General Psychiatry, 30,* 447–451.

Mendlewicz, J., & Rainer, J. D. (1977). Adoption study supporting genetic transmission in manic depressive illness. *Lancet, 268,* 327–329.

Murphy, G. E. (1975). The physician's responsibility for suicide I and II. Errors of commission and omission. *Annals of Internal Medicine, 82,* 301–309.

Paykel, E. S. (1976). Life stress, depression, and attempted suicide. *Journal of Human Stress, 2,* 3–12.

Perris, C. A. (1966). A study of bipolar (manic-depressive) and unipolar recurrent depressive psychoses. *Acta Psychiatrica Scandinavica, 42* (Suppl.), 7–188.

Prange, A. J., Wilson, I. C., Rabon, A., & Lipton, M. A. (1969). Enhancement of imipramine antidepressant activity by thyroid hormone. *American Journal of Psychiatry, 126,* 457–468.

Price, J. (1968). The genetics of depressive behavior. In A. Coopen & A. Walk (Eds.), Recent developments in affective disorders. *British Journal of Psychiatry* (spec. publ.), *2,* 37–54.

Rabkin, J. G., & Struening, E. L. (1976). Life events, stress and illness. *Science, 194,* 1013–1020.

Recamier, P. C., & Blanchard, M. (1957). De l'angiosse a la manie. *L'Evolution Psychiatrique, 3,* 558–587.

Robinson, D. S., Davis, J. M., Nies, A., Ravaris, C. L., & Sylvester, D. (1971). Relation of sex and aging to monoamine oxidase activity of human brain, plasma, and platelets. *Archives of General Psychiatry, 24,* 536–539.

Rosenthal, N. E., Sack, D. A., Gillin, J. C., Lewy, A. J., Goodwin, F. K., Davenport, Y., Mueller, P. S., Newsome, D. A., & Wehr, T. A. (1984). Seasonal affective disorder. *Archives of General Psychiatry,* 72–80.

Rosenthal, T. L., Akiskal, H. S., Scott-Strauss, A., Rosenthal, R. H., & David, M. (1981). Familial and developmental factors in characterological depressions. *Journal of Affective Disorders, 3,* 183–192.

Seligman, M. D. (1975). *Helplessness: On depression, development, and death.* San Francisco: Freeman.

Spitz, R. (1942). Anaclitic depression: An inquiry into the genesis of psychiatric conditions in early childhood. *Psychoanalytic Study of the Child, 2,* 313–342.

Thomson, K. D., & Hendrie, H. C. (1972). Environmental stress in primary depressive illness. *Archives of General Psychiatry, 26,* 139–132.

Vogel, G. W. (1975). A review of REM sleep deprivation. *Archives of General Psychiatry, 32,* 749–761.

vonKnorring, A. L., Cloninger, C. R., Bohman, M., & Sigvardsson, S. (1983). An adoption study of depressive disorders and substance abuse. *Archives of General Psychiatry, 40,* 943–950.

Warheit, G. H. (1979). Life events, coping, and depressive symptomatology. *American Journal of Psychiatry, 136,* 943–950.

Weissman, M. M., & Akiskal, H. S. (1984). The role of psychotherapy in chronic depressions: A proposal. *Comprehensive Psychiatry, 25,* 23–31.

Winokur, G. (1981). *Depression: The facts.* New York: Oxford University Press.

16

The Future of Depression
Prevention Research

Ricardo F. Muñoz
University of California, San Francisco

"Can depression be prevented?
*In general, the onset of a clinical depression cannot be prevented."**

A more accurate response to the above question would be: "We have not yet done the necessary research to know whether depression can be prevented." Until we have evaluated preventive interventions based on the state of the science, we are misleading the public when we categorically state that depression cannot be prevented. The answer cited above implies that we have tried to do so and failed. As of 1984, when the NIMH public education pamphlet was published, no prevention intervention trial focused on reducing the incidence of clinical depression had been completed.

Hopefully, by the early part of the twenty-first century, the answer to the above question will be: "Certain kinds of depression *can* be prevented." In order to achieve this goal, the mental health field must gain experience with prevention and carry out prevention trials.

AVENUES DISCUSSED
IN THE PRECEDING CHAPTERS

The contributors to this book have presented the following concepts and research directions which they have felt to be of importance to the prevention enterprise:

1. Defining the type of depression which is the target of the intervention (see chaps. 1 and 2, this volume).
2. Utilizing epidemiological data to identify high risk factors and high risk groups (see chaps. 1 and 3, this volume).
3. Adopting a life cycle perspective; tailoring preventive approaches to different age groups and to persons going through specific milestones in life (see chaps. 4, 5, 6, 8 and 11, this volume).
4. Taking into account cultural factors (see chaps. 3, 8, 12 and 13 this volume).
5. Evaluating the role of physical exercise (see chap. 7, this volume).
6. Developing and evaluating preventively focused interventions (see chaps. 9, 10 and 11, this volume).

*From: *Depression: What we know.* A public information pamphlet from the National Institute of Mental Health (Lobel & Hirschfeld, 1984, p. 4).

7. Carrying out randomized controlled prevention trials focused on reduction of the incidence of clinical depression (see chaps. 12 and 13, this volume).

8. Developing appropriate data analytic techniques to increase the informational yield of prevention trials (see chap. 14, this volume).

9. Taking into account biological factors in the planning of preventive programs (see chap. 15, this volume).

ADDITIONAL DIRECTIONS WHICH SHOULD ALSO BE EXPLORED

There are a number of possible directions that have not been covered in this book and which should be considered:

1. The impact of economic approaches to the prevention of depression.

2. The role of ideology in the occurrence of depression. (Do religious beliefs, social and political commitments, or philosophies of life exert an influence on risk for depression?)

3. The role of nutrition.

4. The potential preventive effect of purposeful social change.

LIMITATIONS OF OUR KNOWLEDGE

Current limitations to the study of the prevention of depression have to do with the state of the science of depression in general. For example, Gershon et al. (1982) point out that there may be no "true" rate of diagnosable affective disorders. This rate is a function of procedures, criteria used, and the culture of the population being sampled. This inherent variability in rates of depression will obviously hamper studies which assume the existence of a reliably identifiable disorder.

Similar issues can be raised regarding the nature of many of the concepts that have been related to depression. Such factors as social support, life events, dysfunctional beliefs, inadequate levels of pleasant activities, and so on, are theoretically convincing, but hard to operationalize. Obtaining norms for such variables across the many subgroups in the population for whom prevention programs would be advisable is also problematic.

SPECULATIVE SOURCES FOR FUTURE PROGRESS

Conceptual Suggestions

Kindling and Behavioral Sensitization Models

Post, Rubinow, and Ballenger (1984) have reviewed several models based on animal experimental work which may have relevance for the course of affective disorders in humans. Kindling refers to "the eventual development of motor seizures to repeated electrical stimulation of the brain with current which was originally insufficient to produce overt behavioral effects." Similarly, pharmacological agents can gradually produce such seizures at initially subthreshold doses. Neural excitability may increase even without motor seizures. Behavioral sensitization refers to increasing effects on behavior of low doses of psychomotor stimulants and dopamine agonist agents.

Post et al. (1984) suggest that phenomena similar to kindling or behavioral sensitization may be at work in the observed increase in recurrences of affective episodes and the gradually more rapid and apparently autonomous onset of episodes. Perhaps the human organism is altered in terms of neuronal excitability in selected brain areas by the occurrence of single episodes. In addition, conditioned psychological, physiological, and neurotransmitter responses caused by such episodes may increase the probability of affective dysfunctions in the future. Silverman (1985) has suggested that if processes such as kindling are involved in depression, preventive approaches which reduce the probability of first onset, or even prevent early recurrences of depressive episodes, may reduce the likelihood of severe recurrent depressions. This model provides a very interesting rationale for interventions focused on subclinical depressions.

Self-control Approaches

The theoretical model of self-control found in the writings of social learning theorists (Bandura, 1969, 1977; Mahoney & Thoresen, 1974) and specifically applied to depression by Rehm (1977) predicts that persons who learn cognitive and behavioral patterns to change their own feelings and behavior are less likely to become depressed. A longitudinal, controlled study in which these skills are taught to young children, and in which the children are followed into adulthood, would be of great importance. Whether such a study is feasible and ethical remains in question. It is interesting to note that in a treatment outcome study comparing pharmacotherapy to cognitive therapy (Murphy, Simons, Wetzel, & Lustman, 1984), the only measure which predicted to differential effectiveness between the two approaches was a measure of "learned resourcefulness" (Simons, Lustman, Wetzel, & Murphy, 1985). This measure (Rosenbaum, 1980) taps what appear to be beliefs in self-control or self-efficacy. Perhaps holding such attitudes increases the chances that interventions relying on self-change will be effective. There would be two implications to this finding: First, training children to develop such an attitude (see chap. 4, this volume) may be in itself a preventive intervention because it is likely that self-change will be necessary at various times in their life. Secondly, such a relationship would be of use in tailoring interventions to different populations. Studies designed to answer the question "which interventions prevent which type of disorder in which populations?" could be carried out using strategies which take into account such learned characteristics.

Varied Methods for Intervention

An important element necessary to make prevention approaches feasible is the broadening of the concept of mental health intervention from that of a professional having personal contact with a client or clients. There are a number of ways in which mental health service delivery can be expanded: utilization of paraprofessionals trained in specific interventions, the use of volunteer helpers, self-help groups, electronic and mass media, and print have been suggested (Christensen, Miller, & Muñoz, 1978). Evaluation of *each* of these modalities for prevention is still a necessity, even if the intervention has been found effective when performed with another modality. Nor is it necessary to assume that more costly modalities are necessarily more effective.

The use of the mass media is a particularly important area that should be developed in the future (Maccoby & Alexander, 1979; Muñoz, Glish, Soo-Hoo, & Robertson, 1982).

Ecological Approaches

The community psychology movement has repeatedly warned clinicians that population-wide interventions, particularly preventive interventions, must be carried out taking into account the context in which they occur and the relationships of all segments of the environment in which they take place. Kelly (1966, 1968, 1969, 1971, 1977) has suggested research methods from an ecological perspective. The point of these suggestions is that for interventions to be effective and to endure, they must be integrated into the fabric of the community. Technological interventions, no matter how powerful in the laboratory, will not be effective in the field without taking into account the culture into which they are introduced.

Rappaport, Seidman, & Davidson (1979) present a case study of an innovation which was "successful" when under the control of the researchers who developed and evaluated it, but which was radically altered once it was adopted by the institution for which it was developed. The translation of preventive programs from theory, to research-oriented practice, and finally to ongoing prevention services must be done carefully. An assessment of community influences on programs should be an integral part of preventive intervention research.

The Stressful Life-Event Paradigm

Bloom (1985) has recommended that instead of focusing on prevention interventions for specific disorders, a more realistic and ultimately practical approach would be to focus on interventions which attempt to reduce the impact of stressful life events. His argument is that such events are known to have a myriad of negative effects, producing many types of physical and emotional disorders. For example, an intervention that is designed for newly divorced individuals, would be expected to prevent not just depression, but a number of other dysfunctions (Bloom, Hodges, & Caldwell, 1982).

Clinical researchers are generally wedded to specific disorders, and believe that progress is greater when one focuses on studying the processes contributing to well-delineated clinical entities. There is no reason, however, why both approaches could not be implemented at the same time. Depression prevention research could emphasize interventions which have been developed in the context of depression, while at the same time documenting effects on other dysfunctional patterns. Stress reduction and coping research could evaluate its effects on depression, among other variables, and thus also contribute to the depression prevention field.

Empowerment

Rappaport (1981) has criticized the prevention movement for being too clinical in its conceptualization. Rappaport argues that such a clinical perspective derives from a needs/dependency model, which views people as children, and professional experts as leaders who know the answers and provide them for their clients. He proposes a model of empowerment, which suggests collaboration and implies that many competencies are already present in members of the community. Poor functioning is a result of social structure and lack of resources which make it impossible for the existing competences to operate. His paper (Rappaport, 1981) is a very challenging document which should be read by prevention practitioners and researchers.

Albee has made a similar argument regarding the negative consequences of too much power in the hands of the few (Albee, 1981; Kessler & Albee, 1975). He argues that much of what we label psychopathology stems from the unhealthy concentrations of power throughout society.

Although both of these arguments may seem too far afield for traditional clinicians and clinical researchers, professionals considering careers in prevention should take them seriously. Prevention is inherently a population-based intervention. As such, it must take into account social and community factors which often exert great influence on behavior.

IF PREVENTION IS SUCH A LOGICAL APPROACH, WHY IS IT NOT BEING IMPLEMENTED?

The biggest stumbling block in the path of prevention is the lack of societal interest in the area. Perhaps by looking at the history of prevention in other fields (Freymann, 1975; Terris, 1975) we can gain some insight into what is needed to foster prevention-mindedness.

Freymann (1975) asserts that even the most primitive societies demand curative services, that is, clinical treatment. On the other hand, public health and prevention efforts are possible only when six societal requirements are satisfied:

1. a future orientation.
2. a positive attitude toward health as a controllable asset.
3. valuing of other individuals' life and health instead of a spirit of "every man for himself."
4. the existence of epidemiological and demographic data which define the health problems of a society.
5. an effective administrative organization.
6. personnel qualified for the task.

Of the six items Freymann suggests, the last two are perhaps the farthest from existence at this time. There is no organization whose primary job it is to implement and coordinate primary prevention in mental health. And there is no cadre of professionals trained specifically to develop, carry out, and evaluate primary prevention programs. Until these two needs are met, primary prevention progress is in the hands of the few interested clinicians, community mental health professionals, and medical and social scientists who can come up with individual sources of support (Muñoz, 1976).

Glidewell (1983) has commented on several related reasons why prevention does not receive sufficient public and professional support: preventive actions are rarely perceived as urgent by individuals; expertise about prevention is less convincing than expertise about, say, surgery; successful prevention is invisible, that is, one never knows who would have become a case had there been no prevention; and, as long as this is the case, no one knows whom to thank (or pay): "The most brilliant preventive interventionist simply cannot expect a bequest from a deeply grateful rich family" (Glidewell, 1983, p. 311).

A probabilistic view of life is the most conducive to preventive thinking and action. The chances that one will become clinically depressed, as well as the duration and intensity of the depressive episode, are influenced by a host of factors. By systematically manipulating those factors which are under our control, we can reduce the probability of becoming depressed, and, if we do become depressed, we can increase the chances that the episode will be short and relatively less severe. This is what prevention can offer. The challenge is convincing our society that this offer is worth supporting.

POTENTIAL SOURCES OF SUPPORT

The Role of Professionals Serving Underserved Populations

Some of the impetus for prevention comes from the experiences of professionals serving underserved groups. The underutilization of traditional treatment services, partly because of cultural stigma regarding psychiatric care, and partly because of inappropriate types of services, has led professionals to seek other kinds of service provision. It is probably not just a matter of chance that the first two randomized controlled prevention trials focused on clinical depression are being conducted by minority teams (see chaps. 12 and 13, this volume).

It has been argued that Hispanics, for example, might respond better to prevention services than to treatment services. A great proportion of Hispanics are immigrants, with interest in learning as much as possible about how to get along in their new country. They value education highly, and might be quite willing to take advantage of educationally oriented interventions (Muñoz, 1982). The small number of Spanish-speaking professionals in relation to the large Hispanic population also points to the wisdom of developing interventions that can reach large numbers of persons, such as mass media approaches.

The opportunities for research which are available once one considers language and cultural minorities as an integral part of the community have only begun to be tapped. It would be possible, for example, to carry out quasi-experimental studies in communities which have large proportions of Spanish-speaking individuals by presenting the intervention in Spanish. The non-Spanish-speaking population living in the same area (even in the same city blocks) could then serve as a comparison group. Their geographical contiguity would be likely to distribute such major variables as socioeconomic status, environmental stresses, and so on, across both groups.

Should Both Practice and Research Be Supported?

An important decision that the field must make is whether to limit resources for prevention to research alone or to also fund the practice of prevention. The argument has been made that we do not know enough at present to engage in prevention as a service, and thus that funding for prevention programs is premature

(Lamb & Zusman, 1981). I have made the argument (Muñoz, 1985) that preventive programs have the potential to teach the field what the issues are in the delivery of preventive interventions. Just as much of what we have learned from clinical research has come from hypotheses derived from well-documented clinical experience, so also will the prevention researcher be better able to plan useful research programs based on the experiences of practitioners in the field.

Advocates of prevention programs point out that such programs should be supported by the public sector as part of its public health responsibility. However, prevention programs have traditionally received the least amount of funding, even during the period when community mental health centers were better supported (Snow & Newton, 1976). It is possible that if prevention intervention research were to show solid evidence that specific programs reduce the incidence of depression and concommittant problems governmental bodies might provide support for them. Unfortunately, their present lack of support is likely to delay such advances.

Other likely sources of funding for prevention in years to come are corporations and other private institutions which cannot afford the reduction in productivity resulting from depression and other psychological problems. Employee health programs are likely to begin with a treatment stance, and gradually move to prevention and health enhancement because they soon find that relatively mild problems can create significant hidden costs (Manuso, 1981). It is not just absenteeism, lateness, and severely disruptive behavior which causes problems in an organization. Depressed employees may work hard, be punctual, and even put in overtime, and still function below adequate levels.

Health maintenance organizations and insurance companies may also find it profitable to provide relatively low cost preventive services if by doing so they can reduce utilization of prolonged and expensive treatment services.

The Role of Prevention in the Health Care Delivery System

As we move toward careful development of preventive interventions, we ought to consider the context within which they might be utilized.

Ideally, preventive interventions would be embedded in a number of community settings. Preventive programs would be available for all persons who find themselves in such settings, though special efforts would be made to attract those at high risk. Those who are already suffering from clinical depression would be referred directly to the treatment system. (Brief screening measures would be used to identify those at risk, and measures of depression would flag those who might already need treatment).

Those referred to treatment would be assigned to treatments shown to be effective and efficient. In cases where there is no demonstrated difference in effectiveness, the patient's preference should determine which approach is tried first (for example, pharmacotherapy or cognitive-behavioral therapy). If, after a reasonable trial, there is little improvement, the other approach would be recommended.

For cases of recurrent depression, maintenance programs would be implemented. Thus, the entire spectrum of interventions, from prevention, through treatment, and into maintenance (Christensen, Miller, & Muñoz, 1979), would be orchestrated to produce the lowest incidence and prevalence possible in the population.

To concretize the above suggestions, let us delineate a specific example. All expectant mothers in a community might be invited to take part in a depression prevention program as part of their prenatal care. A brief screening instrument would be administered to determine if any of them fit into already known high risk profiles (for example, a history of depression in their families, early parental loss, marital problems, lack of social support, and so on). Those with a high risk profile would be contacted individually to increase the chances of attendance. The screening instrument would also include a self-report depression scale. Those scoring above a predetermined cut-off score would be invited in for a face-to-face diagnostic interview, and, if they meet criteria for clinical depression, invited to enter treatment. The prevention program would include meetings of participants after their babies are born, to provide continued support during a stressful period, as well as to evaluate the effect of the prenatal program. Followups at specified intervals, including measures of child functioning, would provide invaluable information designed to continue to improve the preventive intervention.

ETHICAL ISSUES IN THE PREVENTION
OF DEPRESSION

The identification and notification of individuals at high risk for depression, or the recommendation that individuals who meet criteria for clinical depression obtain treatment involve sensitive issues that should not be glossed over lightly.

Only 20% of those who meet criteria for clinical depression go to a mental health specialist for treatment. Yet about 70% of them go to non-psychiatric clinicians to be treated for ailments which may or may not be presented as depression (Shapiro et al., 1984). Although it is likely that this is partly due to lack of knowledge, it is probably also due to the stigma of psychological problems. Even professional health care providers find it hard to talk with patients regarding clinical depression, tend to "explain away" the depression because there is a "reason" for their being depressed, and often do not refer them for treatment (Murphy, 1975a, 1975b).

Social stigma can have nontrivial consequences on people's lives. Therefore, the benefits of early identification of depressed persons, or even of persons who fit high-risk profiles must be considered in relation to the possible costs to these persons. These costs include the personal emotional turmoil that might be engendered in knowing that one has a "mental illness," or the possible negative effect on interpersonal relationships that might result from being identified as being "at risk" for depression.

Depression is a self-limiting disorder in most cases. The fact that so few persons who meet criteria for the disorder go for treatment brings to mind the following question: What proportion of those who are clinically depressed need treatment? Is it possible that a sizable proportion of them could experience episodes which, though debilitating to some extent, do not produce sufficient disruption in their lives to merit the cost (in time, money, and self-perception as someone with an illness) involved in obtaining treatment?

In the case of identification of high risk groups, we must remember that, unless the risk factors predict a probability of over 50% of developing clinical depression (and few presently known factors do), most of those at risk will never have a full blown depressive episode. The psychological cost of knowing that one is at risk and the cost in time and money in attending the prevention intervention must be compared to the effectiveness of the intervention. That is, a very effective intervention might clearly justify the cost to the participants of a prevention program, whereas a relatively weak intervention would not.

These ethical questions often involve dilemmas, that is choices involving equally unsatisfying solutions. These predicaments are not just the result of lack of information. Even with all needed information, a decision would still be difficult to make. For example, preventive interventions with strong effects might themselves be subject to criticism. If these interventions involved changes in thinking or behavior of individuals, such as those involved in cognitive-behavioral therapies, it would be possible to ask whether such interventions might be manipulating, coercive, or considered "brainwashing" by those who objected to them.

Behavior modification techniques received bad press partly because they were relatively more effective in actually changing individual's behavior than more traditional approaches. If we find that a certain approach works on almost all the people it reaches, we tend to attribute the cause of the changes brought about to the power of the method, and less to the volition of the people whose behavior has changed. A less effective method, say one which only caused changes in 50% of the population receiving it, would be seen as more appropriate from the point of view of individual freedom. (At the other end of the continuum, a method which changed very few target behaviors would be just considered a failure, of course).

One way around these possible criticisms of imposing the values of prevention professionals on the public is to advocate for programs that are voluntary. But is it ethical to focus our efforts only on volunteers?

A number of critics of the mental health system have accused it of serving only the white middle class or those members of minority groups who either have adopted middle class values or have been made dependent upon the system. These critics have advocated for services for minority populations which are relevant, accessible and acceptable to them, and which are delivered by people who either belong to those groups, or who are at least sensitive to their values. Inherent in these arguments is the point that people can be systematically excluded from services without overt discrimination. Preventive programs could fall into the same trap. In our well-intended attempts not to coerce people to accept unwanted influences in their lives, we may actually be keeping valuable resources away from them.

There are at least three ways in which services might be inadvertently denied: channels of communication might be used which do not reach certain segments of the population, insufficient resources might be allocated to reach specific groups, and the groups themselves might be resistant to even emergency messages. The first instance is relatively simple to explain: certain groups are more likely to listen to or read specific types of media. Assessment of which audience is being reached is imperative to avoid excluding participants merely by not letting them know that the program is available. Availability of such programs in languages other than English is imperative in many communities.

The second instance is depicted very strikingly in a chapter by Maccoby and Alexander (1979, pp. 94–96) in which they recount how the Stanford Heart Disease Prevention Study finally included a Spanish-speaking component. Their initial grant did not include funds for such a sample, even though the towns in the study were 15% to 20% Spanish-speaking. If it had not been for a member of the team who felt strongly that their study would not be done properly without a Spanish-speaking sample, either from a scientific or ethical point of view, the study would have been conducted entirely in English. This is an ethical issue which becomes compounded by the relatively small numbers of Spanish-speaking professionals.

The third way in which services might be denied has to do with differential response characteristics. Perry, Lindell, and Greene (1982) report that when they looked at a probability sample of flood evacuation warning recipients, they found that Mexican-Americans 1) were more skeptical than whites about believing warning messages, no matter how specific the message; 2) interpreted the same warning messages as indicating lower levels of personal danger; and 3) were less likely to take protective action (that is, evacuate) than whites. If these differences can be found even in cases of immediate danger, what kind of effects are we likely to find with preventive messages? If such effects are found consistently, we must rethink the strategy of using only volunteer groups, which might result in a policy of benign neglect with not-so-benign consequences. The dilemma is that the other side of the coin involves the danger of coercing populations which have less power in this society into taking part in programs which the more powerful, no matter how good their intentions, consider to be beneficial to them.

Interventions which are best implemented wholesale on already-existing groups, such as classroom-wide interventions, also have the problem of volunteer versus mandatory formats. If one asks for volunteers in this case, there are two possible negative consequences. Those children who are in the program run the risk of being labeled as being "at risk," or as already in need of extra help. In addition, by serving a biased segment of the population, evaluations of the service are limited in terms of their generalizability, and the service itself might turn out to serve only those who need it least. On the other hand, if one wants to include the entire classroom, should parents be asked to give permission for their children to participate? If so, how much information should the parents have regarding the intent of the intervention? In other words, should they be told that it is an education intervention that is meant to give their children useful living skills, or should they be told that it is a psychological intervention, designed to have preventive effects regarding actual clinical disorders?

As our interventions become more reliably effective, there will be ethical issues involving the decision whether or not to intervene. In the far distant future, it is possible that we will have sufficient documentation to know what types of intervention reduce certain disorders, as well as what "side-effects" they produce, particularly in terms of which other disorders might be increased by the interventions in question. At that time, humanity may be called upon to decide which disorders it is willing to live with, in order to reduce the prevalence of others.

THE ULTIMATE GOAL OF PREVENTION: THE REDUCTION OF UNNECESSARY SUFFERING

There is much suffering in the world which stems from sources beyond human control, such as earthquakes and other natural disasters. There is also suffering perpetrated by human beings. Some such suffering is perpetrated on others, such as war, racism, and unjust or unwise distribution of resources (so that, for example, human beings starve when food elsewhere is destroyed or purposefully not grown to keep prices up). But much suffering is also perpetrated on individuals by their own hand. Few people realize, for example, that more people in the United States die from suicide than from being killed by others (U.S. Bureau of the Census, 1984). If, in addition to suicide, we consider deaths from self-imposed causes which are known to be deleterious (such as the use of tobacco, alcohol, and other drugs, and other high-risk behaviors, such as driving too fast) we begin to realize that much human suffering is self-imposed.

It would be difficult to determine how much human suffering comes from sources not within human control, but I would not be surprised if the majority is directly attributable to human attitudes, human choices, and human actions.

Even in cases of death "from natural causes," one can conceive of better and worse kinds of death experiences. In a very real way, death is not the enemy. Rather, unnecessary deaths, lonely deaths, deaths after lives without purpose are the proper target for human intervention.

In a challenging treatment of this concept, Fries and Crapo (1981) suggest that, given the fact that death is inevitable, and that the likelihood of prolonging human life much past our present life expectancies is unrealistic, our goal should be to increase the proportion of time that human beings are healthy. In effect, they propose that we should aim to delay debilitating conditions so that their expected onset can be gradually pushed further and further back, perhaps until after the average life expectancy. Their message is a clearly preventive one, and one which, if accepted by the majority of the population, would bring about a radically different and positive philosophy of life.

The reduction of unnecessary suffering is at the core of the depression prevention effort. Many of the factors that have been implicated in the development of depression involve human actions: stressful life events often have to do with interpersonal conflict, lack of social support is clearly of human making, dysfunctional attitudes are learned, taught, and often carefully nourished. How much could depression be reduced if we limited our interventions merely to human actions and ways of thinking?

Research into the prevention of depression is a bonafide social, psychological, and biological scientific endeavor, with specifiable methodologies, and quantifiable goals (such as the reduction in the incidence of clinical depressive episodes). In a larger sense, however, the prevention of depression is a task which encompasses larger realms of human activities, including philosophical, theological, political, and economic fields.

Recognition of this universal human goal and a conscious, purposeful striving to achieve it, may accelerate our progress. The goal is clearly an asymptotical one: we may come closer and closer to it, but we can not expect ever to reach complete reduction in human-caused suffering. Nevertheless, we will be able to quantify reduction in specific areas.

The aim of prevention can be described as pushing back the boundaries of what is unavoidable and inescapable. How far will we be able to push back those boundaries? The answer will hopefully never be known. Each generation will start where the old one left off and continue the process. There is some sadness in that thought, for none of us will be alive to see the ultimate preventive step. But there is hope, too, that our descendants will enjoy the fruits of our labor, and still have challenges left to fill their lives with a sense of meaning and purpose.

The aims of the research efforts advocated in this book are to investigate interventions which may protect us from depression. In doing so, we will not be just discovering reality in a scientific sense: we will be changing reality so that human suffering that is inevitable now will not be inevitable in the future.

REFERENCES

Albee, G. W. (1981). Politics, power, prevention, and social change. In J. M. Joffe, & G. W. Albee (Eds.), *Prevention through political action and social change* (pp. 5–25). Hanover, NH: University Press of New England.

Bandura, A. (1969). *Principles of behavior modification.* New York: Holt, Rinehart, & Winston.

Bandura, A. (1977). *Social Learning Theory.* Englewood Cliffs, NJ: Prentice-Hall.

Bloom, B. L. (1985). *Stressful life event theory and research: Implications for primary prevention.* (DHHS Publication No. ADM 85-1385). Washington, DC: U.S. Government Printing Office.

Bloom, B. L., Hodges, W. F., & Caldwell, R. A. (1982). A preventive intervention program for the newly separated: Initial evaluation. *American Journal of Community Psychology, 10,* 251–264.

Christensen, A., Miller, W. R., & Muñoz, R. F. (1978). Paraprofessionals, partners, peers, paraphernalia, and print: Expanding mental health service delivery. *Professional Psychology, 9,* 249–270.

Freymann, J. G. (1975). Medicine's great schism: Prevention vs. cure: An historical interpretation. *Medical Care, 13,* 525–536.

Fries, J. F., & Crapo, L. M. (1981). *Vitality and aging: Implications of the rectangular curve.* San Francisco: W. H. Freeman and Co.

Gershon, E. S., Hamovit, J., Guroff, J. J., Dibble, E., Leckman, J. F., Sceery, W., Targum, S., Nurnberger, J. I., Goldin, L. R., & Bunney, W. E. (1982). A family study of schizoaffective, bipolar I, bipolar II, unipolar, and normal control probands. *Archives of General Psychiatry, 39,* 1157–1167.

Glidewell, J. C. (1983). Afterword: Prevention—The threat and the promise. In R. D. Felner, L. A. Jason, J. N. Moritsugu, & S. S. Farber (Eds.), *Preventive psychology: Theory, research, & practice* (pp. 310–312). New York: Pergamon.

Kelly, J. G. (1966). Ecological constraints on mental health services. *American Psychologist, 33,* 535–539.

Kelly, J. G. (1968). Towards an ecological conception of preventive interventions. In J. W. Carter, Jr. (Ed.), *Research contributions from psychology to community mental health* (pp. 75–99). New York: Behavioral Publications.

Kelly, J. G. (1969). Naturalistic observations in contrasting social environments. In E. P. Willems, & H. L. Raush (Eds.), *Naturalistic viewpoints in psychological research* (pp. 183–199). New York: Holt, Rinehart & Winston.

Kelly, J. G. (1971). The quest for valid preventive interventions. In G. Rosenblum (Ed.), *Issues in community psychology and preventive mental health* (pp. 109–139). New York: Behavioral Publications.

Kelly, J. G. (1977). The search for ideas and deeds that work. In G. W. Albee & J. M. Joffe (Eds.), *Primary prevention of psychopathology: Vol. 1. The issues* (pp. 7–17). Hanover, NH: University Press of New England.

Kessler, M., & Albee, G. W. (1975). Primary prevention. *Annual Review of Psychology, 26,* 557–591.

Lamb, H. R., & Zusman, J. (1981). A new look at primary prevention. *Hospital and Community Psychiatry, 32,* 843–848.

Lobel, B., & Hirschfeld, R. M. A. (1984). *Depression: What we know* (DHHS Publication No. ADM 85-1318). Washington, DC: U.S. Government Printing Office.

Maccoby, N., & Alexander, J. (1979). Reducing heart disease risk using the mass media: Comparing the effects on three communities. In R. F. Muñoz, L. R. Snowden, & J. G. Kelly (Eds.), *Social and psychological research in community settings* (pp. 69–100). San Francisco: Jossey-Bass.

Mahoney, M. J., & Thoresen, C. E. (1974). *Self-control: Power to the person.* Monterey, CA: Brooks/Cole.

Manuso, J. S. J. (1981). Psychological services and health enhancement: A corporate model. In

A. Broskowski, E. Marks, & S. H. Budman (Eds.) *Linking health and mental health* (pp. 137–158). Beverly Hills: Sage.

Muñoz, R. F. (1976). The primary prevention of psychological problems: A review of the literature. *Community Mental Health Review, 1,* 1–15.

Muñoz, R. F. (1982). The Spanish-speaking consumer and the community mental health center. In E. E. Jones, & S. J. Korchin (Eds.), *Minority mental health* (pp. 362–398). New York: Praeger.

Muñoz, R. F. (1985). Primary prevention: Should we support both practice and research? *Journal of Primary Prevention, 5,* 284–292.

Muñoz, R. F., Glish, M., Soo-Hoo, T., & Robertson, J. (1982). The San Francisco Mood Survey Project: Preliminary work toward the prevention of depression. *American Journal of Community Psychology, 10,* 317–329.

Murphy, G. E. (1975a). The physician's responsibility for suicide. I. An error of commission. *Annals of Internal Medicine, 82,* 301–304.

Murphy, G. E. (1975b). The physician's responsibility for suicide. II. Errors of ommission. *Annals of Internal Medicine, 82,* 305–309.

Murphy, G. E., Simons, A. D., Wetzel, R. D., Lustman, P. J. (1984). Cognitive therapy and pharmacotherapy: Singly and together in the treatment of depression. *Archives of General Psychiatry, 41,* 33–41.

Perry, R. W., Lindell, M. K., & Greene, M. R. (1982). Crisis communications: Ethnic differentials in interpreting and acting on disaster warnings. *Social Behavior and Personality, 10,* 97–104.

Post, R. M., Rubinow, D. R., & Ballenger, J. C. (1984). Conditioning, sensitization, and kindling: Implications for the course of affective illness. In R. M. Post & J. C. Ballenger (Eds.), *Neurobiology of mood disorders* (pp. 432–466). Baltimore: Williams & Wilkins.

Rappaport, J. (1981). In praise of paradox: A social policy of empowerment over prevention. *American Journal of Community Psychology, 9,* 1–25.

Rappaport, J., Seidman, E., & Davidson, W. S., II. (1979). Demonstration research and manifest versus true adoption: The natural history of a research project to divert adolescents from the legal system. In R. F. Muñoz, L. R. Snowden, & J. G. Kelly (Eds.), *Social and psychological research in community settings* (pp. 101–144). San Francisco: Jossey-Bass.

Rehm, L. P. (1977). A self-control model of depression. *Behavior Therapy, 8,* 787–804.

Rosenbaum, M. (1980). A schedule for assessing self-control behaviors: Preliminary findings. *Behavior Therapy, 11,* 109–121.

Shapiro, S., Skinner, E. A., Kessler, L. G., Von Korff, M., German, P. S., Tischier, G. L., Leaf, P. J., Benham, L., Cottler, L., & Regier, D. A. (1984). Utilization of health and mental health services: Three Epidemiological Catchment Area sites. *Archives of General Psychiatry, 41,* 971–978.

Silverman, M. M. (1985, May). Preventing depression: A federal perspective. In A. Stoudemire (Chair.), *Perspectives in the prevention of depression.* Symposium conducted at the meeting of the American Psychiatric Association, Dallas, Texas.

Simons, A. D., Lustman, P. J., Wetzel, R. D., & Murphy, G. E. (1985). Predicting response to cognitive therapy of depression: The role of learned resourcefulness. *Cognitive Therapy and Research, 9,* 79–89.

Snow, D. L., & Newton, P. M. (1976). Task, social structure, and social process in the community mental health center movement. *American Psychologist, 31,* 582–594.

Terris, M. (1975). Evolution of public health and preventive medicine in the United States. *American Journal of Public Health, 65,* 161–169.

U.S. Bureau of the Census. (1984). *Statistical Abstracts of the United States* (104th ed.). Washington, DC: U.S. Government Printing Office.

Index